Neurosurgery for Neurologists

Editors

DANIEL K. RESNICK
RUSSELL R. LONSER

NEUROLOGIC CLINICS

www.neurologic.theclinics.com

Consulting Editor
RANDOLPH W. EVANS

May 2022 • Volume 40 • Number 2

ELSEVIER

1600 John F. Kennedy Boulevard • Suite 1800 • Philadelphia, Pennsylvania, 19103-2899

http://www.theclinics.com

NEUROLOGIC CLINICS Volume 40, Number 2
May 2022 ISSN 0733-8619, ISBN-13: 978-0-323-89708-2

Editor: Stacy Eastman
Developmental Editor: Hannah Almira Lopez

Neurologic Clinics (ISSN 0733-8619) is published quarterly by Elsevier Inc., 360 Park Avenue South, New York, NY 10010–1710. Months of issue are February, May, August, and November. Periodicals postage paid at New York, NY, and additional mailing offices. Subscription prices are $343.00 per year for US individuals, $916.00 per year for US institutions, $100.00 per year for US students, $420.00 per year for Canadian individuals, $953.00 per year for Canadian institutions, $475.00 per year for international individuals, $953.00 per year for international institutions, $210.00 for foreign students/residents, and $100.00 for Canadian students/residents. To receive student/resident rate, orders must be accompanied by name of affiliated institution, date of term, and the *signature* of program/residency coordinator on institution letterhead. Orders will be billed at individual rate until proof of status is received. Foreign air speed delivery is included in all *Clinics* subscription prices. All prices are subject to change without notice. **POSTMASTER:** Send address changes to *Neurologic Clinics*, Elsevier Health Sciences Division, Subscription Customer Service, 3251 Riverport Lane, Maryland Heights, MO 63043. **Customer Service: Telephone: 1-800-654-2452 (U.S. and Canada); 314-447-8871 (outside U.S. and Canada). Fax: 314-447-8029. E-mail: journalscustomerservice-usa@elsevier.com (for print support); journalsonlinesupport-usa@elsevier.com (for online support).**

Reprints. For copies of 100 or more of articles in this publication, please contact the Commercial Reprints Department, Elsevier Inc., 360 Park Avenue South, New York, New York, 10010-1710; Tel.: +1-212-633-3874; Fax: +1-212-633-3820, and E-mail: reprints@elsevier.com.

Neurologic Clinics is also published in Spanish by Nueva Editorial Interamericana S.A., Mexico City, Mexico.

Neurologic Clinics is covered in *Current Contents/Clinical Medicine, MEDLINE/PubMed (Index Medicus), EMBASE/Excerpta Medica, and PsycINFO, and ISI/BIOMED.*

Contributors

CONSULTING EDITOR

RANDOLPH W. EVANS, MD
Clinical Professor, Department of Neurology, Baylor College of Medicine, Houston, Texas

EDITORS

DANIEL K. RESNICK, MD, MS
Professor and Vice Chairman, Department of Neurosurgery, University of Wisconsin-Madison School of Medicine and Public Health, University of Wisconsin Hospital and Clinics, Madison, Wisconsin

RUSSELL R. LONSER, MD
Professor and Chair, Department of Neurological Surgery, The Ohio State University Wexner Medical Center, The Ohio State University, Columbus, Ohio

AUTHORS

ADAM S. ARTHUR, MD, MPH
Professor and Chair, Department of Neurosurgery, Semmes-Murphey Clinic, University of Tennessee Health Science Center, Memphis, Tennessee

NITIN AGARWAL, MD
Department of Neurological Surgery, University of California, San Francisco, San Francisco, California

MANMEET S. AHLUWALIA, MD
Herbert Wertheim College of Medicine, Florida International University, Department of Medical Oncology, Miami Cancer Institute, Baptist Health South Florida, Miami, Florida

AZAM S. AHMED, MD
Associate Professor, Department of Neurological Surgery, University of Wisconsin Hospital and Clinics, Madison, Wisconsin

ASAD S. AKHTER, MD
Department of Neurological Surgery, The Ohio State University Wexner Medical Center, Columbus, Ohio

ALMA RECHAV BEN-NATAN, BA
Department of Neurological Surgery, University of California, San Francisco, San Francisco, California

KELSEY M. BOWMAN, MD
Resident, Department of Neurological Surgery, University of Wisconsin Hospital and Clinics, Madison, Wisconsin

RICHARD W. BYRNE, MD
Department of Neurosurgery, Rush University, Chicago, Illinois

GREGORY J. CANNARSA, MD
Resident Physician, Department of Neurosurgery, University of Maryland Medical Center, Baltimore, Maryland

MAHUA DEY, MD
Department of Neurosurgery, University of Wisconsin-Madison School of Medicine and Public Health, Madison, Wisconsin

DAVID DORNBOS III, MD
Assistant Professor, Department of Neurosurgery, University of Kentucky College of Medicine, Lexington, Kentucky

RYAN G. EATON, MD
Department of Neurological Surgery, The Ohio State University Wexner Medical Center, The Ohio State University, Columbus, Ohio

TURKI ELARJANI, MD
Neurosurgery Resident, Department of Neurological Surgery, University of Miami Miller School of Medicine, Miami, Florida

JOHN D. HEISS, MD
Head, Clinical Unit, National Institutes of Health, National Institute of Neurological Disorders and Stroke, Surgical Neurology Branch, Bethesda, Maryland

JEREMY HUANG, BS
Department of Neurological Surgery, University of California, San Francisco, San Francisco, California

HILLIARY E. INGER, MD
Clinical Assistant Professor, Department of Ophthalmology, The Ohio State University Wexner Medical Center, Department of Ophthalmology, Nationwide Children's Hospital, Columbus, Ohio

MEGAN M. JACK, MD, PhD
Mayo Clinic, Department of Neurologic Surgery, Rochester, Minnesota

RUPESH KOTECHA, MD
Department of Radiation Oncology, Miami Cancer Institute, Baptist Health South Florida, Herbert Wertheim College of Medicine, Florida International University, Miami, Florida

JONATHAN LEE, MD
Imaging Institute, Cleveland Clinic Foundation, Cleveland, Ohio

ALLAN D. LEVI, MD, PhD
Professor and Chairman, Department of Neurological Surgery, University of Miami Miller School of Medicine, Miami, Florida

RUSSELL R. LONSER, MD
Professor and Chair, Department of Neurological Surgery, The Ohio State University Wexner Medical Center, The Ohio State University, Columbus, Ohio

MICHAEL W. MCDERMOTT, MD
Herbert Wertheim College of Medicine, Florida International University, Division of Neurosurgery, Miami Neuroscience Institute, Baptist Health South Florida, Miami, Florida

KYLE McGRATH, BS
Center for Spine Health, Department of Neurosurgery, Neurologic Institute, Cleveland Clinic Foundation, Cleveland, Ohio

JOHN M. McGREGOR, MD
Associate Professor, Clinical Neurosurgery, Vice Chair for Strategic Initiatives, Director of Trauma Services, Department of Neurological Surgery, The Ohio State University Wexner Medical Center, Columbus, Ohio

DANA MITCHELL, MS
Department of Pediatrics, Indiana University, Indianapolis, Indiana

PRAVEEN V. MUMMANENI, MD, MBA
Department of Neurological Surgery, University of California, San Francisco, San Francisco, California

I. JONATHAN POMERANIEC, MD, MBA
Senior Neurosurgery Resident, National Institutes of Health, National Institute of Neurological Disorders and Stroke, Surgical Neurology Branch, Bethesda, Maryland

DANIEL K. RESNICK, MD, MS
Professor and Vice Chairman, Department of Neurosurgery, University of Wisconsin-Madison School of Medicine and Public Health, University of Wisconsin Hospital and Clinics, Madison, Wisconsin

R. MARK RICHARDSON, MD, PhD
Director, Functional Neurosurgery, Massachusetts General Hospital, Charles A. Pappas Associate Professor of Neurosciences, Harvard Medical School, Visiting Associate Professor of Brain and Cognitive Sciences, Massachusetts Institute of Technology, Boston, Massachusetts

JARED S. ROSENBLUM, MD
Post-Doctoral Fellow, National Institutes of Health, National Cancer Institute Neuro-Oncology Branch, Bethesda, Maryland

ROBERT J. ROTHROCK, MD
Assistant Professor of Translational Medicine and Neurosurgery, Herbert Wertheim College of Medicine, Florida International University, Baptist Health South Florida, Miami, Florida

SEPEHR B. SANI, MD
Department of Neurosurgery, Rush University, Chicago, Illinois

BRADLEY T. SCHMIDT, MD
Chief Resident, Department of Neurosurgery, University of Wisconsin Hospital and Clinics, Madison, Wisconsin

LAUREN N. SCHULZ, MD
Department of Neurological Surgery, The Ohio State University Wexner Medical Center, Columbus, Ohio

SAMAN SHABANI, MD
Department of Neurological Surgery, University of California, San Francisco, San Francisco, California

JAY L. SHILS, PhD
Department of Neurosurgery, Rush University, Chicago, Illinois

JACK M. SHIREMAN, BS
Department of Neurosurgery, University of Wisconsin-Madison School of Medicine and Public Health, Madison, Wisconsin

J. MARC SIMARD, MD, PhD
Professor, Departments of Neurosurgery, Pathology, and Physiology, University of Maryland Medical Center, Baltimore, Maryland

VITALY SIOMIN, MD
Herbert Wertheim College of Medicine, Florida International University, Division of Neurosurgery, Miami Neuroscience Institute, Baptist Health South Florida, Miami, Florida

BRANDON W. SMITH, MD
Mayo Clinic, Department of Neurologic Surgery, Rochester, Minnesota

ROBERT J. SPINNER, MD
Mayo Clinic, Department of Neurologic Surgery, Rochester, Minnesota

MICHAEL STEINMETZ, MD
Center for Spine Health, Department of Neurosurgery, Neurologic Institute, Cleveland Clinic Foundation, Cleveland, Ohio

ANDREW K. WONG, MD
Department of Neurosurgery, Rush University, Chicago, Illinois

Contents

Multiple sclerosis (MS) is an autoimmune inflammatory disease that results in demyelination of the central nervous system (CNS). MS affects as many as 350,000 individuals in the United States and commonly presents before the age of 45 years. Patients with MS, as the general population, are likely to encounter degenerative changes of the spine as they age, and this can pose a unique challenge to both patients with MS and physicians, as both conditions can have a great deal of symptomatic overlap despite stark differences in management. Currently there is no definitive approach that allows physicians to distinguish between the two conditions; however, specific clinical and radiologic findings have been identified as being useful in evaluating these patients.

Spinal fusion is frequently performed for a variety of indications. It is performed to treat instability due to trauma, infection, or neoplasm. It may be used to treat regional or global spinal deformity. There are even occasions when it is appropriate as a treatment of low back pain without overt instability or deformity. One common indication for fusion is as an adjunct to decompression for patients with neurogenic claudication or radiculopathy caused by stenosis associated with spondylolisthesis. There have been a number of high-quality publications in high-quality journals that have reported conflicting results regarding the utility of fusion in this patient population. The existence of conflicting data from seemingly similarly designed trials has resulted in some confusion as to when a fusion should be used. This chapter will describe the controversy, discuss the likely basis for the disparate results reported in the literature, and recommend a reasonable treatment strategy. Going forward, the SLIP II study is an ongoing randomized, controlled trial designed to help clarify the situation. Preliminary findings drawn from this study will be discussed.

The use of intraoperative neuromonitoring (IONM) can improve surgical outcomes. Although inclusion of IONM is considered standard practice in more complicated spine surgeries, there are no national-level guidelines for the usage of IONM in spine surgery. Technical advancement in IONM has increased both its sensitivity and specificity, and with a recently developed algorithmic checklist it can be more easily adopted by the surgical team in their practice.

This chapter will review the current management of patients with peripheral nerve injuries and nerve compression syndromes that result in favorable surgical outcomes when appropriately evaluated and referred in a timely fashion. Given the fact that neurologists frequently evaluate patients with these conditions and refer patients to neurosurgeons, it is important for them to be aware of the indications for, types and timing of surgical procedures, and expected outcomes with the various types of interventions.

Chiari Malformation Type I (CMI) is a congenital malformation diagnosed by MRI findings of at least 5 mm of cerebellar ectopy below the foramen magnum. CM1 is frequently associated with syringomyelia. Herein, we discuss the history of CMI and syringomyelia, including early pathological and surgical studies. We also describe recent investigations into the pathogenesis and pathophysiology of CMI and their practical implications on management and surgical intervention. We also highlight the recent development of the Common Data Elements for CMI, providing a framework for ongoing investigations. Finally, we discuss current controversies of surgical management in CMI.

Following the successful completion of 5 major trials establishing the clinical efficacy of endovascular thrombectomy for ELVO in the setting of AIS, there has been a tremendous focus on identifying additional patient populations that may benefit from the intervention. Improved imaging modalities and subsequent trials found thrombectomy to be highly efficacious in patients presenting up to 24 hours after stroke onset, particularly with good collaterals and large penumbral regions. Iterative catheter and device development have improved the safety profile and enhanced the efficacy of the procedure with the introduction of balloon-guide catheters, larger bore navigable aspiration catheters, and smaller catheters and devices to access medium and distal vessel occlusions. While trials are ongoing to assess the utility of thrombectomy in patients presenting with large core infarcts, distal occlusions, and direct aspiration as a first-line approach, the highly effective nature of thrombectomy for ELVO is continuing to drive the field of endovascular stroke care forward.

Malignant cerebral edema after large hemispheric infarct is a highly morbid condition, and major, randomized trials over the last 2 decades have affirmed the beneficial effect of surgical intervention in the form of decompressive craniectomy. Early (<48 hours) decompressive craniectomy increases good functional outcomes (mRS 0–3) and reduces mortality. Additionally, trials have found the benefit of surgery to persist in those patients more than 60 years, though the apparent benefit is of lesser magnitude. A summary table of the major randomized trials of decompressive craniectomy is included. A detailed description and figures of the decompressive craniectomy procedure is included. The complications of decompressive craniectomy are also discussed, and recent literature on promising alternatives, both surgical and medical, is reviewed.

The morbidity and mortality associated with spontaneous intracerebral haemorrhage high, with 40% reported mortality at 1 month and fewer than 40% of patients regaining functional independence. Despite advances made in the treatment of ischemic stroke, similar improvements have not been seen with intracerebral hemorrhage. Medical control of blood pressure and intracranial pressure, among other factors, are key to management. The impact of surgical intervention is less clear. This article reviews the data surrounding the surgical management of intracerebral hemorrhage, including open and minimally invasive techniques and discusses the controversies and future directions surrounding surgical management.

Advances in device technology have created greater flexibility in treating seizures as emergent properties of networks that exist on a local to global continuum. All patients with drug-resistant epilepsy are potential surgical candidates, given that intracranial neuromodulation through deep brain stimulation and responsive neurostimulation can reduce seizures and improve quality of life, even in multifocal and generalized epilepsies. To achieve this goal, indications and strategies for diagnostic epilepsy surgery are evolving. This article describes the state-of-the-art in epilepsy surgery and related changes in how we define indications for diagnostic and therapeutic surgical intervention.

Intraoperative neuromonitoring encompasses a variety of different modalities in which different neuropathways are monitored either continuously or at defined time points throughout a neurosurgical procedure. Surgical morbidity can be mitigated with careful patient selection and thoughtful implementation of the appropriate neuromonitoring modalities through the identification of eloquent areas or early detection of iatrogenic pathway disruption. Modalities covered in this article include somatosensory and motor evoked potentials, electromyography, electroencephalography, brainstem auditory evoked responses, and direct cortical stimulation.

innovative therapeutic trials that take advantage of intracavitary delivery of therapeutic agents after resection. In this article, we review the role of surgical intervention for both low- and high-grade gliomas as well as the innovations that are driving and expanding the role of surgery in this therapeutically challenging group of malignancies.

Robert J. Rothrock, Turki Elarjani, and Allan D. Levi

The goal of the following article is to help the practicing physician learn to recognize conditions that mimic conditions requiring neurosurgical intervention. Each case vignette is presented with relevant clinical history and examination, imaging studies and findings, as well as other testing results. The management for the corresponding diagnosis is presented. Finally, the relevant mimics and differentiating features are discussed.

NEUROLOGIC CLINICS

ISSUES OF RELATED INTEREST

Neurosurgery Clinics
https://www.neurosurgery.theclinics.com/
Neuroimaging Clinics
https://www.neuroimaging.theclinics.com/
Psychiatric Clinics
https://www.psych.theclinics.com/
Child and Adolescent Psychiatric Clinics
https://www.childpsych.theclinics.com/

THE CLINICS ARE AVAILABLE ONLINE!
Access your subscription at:
www.theclinics.com

Preface

Neurosurgery for Neurologists

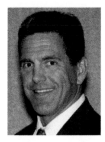 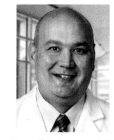

Daniel K. Resnick, MD, MS   Russell R. Lonser, MD
Editors

This issue of *Neurology Clinics* is dedicated to exploring critical clinical links between neurology and neurosurgery. Because both specialties focus on disorders of the nervous system, there are obvious areas of collaboration and numerous opportunities for productive synergism. This issue describes the more common interfaces between the specialties, including epilepsy, intraoperative monitoring, cerebrovascular treatment, neuro-oncology, and neuro-critical care. We hope to provide pithy updates on topics not typically managed by a neurologist but are clinical points of intersection between specialties and are associated with evolving management paradigms. Finally, a discussion of neurosurgical mimics of neurologic disorders is presented along with discussions of the management of patients with multiple disorders (such as multiple sclerosis and cervical myelopathy) who require collaborative management by both specialties.

Daniel K. Resnick, MD, MS
Department of Neurosurgery
University of Wisconsin Madison
School of Medicine and Public Health
K4/834 Clinical Science Center
600 Highland Avenue
Madison, WI 53792, USA

Russell R. Lonser, MD
Department of Neurosurgery
Ohio State University
Wexner Medical Center
410 West 10th Avenue, Doan 1047
Columbus, oh 43210, USA

E-mail addresses:
resnick@neurosurgery.wisc.edu (D.K. Resnick)
russell.lonser@osumc.edu (R.R. Lonser)

https://doi.org/10.1016/j.ncl.2021.11.014
0733-8619/22/© 2021 Published by Elsevier Inc.
neurologic.theclinics.com

Degenerative Spine Disorders and Multiple Sclerosis

Kyle McGrath, BS[a],*, Jonathan Lee, MD[b], Michael Steinmetz, MD[a],
Russell R. Lonser, MD[c], Daniel K. Resnick, MD, MS[d]

KEYWORDS

- Multiple sclerosis • Degenerative spine • Spondylosis • Myelopathy

KEY POINTS

- Multiple sclerosis (MS) is an autoimmune inflammatory disease of the central nervous system that results in demyelination of the brain and spinal cord.
- Degenerative disease of the spine is a common imaging finding with increasing age and when symptomatic, may present similarly to an MS exacerbation.
- Patients with concomitant MS and degenerative disease of the spine must be assessed carefully, as the two conditions are treated very differently despite symptomatic overlap.
- MRI is currently the gold standard for identifying spinal cord lesions caused by both MS and degenerative disease, and specific characteristics can help physicians distinguish between the two.
- Physicians must consider patient history, physical examination, and imaging when deciding on the best course of treatment of patients with MS presenting with ambiguous symptomatology.

INTRODUCTION

Multiple sclerosis (MS) is an autoimmune inflammatory disease that results in demyelination of the central nervous system (CNS). As many as 350,000 individuals in the United States and 2.5 million individuals worldwide are affected by this disease. MS often presents between the ages of 18 and 45 years and is more common in women. Currently there are several known and proposed pharmacologic treatments of MS, including immunomodulation with corticosteroids and interferon beta. There is currently no known cure for the disease however, meaning patients often require life-long intervention.[1–3]

[a] Department of Neurosurgery, Center for Spine Health, Neurologic Institute, Cleveland Clinic Foundation, 9500 Euclid Avenue, S40, Cleveland, OH 44195, USA; [b] Imaging Institute, Cleveland Clinic Foundation, 9500 Euclid Avenue Cleveland, OH 44195, USA; [c] Department of Neurosurgery, The Ohio State University College of Medicine, 410 W. 10th Ave, Columbus, Ohio 43210, USA; [d] Department of Neurosurgery, University of Wisconsin School of Medicine and Public Health, 600 Highland Ave, Madison, WI 53792, USA
* Corresponding author.
E-mail address: Kb725416@ohio.edu

Neurol Clin 40 (2022) 249–259
https://doi.org/10.1016/j.ncl.2021.11.004
0733-8619/22/© 2021 Elsevier Inc. All rights reserved.
neurologic.theclinics.com

Abbreviations	
MS	Multiple Sclerosis
CSM	Cervical Spondylotic Myelopathy
OPLL	Ossification of the Posterior Longitudinal Ligament

Degenerative disorders of the spine, or degenerative spine disease, pose a unique challenge to patients with MS, as both conditions can have a great deal of symptomatic overlap despite stark differences in management. Herein the authors discuss some of the challenges that those with concomitant MS and degenerative spine disorders face and current data, as they pertain to successfully navigating this clinical dilemma.

DISCUSSION
Degenerative Disorders of the Spine

Degenerative disorders of the spine refer to a broad range of abnormalities that occur over the course of one's life in response to loading on the spine as well as genetics. Mild degeneration of the spine is normal in the aging process and is only considered pathologic if responsible for associated symptoms. Degenerative spine disorders may arise from overuse and chronic trauma, although there are many known pathologic inciting factors that can compound over time ultimately requiring intervention. This topic includes a myriad of different diagnoses, many of which have different clinical presentations and management strategies. The authors discuss many of these diagnoses in brief and their neurologic presentation, as it pertains to patients with MS.[4]

Spondylosis is the most common degenerative change seen in aging spines, being present in 60% of women and 80% of men after 50 years of age. Signs of spondylosis include the presence of osteophytes and signs of intervertebral disc degeneration, both of which can compress the spinal cord or exiting nerve roots resulting in symptoms. Disc degeneration occurs with age, as circumferential tears occur in the annulus fibrosis due to the replacement of collagen and proteoglycans with fibrous tissue. Eventually if the tears become substantial enough, axial pressure can result in the herniation or prolapse of the nucleus pulposus through the annulus into the spinal canal or foramen.[4,5]

The cervical and lumbar spine, specifically C5–C7 and L4–S1, are the most common locations for degenerative changes due to unique biomechanical stressors at these levels.[4] Because of this increase in incidence, patients with symptomatic degeneration of the spine are most likely to present with symptoms related to the cervical and lumbar regions. MS-related lesions in these areas may be difficult to distinguish from more common degenerative processes.

Cervical Spine

The prevalence of cervical spine–derived disability is as high as 4.6% in general population.[6] Patients with symptomatic degeneration of the cervical spine are likely to present with neck pain, radiculopathy, myelopathy, or a combination thereof depending on what neurologic components are being affected.[7,8]

Cervical radiculopathy commonly results from foraminal encroachment of a spinal nerve root, which can present with more localized symptoms to a specific dermatome or myotome. These symptoms include neck pain with or without radiating upper extremity pain, a positive Spurling sign, numbness or paresthesias, weakness, and hyporeflexia.[8] Conversely, myelopathy can occur when the cervical spinal cord is affected directly. In addition to sensory abnormalities, myelopathy can present with clinical signs of upper motor neuron dysfunction not seen in radiculopathy. These include hyperreflexia, Hoffmann sign, Babinski sign, clonus, increased muscle tone and spasticity, gait abnormalities, upper extremity loss of fine motor dexterity, and bowel or bladder dysfunction.[7,9]

Spondylosis is the most common cause of cervical spine degeneration. It can result in all of the aforementioned symptoms; however, when inciting myelopathy, the patient is given the clinical diagnosis of cervical spondylotic myelopathy (CSM).[10,11] CSM is the diagnosis of interest for most of the literature assessing patients with concomitant MS due to the degree of clinical overlap between the 2 disorders with respect to presenting symptoms. Other common causes of cervical spine degeneration include cervical disc herniation (**Fig. 1**) and ossification of the posterior longitudinal ligament (OPLL). OPLL can result in spinal stenosis and incite cervical myelopathy, whereas cervical disc herniation can present with a combination of myelopathy and radiculopathy depending on the level and direction of the herniation.[12–14]

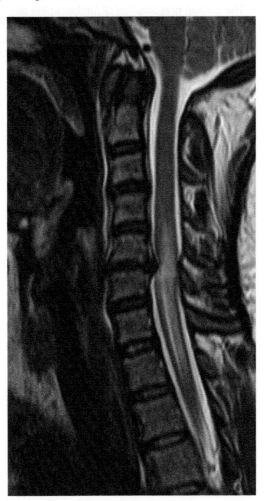

Fig. 1. Sagittal T2-weighted MRI of the cervical spine exhibiting a C5–C6 disc bulge, resulting in spinal cord compression and signal hyperintensity.

Although most of the patients do not require surgical intervention,[7] it may be offered to those who fail conservative treatment or those experiencing myelopathy, severe radiculopathy, or axial neck pain that limits range of motion.[15] Decompression procedures in the form of anterior discectomy and fusion, posterior fusions, laminectomies, and laminoplasties, among others can arrest progressive neurologic deterioration and restore function in these patients.[10,12,15,16]

Lumbar Spine

Degenerative disorders of the lumbar spine, similar to that of the cervical spine, are common among older populations. Hallmark symptoms of degenerative lumbar spine disorders occur due to compression of the neurologic elements within the central canal or exiting foramen (**Fig. 2**). Spinal stenosis, the narrowing of the central canal, most commonly results from degenerative lumbar disc disease or spondylolisthesis, the anterior displacement of one vertebral body on another.[17] Lateral recess or foraminal stenosis classically results from arthritic changes of the facet joints and degeneration of the lumbar discs. The clinical presentation of lumbar spine degeneration typically includes low back pain, radiculopathy, and neurogenic claudication.[18] Because the spinal cord ends at the rostral extent of the lumbar spine, upper motor neuron signs are uncommon and differentiation from MS is more straightforward. The classic

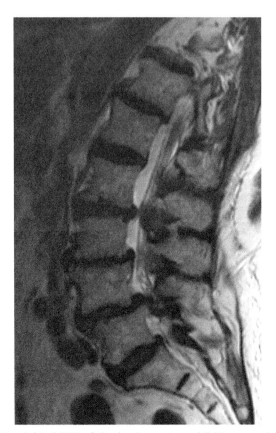

Fig. 2. Sagittal T2-weighted MRI of the lumbar spine exhibiting spondylosis, resulting in compression of the spinal canal.

symptoms of lumber radiculopathy and neurogenic claudication are usually easily distinguished from MS. However, patients may present with more complex gait disturbances and complaints, and determining the relative contribution of different pathologies can be challenging.

Although up to 90% of patients with symptomatic lumbar disc disease will have symptom relief with conservative management, it was still responsible for 342,000 disc-related procedures in 2010 alone, emphasizing that degenerative changes are a major factor driving surgery in the United States.[19,20]

Surgical treatment of degenerative disorders of the lumbar spine can include posterior decompression (eg, foraminotomy, laminotomy, and laminectomy procedures) and fusion procedures with and without instrumentation such as pedicle screw and rod constructs. These can be achieved from a variety of different approaches but are traditionally done posteriorly. Discectomies can also be done in the case of an isolated disc herniation without the need for additional stabilization.[18]

CLINICAL RELEVANCE
Degenerative Disorders of the Spine in Patients with Multiple Sclerosis

The cervical region of the spine is the most frequently affected region of the spinal cord in MS. The clinical presentation of cervical spine MS lesions can be identical to that of CSM, including hyperreflexia, spasticity, motor weakness, bowel and bladder dysfunction, gait abnormalities, and sensory changes.[1,3,21] MS of the cervical spine and CSM are so similar in presentation that patients with undiagnosed MS have undergone unnecessary cervical decompression surgery for misdiagnosed CSM.[22] In patients with MS, the incidence of spondylosis and CSM is similar to that of the general population. One study even demonstrated that degenerative changes in the discs of the cervical and lumbar spine were present in 19% of patients with MS regardless of symptomatology.[23] As incidence increases with age regardless of MS status, this becomes a clinical dilemma that many patients with MS older than 50 years are likely to encounter.[24]

Although the symptomatic overlap between MS and degenerative lumbar spine disorders is not as widely studied as that between MS and CSM, it is possible that MS lesions can be misdiagnosed as a lumbar spine disease. MS can affect any level of the spinal cord and present with bowel and bladder dysfunction, radiculopathy, and low back pain, which can be identical in presentation to many lumbar spine pathologies. It has been reported that localized back and neck pain is reported as a major complaint in up to 55% of patients with MS, and among patients with MS reporting back pain 97% have spinal cord MS lesions.[25] If imaging suggested concomitant lumbar spine pathology in these patients, their MS may go untreated or they may even be offered unnecessary surgery.

Although there is significant overlap in the symptomatology between those with isolated MS and degenerative spine disorders, valuable data have been gathered on patient presentation that can help physicians discern between the 2 conditions. It has been found that neck pain and radiculopathy are more specific indicators of cervical spondylosis than MS,[26] and among patients undergoing surgical decompression for CSM, those without a diagnosis of MS are more likely to have neck pain and radiculopathy than those with MS.[27] Furthermore, if a patient with MS presents to the clinic with neck pain and radiculopathy, it is reasonable to work them up for cervical spondylosis.

Imaging

Imaging along may be suboptimal for distinguishing between neurologic lesions caused by MS and those caused by degenerative spine disorders. MRI is the gold standard for evaluation of patients experiencing myelopathy or radiculopathy, as it allows for detailed visualization of soft tissue and fluid as seen in the intervertebral discs, spinal cord, and the cerebrospinal fluid[7,18] (**Fig. 3**), and this allows for detailed visualization of stenosis within the central canal and foraminal, as well as spinal cord and nerve root compression in the cervical and lumbar spine. Regarding the spinal cord specifically, both CSM and MS lesions can be identified on MRI as signal hyperintensity on T2-weighted (T2W) images and low intensity on T1 images.[3,7] Furthermore, gadolinium contrast in MRI is useful in visualizing inflammation and demyelination and may be very useful in identifying active MS activity.[28]

As was mentioned, both CSM and MS can present very similarly on T2W MRI images even in the presence of gadolinium contrast (**Fig. 4**). However, a recent study

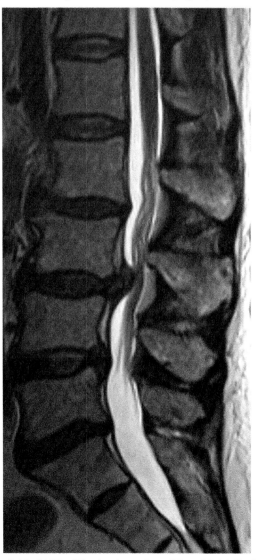

Fig. 3. Sagittal T2-weighted MRI of the lumbar spine with an L3–L4 disc herniation showing detailed distinction between bone, soft tissue, and cerebral spinal fluid.

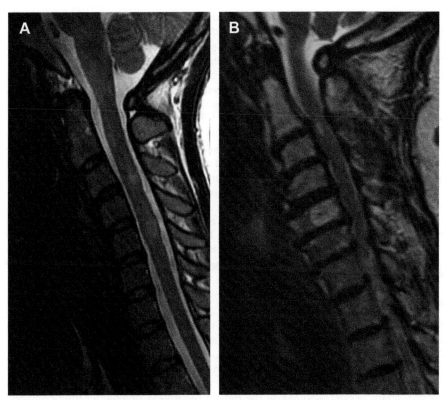

Fig. 4. Sagittal T2-weighted MRI of the cervical spine exhibiting (*A*) multiple sclerosis lesions of the spinal cord at approximately the C3–C4 and C5 levels and (*B*) cervical spondylosis. Notice the spinal cord hyperintense lesions present in both pathologies.

by Givon and colleagues proposed a grading system based on axial and sagittal T2W MRI that allows physicians to reliably differentiate between CSM lesion and MS lesions of the cervical spine (**Table 1**). Based on imaging, it was determined that MS lesions are more likely to be found in higher cervical levels than CSM lesions. MS lesions

Table 1
Cervical spondylotic myelopathy-multiple sclerosis scoring system

	Point Score		
Variables	0	1	2
Cord level	C4–C7	Cl–C3	—
Cord thickness	Decreased	Increased	Normal
Location in axial view	Lateral	Central	—
Location in sagittal view	Anterior/central/combination	Posterior	—
Lesion deliniation	Ill-defined	—	Well-defined

Score 0–3: suggests the lesion in question is due to CSM
   Score 4–7: suggests the lesion in question is due to the given diagnosis of MS
   (*From* Givon U, Hoffman C, Friedlander A, Achiron A. Cervical MRI Rating Scale: Innovative Approach to Differentiate between Demyelinating and Disc Lesions. Clin Neuroradiol. 2019;29(4):639-644. https://doi.org/10.1007/s00062-018-0721-1 with permission.)

are likely to present as well-defined lesions located centrally in axial imaging and posteriorly on sagittal imaging with a normal cord thickness. Conversely, CSM lesions are more likely to be found below the level of C3, presenting as a lesion with poorly defined borders located centrally or laterally in axial imaging and centrally in sagittal imaging. They also found no significant difference between gadolinium enhancement and edema between both types of lesions. Their initial study demonstrated that this scoring system has both high interreader reliability among physicians and reliability in identifying the correct diagnosis (CSM or MS lesion).[3]

Although MRI is able to provide valuable diagnostic information in discerning compressive myelopathy from MS, information gathered from imaging alone will inevitably leave physicians with unanswered questions. In patients with degenerative spine disease, the degree of compression and stenosis seen on MRI often does not correlate directly to a patient's symptom severity.[18] Similarly, there is a phenomenon known as the clinical-radiological paradox seen in patients with MS in which the radiological findings are not supported by clinical symptomatology.[29] The disconnect between imaging and clinical findings in patients experiencing one or both of these conditions reinforces the need for physicians to incorporate patient history and physical examination with imaging findings to determine the best course of treatment.

Management

Patients diagnosed with MS who present with both clinical and imaging findings that suggest degenerative spine disorders still face therapeutic challenges. Although the presenting symptoms may be ambiguous toward a diagnosis, the treatment options for an MS exacerbation and degenerative spine disease vary widely. If surgery is ultimately offered as a viable option, it imposes additional trauma, financial cost, and risk to the patient regardless of whether their condition is correctly diagnosed.[3] Furthermore, patients with MS may be particularly vulnerable when undergoing surgery. Studies have demonstrated that surgery and physical trauma, in addition to postoperative fever can increase a patient's risk for an acute MS exacerbation although additional studies have failed to demonstrate this same correlation.[27,30,31]

Most of the postoperative outcome data on patients diagnosed with MS receiving surgery for degenerative spine disease are on cervical decompression for CSM, although some data do exist on postoperative outcomes for lumbar decompression.[21] Brain and colleagues were the first to evaluate 17 patients with concurrent MS and cervical spondylosis.[32] They found surgery to be of marginal benefit; however, more recent data suggest otherwise. Since the first study in 1957, 5 additional studies have been done including the largest study to date by Lubelski and colleagues assessing postoperative outcomes in both patients with and without MS undergoing decompressive procedures for degenerative spine disorders. These studies collectively have determined that when a patient with MS presents with signs and symptoms that suggest degenerative disease of the spine supported by MRI, surgery is an effective and safe method of helping these patients.[21,26,33,34] However, it was also demonstrated that patients with MS are significantly less likely to experience resolution of cervical myelopathic symptoms in both the short- and long-term follow-up period than those patients without MS receiving the same procedure. In other words, myelopathic patients with MS and cervical spondylosis do improve, albeit to a lesser degree and slower rate than those without MS, and these data should guide physician discussions and patient expectations when receiving surgery for CSM.[27]

SUMMARY

In this article the authors discussed some of the challenges associated with discerning multiple sclerosis from degenerative disease of the spine based on presentation and imaging. Currently there is no definitive approach that allows physicians to distinguish between the two; however, studies have demonstrated that neck pain and radiculopathy are symptoms that may be more specific for cervical spondylosis than MS, and patients with MS presenting with these complaints should be further evaluated for degenerative spine disease.[26,27]

Recently there have been advancements in assessing patients with MS for cervical spondylotic myelopathy based on MRI, which in conjunction with patient history and physical examination can offer valuable insight in determining the best course of treatment.[3] Patients with MS who ultimately undergo decompression surgery for cervical myelopathy may experience symptomatic improvement,[21,26,33,34] although this may be to a lesser degree and at a slower rate than patients without MS.[27] Ultimately a diagnosis of MS makes concomitant degenerative spine disease hard to delineate with current methods; however, effective communication and a comprehensive evaluation of the patient's imaging and presentation can ensure the best chances of a favorable outcome.

CLINICS CARE POINTS

- MS and degenerative disorders of the spine have a significant degree of symptomatic overlap.
- Neck pain and cervical radiculopathy are more specific clinical findings for cervical spondylosis (CS) than MS; therefore, patients with MS presenting with these symptoms should be evaluated for CS.
- MS lesions of the cervical spine will likely present higher in the cervical spine with more well-defined borders than lesions caused by CS. Gadolinium contrast and the presence of edema have not been found to be distinguishing characteristics between the two types of lesions.
- Patients with concomitant MS and CSM undergoing cervical decompression for their CSM are likely to improve at a slower rate and to a lesser extent than patients without MS.

DISCLOSURE

M. Steinmetz, MD, Royalties-Zimmer/Biomet, Elsevier, Globus-Consultant, Globus-Honorarium, Kyle McGrath No Disclosures to report. Jonathan Lee No Disclosures to report; none has an impact on any aspect of this article including content.

REFERENCES

1. Wingerchuk DM, Lucchinetti CF, Noseworthy JH. Multiple sclerosis: Current pathophysiological concepts. Lab Invest 2001;81(3):263–81.
2. Rudick RA, Cohen JA, Weinstock-Guttman B, et al. Management of multiple sclerosis. New Engl J Med 1997;337(22):1604–11. https://doi.org/10.1056/NEJM199711273372207.
3. Givon U, Hoffman C, Friedlander A, et al. Cervical MRI Rating Scale: Innovative Approach to Differentiate between Demyelinating and Disc Lesions. Clin Neuroradiology 2019;29(4):639–44.
4. Gallucci M, Limbucci N, Paonessa A, et al. Degenerative Disease of the Spine. Neuroimaging Clin N Am 2007;17(1):87–103.

5. Weiler C, Schietzsch M, Kirchner T, et al. Age-related changes in human cervical, thoracal and lumbar intervertebral disc exhibit a strong intra-individual correlation. Eur Spine J 2012;21(S6):810–8.
6. Côté P, Cassidy JD, Carroll L. The Saskatchewan health and back pain survey: The prevalence of neck pain and related disability in Saskatchewan adults. Spine 1998;23(15):1689–98. https://doi.org/10.1097/00007632-199808010-00015.
7. Todd AG. Cervical spine: degenerative conditions. Curr Rev Musculoskelet Med 2011;4(4):168–74.
8. Fager CA. Identification and management of radiculopathy. Neurosurg Clin N Am 1993;4(1):1–12. https://doi.org/10.1016/s1042-3680(18)30603-x.
9. Polston DW. Cervical Radiculopathy. Neurol Clin 2007;25(2):373–85.
10. Edwards CC, Riew KD, Anderson PA, et al. Cervical myelopathy: Current diagnostic and treatment strategies. Spine J 2003;3(1):68–81. https://doi.org/10.1016/S1529-9430(02)00566-1.
11. Tracy JA, Bartleson JD. Cervical Spondylotic Myelopathy. Neurologist 2010;16(3):176–87.
12. An HS, Al-Shihabi L, Kurd M. Surgical treatment for ossification of the posterior longitudinal ligament in the cervical spine. J Am Acad Orthopaedic Surgeons 2014;22(7):420–9. https://doi.org/10.5435/JAAOS-22-07-420.
13. Yamazaki S, Kokubun S, Ishii Y, et al. Courses of cervical disc herniation causing myelopathy or radiculopathy: An analysis based on computed tomographic discograms. Spine 2003;28(11):1171–5. https://doi.org/10.1097/00007632-200306010-00017.
14. Matsumoto M, Fujimura Y, Suzuki N, et al. MRI of cervical intervertebral discs in asymptomatic subjects. J Bone Joint Surg - Ser B 1998;80(1):19–24. https://doi.org/10.1302/0301-620X.80B1.7929.
15. Rao RD, Currier BL, Albert TJ, et al. Degenerative cervical spondylosis: Clinical syndromes, pathogenesis, and management. J Bone Joint Surg - Ser A 2007;89(6):1360–78. https://doi.org/10.2106/00004623-200706000-00026.
16. Herkowitz HN, Kurz LT, Overholt DP. Surgical management of cervical soft disc herniation:A comparison between the anterior and posterior approach. Spine 1990;15(10):1026–30. https://doi.org/10.1097/00007632-199015100-00009.
17. Pannell WC, Savin DD, Scott TP, et al. Trends in the surgical treatment of lumbar spine disease in the United States. Spine J 2015;15(8):1719–27. https://doi.org/10.1016/j.spinee.2013.10.014.
18. Ellenbogen RG, Sekhar LN, Kitchen ND, Brito da Silva H. Principles of Neurological Surgery. 2018. doi:10.1176/ajp.99.6.901-a.
19. NHDS. National. Hospital Discharge Survey. Available at: https://www.cdc.gov/nchs/nhds/nhds_tables.htm#procedures. September 15, 2020.
20. Sabnis A, Diwan A. The timing of surgery in lumbar disc prolapse: A systematic review. Indian J Orthopaedics 2014;48(2):127–35. https://doi.org/10.4103/0019-5413.128740.
21. Young WF, Weaver M, Mishra B. Surgical outcome in patients with coexisting multiple sclerosis and spondylosis. Acta Neurol Scand 1999;100(2):84–7.
22. Korovessis P, Maraziotis T, Stamatakis M, et al. Simultaneous three-level disc herniation in a patient with multiple sclerosis. Eur Spine J 1996;5(4):278–80. https://doi.org/10.1007/BF00301334.
23. Drenska Kv, Kaprelyan AG, Tzoukeva AJ. Simultaneous Disc Herniation in Patients With Multiple Sclerosis. J IMAB - Annu Proceeding (Scientific Papers) 2013;19(1):399–401.

24. Ronthal M. On the coincidence of cervical spondylosis and multiple sclerosis. Clin Neurol Neurosurg 2006;108(3):275–7.
25. Moulin DE, Foley KM, Ebers GC. Pain syndromes in multiple sclerosis. Neurology 1988;38(12):1830–4. https://doi.org/10.1212/wnl.38.12.1830.
26. Bashir K, Cai CY, Moore TA, et al. Surgery for cervical spinal cord compression in patients with multiple sclerosis. Neurosurgery 2000;47(3):637–43. https://doi.org/10.1097/00006123-200009000-00022.
27. Lubelski D, Abdullah KG, Alvin MD, et al. Clinical outcomes following surgical management of coexistent cervical stenosis and multiple sclerosis: A cohort-controlled analysis. Spine J 2014;14(2):331–7. https://doi.org/10.1016/j.spinee.2013.11.012.
28. Bradley WG. Use of gadolinium chelates in MR imaging of the spine. J Magn Reson Imaging 1997;7(1):38–46. https://doi.org/10.1002/jmri.1880070107.
29. Pelletier J, Audoin B, Reuter F, et al. Plasticity in MS: From functional imaging to rehabilitation. Int MS J 2009;16(1):26–31.
30. Siemkowicz E. Multiple sclerosis and surgery. Anaesthesia 1976;31(9):1211–6.
31. Mohr DC, Hart SL, Julian L, et al. Association between stressful life events and exacerbation in multiple sclerosis: A meta-analysis. Br Med J 2004;328(7442):731. https://doi.org/10.1136/bmj.38041.724421.55.
32. Brain R, Wilkinson M. The Association of cervical spondylosis and disseminated sclerosis. Brain 1957;80(4):456–78.
33. Arnold PM, Warren RK, Anderson KK, et al. Surgical treatment of patients with cervical myeloradiculopathy and coexistent multiple sclerosis: Report of 15 patients with long-term follow-up. J Spinal Disord Tech 2011;24(3):177–82. https://doi.org/10.1097/BSD.0b013e3181e668d0.
34. Burgerman R, Rigamonti D, Randle JM, et al. The association of cervical spondylosis and multiple sclerosis. Surg Neurol 1992;38(4):265–70. https://doi.org/10.1016/0090-3019(92)90037-N.

Update on Spinal Fusion

Daniel K. Resnick, MD, MS*, Bradley T. Schmidt, MD

KEYWORDS

- Spine • Decompression • Fusion • SLIP

KEY POINTS

- Spinal fusion is commonly performed to treat spinal instability or deformity.
- There is substantial evidence supporting the use of spinal fusion for these indications.
- Spinal fusion is also performed as an adjunct to decompression for patients with neurogenic claudication or radiculopathy associated with degenerative spondylolisthesis.
- The evidence for this practice is substantial yet somewhat controversial and will be the focus of this update.
- The SLIP II study is an ongoing randomized, controlled trial designed to advance our knowledge regarding the role of fusion as an adjunct to decompression and address the controversies which have arisen in the literature.

INTRODUCTION/DEFINITIONS/BACKGROUND

Spinal fusion has long been used as a tool to stabilize the spine in cases of trauma, deformity correction, among others. The role of fusion in the management of patients with low back pain, disc herniations, and symptomatic lumbar spondylolisthesis remains debated. Using spinal fusion as an adjunct in cases adds complexity, cost, length of anesthesia, and other increased potential risks to patients.[1] While medically necessary in many cases, determining guidelines for spinal fusion remains critical to help alleviate some of these confounders when able.

The most recent guideline updates on lumbar spinal fusion were published by a group of experts in the field in 2014.[2] However, despite these guidelines there continues to be a debate in the community regarding techniques to use for optimal fusion as well as indications for fusion itself. Analysis of the variability in the utilization of fusion for the treatment of spondylolisthesis and back pain reveals a wide range of variability between regions of the country and even between hospitals in the same region.[3–5] This phenomenon has led to concerns of over-utilization of fusion without measurable benefit.

Department of Neurosurgery, University of Wisconsin Hospital and Clinics, 600 Highland Avenue, Madison, WI 53792, USA
* Corresponding author.
E-mail address: resnick@neurosurgery.wisc.edu

Neurol Clin 40 (2022) 261–268
https://doi.org/10.1016/j.ncl.2021.11.005
0733-8619/22/© 2022 Elsevier Inc. All rights reserved.

CLINICAL RELEVANCE

Low back pain and disability caused by degenerative changes in the spine are among the most prevalent conditions requiring medical intervention worldwide.[6] Fusion procedures, compared with decompression alone, are associated with increased blood loss, increased costs, and longer postoperative hospital admissions.[1] Therefore, determining the impact fusion has on these pathologies is of great clinical and socioeconomic value.

Spinal fusion is a valuable asset in the spine surgeon's repertoire. Fusion allows for stabilization in the setting of trauma, infection, advanced degeneration, or deformity. Spinal fusion also permits the surgeon to address more challenging pathologies, as these operations often require significant bony removal to deal with the pathologic issue and result in iatrogenic instability that would preclude treatment in the absence of fusion. The basic concepts of spinal fusion have not changed in years as the biomechanics of the spine and the natural history of spinal instability has been well described. There have been dramatic changes in the tools available to the surgeon and a huge shift toward minimally invasive and interbody techniques which have developed directly as the result of improved navigation, implants, and instrumentation (**Fig. 1**). Regardless of how the fusion is performed, however, it should only be performed if it adds to the improvement of patient outcomes.

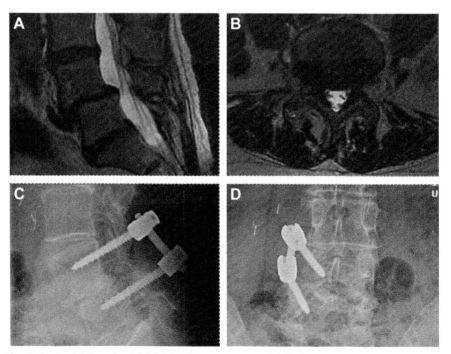

Fig. 1. Sagittal (*A*) and axial (*B*) MRI shows L4-5 spondylolisthesis causing primarily lateral recess and foraminal stenosis in a middle-aged woman with primarily right leg pain which occurs when she stands and walks. She reports 9/10 leg pain and an Oswestry Disability Index (ODI) of 44 prior to intervention. Postoperative radiographs (*C* and *D*) at 6 months show a minimally invasive transforaminal interbody fusion with good healing. Her leg pain is resolved and her ODI has dropped to 8.

A specific area of interest has been the role of fusion as an adjunct to decompression for patients with neurogenic claudication or radiculopathy associated with degenerative lumbar spondylolisthesis. Degenerative spondylolisthesis, especially low grade (Meyerding grade 1) is felt to represent "glacial," or very slowly progressing instability. Because the instability is slowly progressing, because the primary symptoms are caused by nerve compression which is addressed by decompression, and because many of these patients are elderly, the question of how much benefit does fusion provides is an important and relevant issue. Published guidelines for the management of spondylolisthesis published in the last decade currently recommend the performance of fusion but acknowledge the limitations of the available evidence.[7]

Recently, 2 randomized controlled studies looking at the role of fusion in patients with neurogenic claudication due to stenosis associated with grade I degenerative spondylolisthesis were published in the same issue of the *New England Journal of Medicine*. The issue was a great read, particularly because the 2 studies reached opposite conclusions about the utility of fusion as an adjunct to decompression. A North American study authored by Ghogawala and colleagues reported that fusion was associated with better long-term outcomes and a lower long-term reoperation rate than decompression alone. Interestingly, the decrease in reoperation rates resulted in cost savings for the fusion group despite the initial higher costs associated with the performance of fusion.[8] In contrast, a European study authored by Forsth and colleagues found that long-term outcomes were similar between the decompression alone and decompression with fusion groups and that costs and complications were higher in the fusion group.[9]

Why were the results differ between the studies? There are a number of possible explanations related to differences in patient selection, operative techniques, choice of outcome measures, and duration of follow-up.[10] The most important issue, in our opinion, was patient selection. Degenerative spondylolisthesis encompasses a broad range of patients with heterogeneous characteristics that may or may not make them suitable for fusion. It is clear from both the randomized studies that there exist populations of patients who definitely benefit from fusion and there are populations of patients within the same cohort who definitely do not benefit from the performance of fusion. A significant weakness in both randomized trials is that patient selection criteria were exclusively dependent on a classification system (Meyerding) which was developed in the 1930s to aid obstetricians to provide care to pregnant women (ref). This classification system has nothing to do with providing guidance for operative intervention in patients with radiculopathy or neurogenic claudication.

CURRENT GUIDELINES

The AANS/CNS joint section on disorders of the spine and peripheral nerves first published a series of recommendations for spinal fusion for degenerative disease in the lumbar spine in June 2005. These guidelines and the most recent update (published in 2014) are formulated based on a comprehensive analysis of literature (meta-analyses, peer-reviewed studies, etc.).[2] While not comprehensive, these were established the base for treatment protocols.

The most current guidelines regarding spinal fusion were published in 2014 in the Journal of Neurosurgery Spine.[2] In basic summary, these guidelines suggest that there is level II evidence to provide a grade B recommendation for fusion as a suitable treatment plan for low back pain (without disc disease or lumbar stenosis) in patients who are refractory to conservative care.[11] The guidelines suggest spinal fusion should not be used as routine treatment of primary disc excision in patients with isolated disc herniation causing radiculopathy (level IV evidence).[12] Fusion can be used as an adjunct in patients with significant chronic axial back pain and disc herniation and those patients with recurrent disc herniations (level IV evidence).[12] The guidelines recommend surgical decompression and fusion as an effective treatment alternative for patients with symptomatic lumbar stenosis and degenerative spondylolisthesis[7]; however, there is not sufficient evidence to recommend a specific fusion technique. Fusion is recommended against for patients who have lumbar stenosis without spondylolisthesis.[13]

CURRENT RESEARCH

The SLIP II study is currently enrolling patients in a randomized, controlled study looking at the outcomes of these patients following a variety of potential interventions.[14] Patients with grade one degenerative spondylolisthesis are invited to participate in the study. The SLIP II study does not dictate treatment; however, it randomizes patients into either standard care by the referring surgeon, or care by the treating surgeon following review of the case by an expert panel. The review panel contains a set of established senior spine surgeons from varying backgrounds and practice settings.

Those patients who are randomized to the review-panel cohort have clinical vignettes describing symptoms, along with representative images sent out to the panelists. The cohort of senior spine surgeons then review the vignette and images and are asked to provide a treatment recommendation based on the information provided. The recommendations can only be 1 out of 6 categories. Category 1 is a recommendation for no surgery, 2 is a minimally invasive decompression, 3 is for an open decompression, 4 is a decompression with noninstrumented fusion, 5 adds instrumentation, and 6 is a fusion involving an interbody graft with instrumentation. The goal of this study is to examine long-term outcomes to determine if concordance with expert panel recommendations regarding fusion versus decompression-alone provides any significant benefit. A benefit of the study is that clinical images and vignettes may be compared with expert panel recommendations. Therefore, there is the potential to develop a clinically relevant classification system based on patient-specific information to guide the decision to perform a fusion as an adjunct to decompression.

As we began to look into this possibility, it immediately became clear that there were both patient-specific as well as surgeon-specific variables that were important in the expert panel review. **Fig. 2** shows a "heat map" illustrating the recommendations from

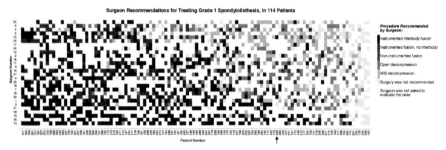

Fig. 2. Heat map summarizing all the recommendations from the 28 review panelists. Rows are ordered by average procedure score for each surgeon, which is a reflection of how aggressive the surgeon tends to be. Columns are ordered by average procedure score per patient, which is a reflection of how invasive the recommended procedures were. Darker colors indicate more aggressive procedures.

a panel of surgeons for a cohort of patients enrolled in the slip study. What the illustration shows is that there are some surgeons who always recommend fusion and some surgeons who very rarely recommend fusion in the same patient cohort. This clearly indicates a training and practice bias intrinsic to the panelist which has little to do with the patent population. The illustration also shows, however, that different patients receive different recommendations from the same expert panelists. This reflects the fact that there are patient-specific factors that guide most of the surgeons in their decision to offer fusion independent of training or practice bias.[5]

We next began to explore the patient characteristics which would lead to a recommendation for fusion. By comparing cohorts of patients in whom there was substantial agreement between the panel members either for or against the performance of fusion, we have been able to identify several key features which differ between the groups (**Fig. 3**). With regard to demographic factors, the fusion cohort was younger and had a lower health state based on EQ-5D scores. With regard to imaging characteristics, we found that greater degree of spondylolisthesis, greater facet angle from horizontal, and movement on dynamic images all predicted a recommendation for fusion. These findings are being incorporated into a proposed classification system for patients with low-grade degenerative spondylolisthesis. This classification will be prospectively applied to the entire SLIP cohort to validate it prospectively. Hopefully, such a classification system will help surgeons more precisely tailor their use of fusion in the spondylolisthesis population to maximize benefit and minimize costs for patients who do, and do not benefit from the addition of fusion following decompression.

DISCUSSION

Fusion is a key component of any spinal surgeon's repertoire. Many indications of fusion are quite clear—unstable spinal trauma, postdecompression restabilization, among others. However, understanding true indications for fusion and which patient factors predict improved outcomes is the key to appropriate patient care. Underutilization of fusion can lead to unnecessary revision surgery, increased pain for the patient, and potentially neurologic injury. Whereas overutilization of fusion can lead to undue anesthesia time, hospital costs, admission lengths, among others.

There is already a significant debate in the medical literature regarding fusion indications and which fusion route to proceed with (instrumented, uninstrumented, interbody, etc.). When concerning patients with neurogenic claudication and grade I degenerative spondylolisthesis there is significant variability in treatment recommendations throughout the literature. There have been multiple studies demonstrating a high degree of variability in fusion treatment recommendations.[3–5] These studies suggest that the degree of disagreement on whether to fuse stems from both patient factors (imaging characteristics, symptomology, etc.) and physician biases (training history, current work environment, etc.).

In fact, one of the most recent studies published by Resnick and Schmidt and colleagues took preliminary data from the SLIP II study and analyzed this variability in more detail.[5] This study sought to investigate the source of the variation in the perceived role of fusion by looking at surgeon as well as patient-specific factors. Their study analyzed the varying treatment recommendations from the expert panel of senior spine surgeons based on 114 patients enrolled in the SLIP II study (all of which had Meyerding grade I degenerative spondylolisthesis). They found that fusion was recommended only 58.5% of the time. And that overall agreement was low with perfect agreement on the need for fusion being seen in only 24 of the 114 patients

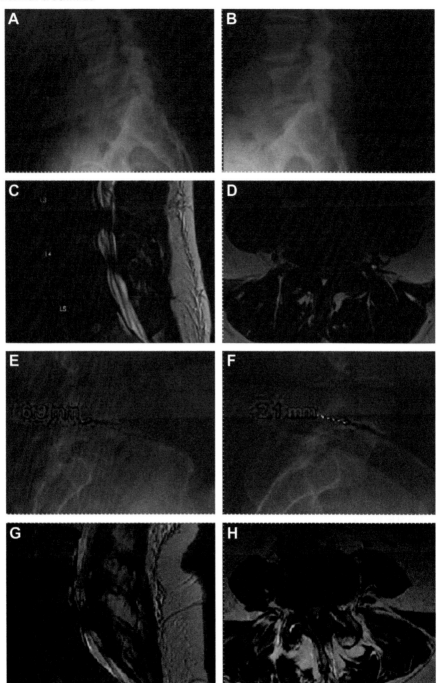

Fig. 3. Example patient from the consensus decompression alone cohort (*A–D*) and consensus decompression and fusion cohort (*E–H*). Note in the decompression alone cohort that there is no motion on dynamic imaging, coronally oriented facets with no T2 signal within the facet, and minimal spondylolisthesis. Upright flexion (*A*) and upright extension (*B*) x-rays, sagittal MRI (*C*) and axial MRI (*D*). Additionally, note that in the decompression and fusion cohort there is obvious motion on dynamic imaging, sagittally oriented facets with T2 signal within the facet, and a moderate degree of spondylolisthesis. Upright flexion (*E*) and upright extension (*F*) x-rays, sagittal MRI (*G*), and axial MRI (*H*).

(21.1%). This study demonstrated the extensive variability among even senior spine surgeon recommendations regarding using fusion as an adjunct with decompression.

Each of these previously described studies demonstrates the complexity and uncertainty in the true utility of fusion in grade I degenerative spondylolisthesis. This uncertainty likely stems from patient-related heterogeneity as well as limitations in the current classification system. Hopefully, continued research in studies like the ongoing SLIP II trial will help elucidate some of the patient characteristics that impact spine surgeon decision making and will help better answer the question as to which patients will have a more substantial response to spinal fusion.

SUMMARY

Spinal fusion is a common strategy used in spinal surgery for a variety of indications. Fusion techniques and materials continue to evolve with time and technological advancements. The use of fusion in the spondylolisthesis population has been extensively yet incompletely examined. The lack of a useful classification system makes comparing across studies difficult. Review of some of the early data from the SLIP II study demonstrates variability in surgeon recommendations due to patient and surgeon-related factors. Examination of patient heterogeneity and the influence of this heterogeneity on the recommendation for fusion is in progress with the intent to develop a rigorous, valid, and useful system to guide the recommendation for fusion in this patient population.

CLINICS CARE POINTS

- Spinal fusion is a valuable asset in the spine surgeon's repertoire. Fusion allows for stabilization in the setting of trauma, infection, degeneration, deformity, or iatrogenic destabilization.
- The use of fusion as an adjunct to decompression is an area of active research and controversy.
- Two simultaneous randomized, controlled studies found opposite conclusions regarding long-term outcomes when using spinal fusion as an adjunct to decompression alone in patients with neurogenic claudication and grade I degenerative spondylolisthesis.
- The SLIP II study is an ongoing randomized, controlled trial looking to help answer the question on the benefit of spinal fusion as an adjunct to decompression alone in patients with neurogenic claudication and grade I degenerative spondylolisthesis.
- Extensive and open discussions with patients regarding all current data are critical to forming an appropriate spinal fusion plan.

DISCLOSURES

Resnick, stock options in NIDUS.

REFERENCES

1. Badhiwala J, Leung S, Jiang F, et al. In-hospital course and complications of laminectomy alone versus laminectomy plus instrumented posterolateral fusion for lumbar degenerative spondylolisthesis: a retrospective analysis of 1804 patients from the NSQIP database. Spine 2021;9:617–23.
2. Groff M. Introduction: guideline update for the performance of fusion procedures for degenerative disease of the lumbar spine. J Neurosurg Spine 2014;21:1.

3. Lubelski D, Williams S, O'Rourke C, et al. Differences in the surgical treatment of lower back pain among spine surgeons in the United States. Spine 2016;41: 978–86.

4. Mroz T, Lubelski D, Williams S, et al. Differences in the surgical treatment of recurrent lumbar disc herniation among spine surgeons in the United States. Spine J 2014;14:2334–43.

5. Resnick D, Schmidt B, Momin E, et al. Interobserver variance and patient heterogeneity influencing the treatment of grade I spondylolisthesis. Spine J 2020;12: 1934–9.

6. Cassidy J, Carroll L, Cote P. The Saskatchewan health and back pain survey. The prevalence of low back pain and related disability in Saskatchewan adults. Spine 1998;23:1860.

7. Resnick D, Watters W, Sharan A, et al. Guideline update for the performance of fusion procedures for degenerative disease of the lumbar spine. Part 9: lumbar fusion for spinal stenosis with spondylolisthesis. J Neurosurg Spine 2014;21: 54–61.

8. Ghogawala Z, Dziura J, Butler W, et al. Laminectomy plus fusion version laminectomy alone for lumbar spondylolisthesis. N Engl J Med 2016;15:1424–34.

9. Forsth P, Olafsson G, Carlson T, et al. A randomized, controlled trial of fusion surgery for lumbar spinal stenosis. N Engl J Med 2016;15:1413–23.

10. Ghogawala Z, Resnick D, Glassman S, et al. Achieving optimal outcome for degenerative lumbar spondylolisthesis: randomized controlled trials. Neurosurgery 2017;64:40–4.

11. Eck J, Sharan A, Ghogawala Z, et al. Guideline update for the performance of fusion procedures for degenerative disease of the lumbar spine. Part 7: lumbar fusion for intractable low-back pain without stenosis or spondylolisthesis. J Neurosurg Spine 2014;21:42–7.

12. Wang J, Dailey A, Mummaneni P, et al. Guideline update for the performance of fusion procedures for degenerative disease of the lumbar spine. Part 8: lumbar fusion for disc herniation and radiculopathy. J Neurosurg Spine 2014;21:48–53.

13. Resnick D, Watters W, Sharan A, et al. Guideline update for the performance of fusion procedures for degenerative disease of the lumbar spine. Part 10: lumbar fusion for spinal stenosis without spondylolisthesis. J Neurosurg Spine 2014; 21:62–6.

14. Ghogawala Z. SLIP II Registry: spinal laminectomy versus instrumented pedicle screw fusion. US National Library of Medicine – Clinical Trials; 2021. Available at: https://clinicaltrials.gov/ct2/show/NCT03570801. September 12, 2021.

Intraoperative Monitoring for Spinal Surgery

Nitin Agarwal, MD*, Saman Shabani, MD, Jeremy Huang, BS,
Alma Rechav Ben-Natan, BA, Praveen V. Mummaneni, MD, MBA

KEYWORDS

- Intraoperative neuromonitoring • Motor evoked potentials
- Somatosensory evoked potentials • Spine surgery

KEY POINTS

- Neuromonitoring has demonstrated effectiveness in particular subsets of spine surgery including spine deformity, spine tumor, and complex multilevel surgical cases.
- Recent improvements in IONM technique have increased the sensitivity and specificity of combined neuromonitoring modalities.
- To aid in IONM, a checklist for responding to intraoperative neuromonitoring alerts has been developed, which could improve effectiveness and efficiency of the neuromonitoring team.

INTRODUCTION

As the average age of the worldwide population grows, so too does the frequency of interventions such as spine surgery to treated degenerative spine disease. However, as with all procedures, risks exist inherent to spine surgery including but not limited to wound infections, hardware failure, cerebrospinal fluid leak, pseudoarthrosis, postoperative hematoma, and postoperative radiculopathy.[1] The use of intraoperative neurophysiological monitoring (IONM) may help to mitigate neurologic risks.[2] As such this article reviews the evolution, indications, pearls, and pitfalls or IONM for spine surgery. The field of IONM continues to grow, bringing additional checks and balances to all parts of the surgical procedure from positioning of trauma and myelopathy cases to complex deformity corrections.

HISTORICAL PERSPECTIVES

The first description of IONM dates to the 1970s, when spinal cord evoked potentials were first used in Japan specifically for spinal cord monitoring. Somatosensory evoked

Department of Neurological Surgery, University of California, San Francisco, 505 Parnassus Avenue, M779, San Francisco, CA 94143, USA
* Corresponding author.
E-mail address: nitin.agarwal@ucsf.edu

potential (SSEP) monitoring was also first explored during this time, with the initial usage described in spine surgery around 1972.[3] In the 1980s, motor evoked potential (MEP) monitoring was first described with the introduction of intravenous anesthesia, which did not have as much of a depressive effect on motor neuron activity as previous gas-based general anesthesia techniques.[4] SSEP and MEP were first combined in the 1990s with the introduction of multiphase techniques and are now considered complementary techniques. Finally, triggered electromyography (tEMG) was first used in neuromonitoring of spine surgery in 1992.[4] At present, multimodal spinal cord monitoring is helpful to improve accuracy, because no single strategy is without drawbacks. Several studies report that combined modality monitoring has increased sensitivity over single-modality monitoring. IONM has historically been used in spine surgery procedures involving spinal neoplasms and scoliosis correction, but it has also recently begun to be incorporated into other spine surgeries, including cervical and lumbar spine surgeries.[5] Ultimately, IONM is becoming more widely used in the perioperative setting to prevent spinal cord injury, increasing surgical safety and efficacy.

DEFINITIONS AND TYPES OF MONITORING MODALITIES
Somatosensory Evoked Potentials

SSEP neuromonitoring measures potentials transmitted through sensory pathways from the peripheral nerve. SSEPs are recorded from the spinal cord and/or the cortex after stimulation of peripheral nerves. SSEP signals are generated by averaging the latency and amplitude of the electrical signals, meaning that signal acquisition time must be considered in surgical reactions. SSEP in spine surgery specifically monitors the dorsal column-medial lemniscus pathway by propagating action potentials from the peripheral nerves to the contralateral sensory cortex.[4] It has been shown that SSEPs can prove useful in detecting peripheral ischemia and potential injury resulting from positioning of the surgical patient.[6,7]

Motor Evoked Potentials

MEP refers to the monitoring of compound corticospinal action potentials initiated by direct axonal activation to track activity of the corticospinal tract.[4] Because these waves do not require signal averaging, there is no acquisition time associated with MEP monitoring. There are several types of MEPs: neurogenic MEPs are stimulated at the spinal cord and recorded at the peripheral nerve, whereas muscle or myogenic MEPs are evoked from transcranial electrodes and recorded at specific muscles depending on the surgical procedure.[4] Muscle MEP does not require an epidural electrode and has a higher generation rate of potentials but may have more signal loss than neurogenic MEP.[4]

D Waves

D (direct) waves are compound corticospinal action potentials generated by direct activation of axons. D waves are obtained by a single transcranial electrical stimulation pulse recorded from the epidural or subdural space of the spinal cord. Therefore, D waves are also known as "spinal motor evoked potentials".[4] D waves usually do not need averaging, although a few averages improve its quality of recording; this provides clinically real-time feedback. Unlike muscle MEPs, it is insensitive to anesthesia and therefore considered simpler to interpret. However, it must be recorded with an epidural electrode, and it is difficult to record stimuli from below the thoracic region. Owing to these limitations, it is often indicated in spine tumor surgeries over deformity surgeries.[8]

Electromyography

EMG does not require stimulation to produce action potentials but monitors prese-
lected muscle groups based on at-risk nerve roots. Although EMG is simple to
monitor, it is also prone to false spontaneous activation and is less effective in patients
with neurologic disorders. There are several types of EMG: spontaneous EMG (sEMG),
also known as free-running EMG, can be monitored continuously but requires a
continuous neuromuscular signal, whereas tEMG can be obtained easily by stimulating the center of the pedicle screw but does not yet have established set thresholds
for neuromuscular alerts.[9]

UTILITY OF NEUROMONITORING

Interpretation of any of the various modalities of IONM mentioned earlier requires analysis of electrophysiological signals to determine deviations from baseline. The most
important properties of the recorded signals are changes in the amplitude, latency,
and wave shape of the response. IONM is highly sensitive to any type of neural
compromise, including from preexisting conditions and physiologic response to anesthetic management, so all members of the surgical team must work together to establish accurate IONM readings.

SSEP can be monitored continuously but relies on signal averaging over time, so
decreases may lag transcranial MEP changes. SSEP signal transmission can be
affected by patient height, temperature, nerve compression, and anesthetic type
and dose.[10] Monitoring of MEP may provide earlier detection of neurologic injury,
but MEP cannot be monitored continuously and may induce patient movement. For
example, a multiphase method of monitoring MEP was developed to address MEP
limitations from anesthesia but created alternative adverse effects in the form of patient tongue and lip lacerations.[10] Both SSEP and MEP are frequently used to monitor
neurologic function during spinal deformity surgery and are useful in evaluating the
functional integrity of the spinal cord. Concurrent use of SSEPs and MEPs to monitor
posterior spinal fusion cases has demonstrated overall improved sensitivity and specificity in neuromonitoring in scoliosis surgery.[11] EMG is less well characterized as a
standalone modality of IONM, because it is usually used in support of SSEP and
MEP. However, it has unique applications in minimally invasive spine surgeries, especially posterior pedicle screw placements. Stimulating the screw can help in determining if there is a medial breach, and it minimizes the use of perioperative
fluoroscopy by allowing for early trajectory correction.[12] EMG is also less susceptible
to the neurologic effects of anesthesia.[10]

Generally, multimodal IONM is recommended in almost all spine surgery cases. The
use of IOMN is inconsistent across the United States. Cole and colleagues[13] performed a study in 2014 of approximately 85,000 single-level spinal procedures, about
11% of which received IONM, and found no trends among IONM inclusion in procedures nationwide. This lack of pattern includes comparisons to geographic region,
overall neurologic complication rates, and with state medical liability environments
as evaluated by the American College of Emergency Physicians.[13] Usually, IONM occurs throughout the entire surgical case, with neuromonitoring leads placed on the patient immediately after administering anesthesia to obtain baseline values for SSEP
and MEP. IONM recommendations have become more refined in recent literature;
for example, Chachan and Bae[14] recommend a multimodal approach consisting of
SSEP, MEP, and EMG in thoracic spine surgeries. The major limitations on widespread IONM use in spine surgery are economic and medicolegal; whereas multimodal IONM is currently the standard of care for spinal deformity surgeries in the

United States and other developed countries, its usage is less consistent elsewhere.[15] For example, the utility of IONM in predicting and mitigating postoperative neurologic deficits in cervical spine surgery is still under debate. In conclusion, the use of IONM is well characterized and is supported for spinal deformity surgeries and spinal tumor surgeries, but its inclusion in less complex degenerative cervical and lumbar spinal procedures is still controversial. Overall, the use of IONM is usually guided by physician preference and local institutional guidelines[9]

INDICATIONS

IONM is not associated with major adverse effects; however, some common complications of IONM include inadvertent stimulation of various nerves, which can lead to tongue bites or patient movement. Steps can be taken to minimize this risk, such as including bite blocks for patients. Patients at risk for seizure or with implanted defibrillators may also face additional risk for neuromonitoring.[8] The major indications for and against IONM for specific spine surgical procedures are the added cost and time of IONM.[15] Setting up IONM does not generally have a significant impact on operative times, taking an average of 5 minutes.[16] However, this average takes into account neither the time needed for the acquisition of preposition baselines nor the time needed to respond to neuromonitoring alerts, which can add significantly to operative time. The use of IONM is largely indicated in multilevel procedures because of increased neurologic operative risk to the patient.[17] Interestingly, Krause and colleagues[18] found that neuromonitoring in a cohort of patients undergoing single-level lumbar discectomies resulted in a significant increase in operative time (174 vs 144 minutes) without differences in clinical outcome between IONM and no IONM groups. However, there was no statistically significant difference in operative times with (532 ± 141 min) and without (492 ± 81 min) IONM in a series of posterior vertebral column resection cases studied by Huang and colleagues.[19]

Indications for specific forms of IONM are generally indicated on an individual case basis, specifically based on case approach, the perceived risk of neurologic injury, and the possibility of injury to anatomic structures.[20] In addition, sEMG and tEMG are advised in the case of risk of nerve root deficits.[20] The higher risk of neurologic injury in revision and deformity cases merits the use of IONM in these cases. Finally, anesthetic requirements and limitations for each form of IONM must be considered. Ultimately, any argument against the use of IONM in spine surgery must consider the long-term costs of managing postoperative neurologic deficits that may have been prevented with perioperative IONM.

DISCUSSION
Sensitivity and Specificity

The sensitivity and specificity of different IONM modalities is critical in deciding which modality, or combination of modalities, to use for various spine surgery procedures. Clark and colleagues[21] found a significant association between IONM MEP alerts and presence of new postoperative deficits. The general sensitivity and specificity they found were 75% and 92%, respectively, with a positive predictive value of 38% for IONM alerts. However, specificity and positive predictive value were higher when the recorded MEP changes did not return to baseline. Without return to baseline Clark and colleagues[21] reported specificity of 98% and positive predictive value of 75%. One notable result from that study is that whereas a subgroup of patients with risk factors for vascular disease and postoperative deficits had a higher rate of neuromonitoring changes compared with those without, they had a lower sensitivity of only

60% compared with the overall patient group (**Figs. 1–3**). In the complementary patient group, those without vascular risk factors, the sensitivity was 100%. Despite these relatively high sensitivity and specificity rates in IONM, postoperative neurologic deficits are observed in patients without significant changes to the monitoring signals during surgery.[22–24]

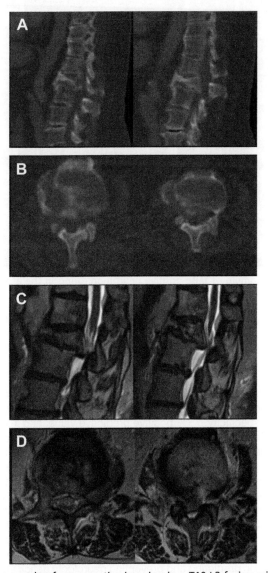

Fig. 1. Illustrative example of preoperative imaging in a T10-L3 fusion with L1 corpectomy for metastatic tumor. (*A*) Sagittal CT with contrast. (*B*) Axial CT with contrast. (*C*) Sagittal MRI with contrast (*left*) and sagittal T2 Turbo Spin Echo (TSE) MRI (*right*). (*D*) Axial T2 images. The CT shows there is an osteolytic mass located mainly at the L1 vertebral body on the left side with involvement of the body and the pedicle. MRI shows extensive loss of height retropulsion of the body causing significant thecal sac compression.

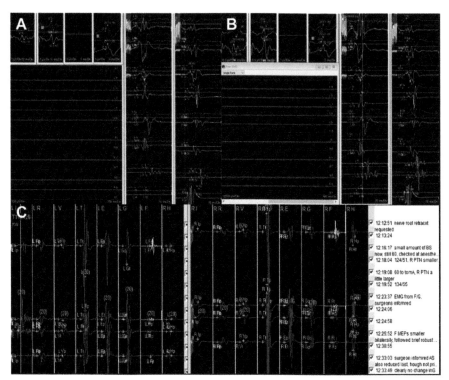

Fig. 2. Illustrative example of false-positive neuromonitoring in the aforementioned case. IONM in this case included SEP, MEP, and EMG. (*A*) Baseline signal for all IONM used. (*B*) IONM signal at the end of case. (*C*) MEP change during the procedure. Despite the suggestion of an adverse event during the procedure, patient was neurologically intact at the end of the case representing a potential false-positive signal. The checklist for MEP alert was used during this procedure.

Performance measures of MEG monitoring in conjunction with SSEP monitoring are found to be superior to those of SSEP monitoring alone. Sensitivity is reported to be 100% with 95.6% specificity, 75% positive predictive value, and 100% negative predictive value.[25] Literature suggests that MEP monitoring is superior to SSEP monitoring, whereas Clark and colleagues argue that it is ultimately better to use both to detect neurologic compromise, spinal cord injury, and potential postoperative deficits.[21,26,27] A partially retrospective, partially prospective study of 200 patients who underwent cervical laminectomy and laminoplasty found that with SSEP monitoring alone C-5 palsy was not predicted.[11,26] However, when MEP monitoring was added prospectively to SSEP monitoring, C-5 palsy was accurately predicted. In addition, a prospective study of 1055 patients who underwent cervical spine surgery who were monitored either with SSEP alone or with SSEP and MEP monitoring concluded that IONM is helpful in predicting and preventing neurologic deficit and that combining IONM methods increases sensitivity significantly.[27] Similarly to Clark and colleagues, this study remarkably found that the diagnostic performance of MEP monitoring was related to certain patient risk factors. The usage of MEP monitoring in these cases is also more likely to partially mitigate the increase in cost associated with neuromonitoring. Such benefits would be able to be confirmed only after the utility of IONM in

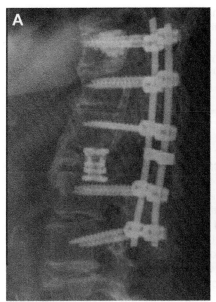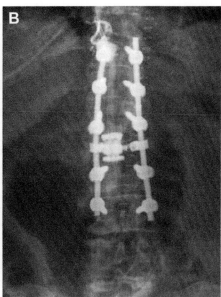

Fig. 3. Postoperative imaging of the aforementioned case. (*A*) Lateral thoracolumbar radiograph. (*B*) Anteroposterior thoracolumbar radiograph. Postoperative images show appropriate placement of the screws with expandable cage at the site of corpectomy at L1. There is restoration of the loss of height. No postoperative magnetic resonance images available.

cervical spine surgery is established, ideally in a multicenter, prospective randomized controlled trial. In a retrospective study of 119 instrumented anterior cervical spine surgery cases, Bose and colleagues[10] found that IONM alerts were more common in multilevel decompression. Their analysis showed that certain physiologic changes like sudden decreases in blood pressure and maneuvers such as unusual arm positioning and hyperextension of the neck likewise led to alerts.

In another study by Agarwal and colleagues,[11] in which patients were likewise monitored by MEP and SSEP, the sensitivity and specificity for new spinal cord deficits were found to be lower, with 75% sensitivity and 83% specificity. The positive predictive value was 60%, and the negative predictive value was 95%. Although these numbers are lower than those reported in the aforementioned study, the combination of MEP and SSEP seems to produce a consistently higher positive predictive value.

During posterior spinal fusions, neurologic insult may occur during several phases of surgery. Injury may be sustained during positioning, during induction of anesthesia, or from direct surgical trauma.[28] Of all levels, the data suggest that the cervical and cervicothoracic levels were most prone to these types of injuries. Given that there is a wealth of literature suggesting that the thoracolumbar region of the spinal cord is the most susceptible to ischemia and hypotension because of limited blood supply and profound watershed effects,[29–31] mechanisms beyond vascular compromise must drive the cervical cord's propensity for injury. It is possible that the cervical cord's distribution of nervous structures renders it vulnerable to injury more frequently during common maneuvers, such as head extension during intubation or manipulation of the neck and upper extremity during positioning. However, 10 of 15 (67%) neuromonitoring changes that occurred at the cervical and cervicothoracic levels were seen in patients with trauma to those regions possibly; this could be because of the soft tissue injury or edema around the cord that renders these patients more susceptible to neuromonitoring changes. Therefore, special attention must be provided when dealing with patients with trauma, especially with positioning and during anesthesia shift changes. Overall, given the risks of neural injury, data support the use of neuromonitoring when performing posterior spinal fusions, at the cervical and cervicothoracic levels.[11]

Cost

Cost has been proved to be a salient factor in decision making regarding the use of IONM in spinal surgery. The cost of the IONM itself and the cost of neurologic injury both need to be taken into consideration in this process. In 2012, Traynelis and colleagues reported no persistent postoperative neurologic deficits in their series of patients with cervical surgeries but estimated that the use of IONM would have cost an hourly rate of $633.32 and incurred a total of US $1,024,754 for reimbursement at the 2011 Medicare rate.[32] Because they found that cervical surgeries without IONM did not significantly impact patient safety, they determined that the cost-benefit analysis supported performing cervical treatments without IONM. However, Ney and colleagues[33] reported cost-effectiveness data of $63,387 in savings per each neurologic injury averted in all spinal surgery. Even though we do not yet have proof that IONM can prevent such injuries, several studies have demonstrated significant benefits in being able to prevent postoperative neurologic deficits as well as spinal cord injury.[10,25–27,34–37]

Algorithm for Positive Monitoring Alerts

A checklist for responding to an intraoperative neuromonitoring alert was devised by Ziewacz and colleagues[38] using an algorithm (**Fig. 4**). The checklist highlights the specific roles of the anesthesiologist, surgeon, and neuromonitoring personnel as well as encourages communication between teams. The checklist focuses on the items critical for identifying and correcting reversible causes of neuromonitoring alerts. Following initial design, the checklist draft was reviewed and amended with stakeholder input. The checklist was then evaluated in a small-scale trial and revised based on usability and feasibility.

The logical algorithm to design, develop, and implement the neurosurgery checklist was based on aviation and general surgery experience in creating checklists used for similar purposes. The algorithm includes 14 key steps, beginning with thinking about and explaining the goals of the project and the philosophy behind it, going through the process of obtaining support and involving all stakeholders to work collaboratively on determining the structure and content of the checklist. After the initial checklist is drafted and reviewed small-scale trials are conducted, which are followed by modifications, repeated training, and the gradual rollout of the checklist to the perioperative staff. After the checklist is implemented, periodic retraining accommodates new hires and ensures checklist compliance and completion is maintained. The checklist is specifically designed for patients with spinal deformity or myelopathy.

When tested in 3 cases, the checklist was found effective in identifying the factors responsible for the neuromonitoring alerts. In all 3 cases the responsible factor was identified as anesthetic regime changes. Importantly, the checklist guides all teams to ensure the change in monitoring is not due to instrumentation failure or artifact by instructing the team to ensure that all leads are correctly placed and repeat the signals.

Checklist for Neuromonitoring (MEP) Alert in Patients with Myelopathy or Deformity

Spine Surgeon:

☐   Stop current manipulation

☐   Assess field for structural cord compression (misplaced hardware or bone graft, osteophytes, or hematoma)

    ☐   Perform further decompression if stenosis is present

☐   Consider reversing correction of a spinal deformity

Neurophysiologist:

☐   Repeat trials of MEPs and SSEPs to rule out potential false positive

☐   Check all leads to make sure no pull-out, may add leads in proximal muscle groups if possible

☐   Assess the pattern of changes

    ☐   Asymmetric changes (associated with cord or nerve root injury)

    ☐   Symmetric changes (associated with anesthetic or hypotension issues)

☐   Quantify improvement and communicate to the surgical team

Anesthesiologist:

☐   Check if neuromuscular blockade (muscle relaxant) given

    If yes, ☐ Check train of four (TOF)

☐   Verify that no change in anesthetic administration occurred

☐   Assess anesthetic depth

    ☐ BP   ☐ RR   ☐ HR   ☐ BIS monitor (if available)

☐   Restore or maintain blood pressure (goal mean arterial pressure of 90-100)

☐   Check Hemoglobin/Hematocrit (goal hemoglobin >9-10)

☐   Check temperature and I/O's for adequate resuscitation

☐   Check extremity position in case of plexus palsy

☐   Lighten depth of anesthesia

    ☐   Reduce to 1/3 MAC or temporarily eliminate inhaled agents (i.e. desflurane)

    ☐   Reduce intravenous anesthetics such as propofol (which may accumulate systemically during the case and blunt MEPs)

    ☐   Add adjuvant agents such as Ketamine to permit reduction of MEP suppressive agents (i.e. propofol and inhalational anesthetics)

IF No Change:

☐ Increase MAP >100

☐ Consider Steroid Administration

☐ Consider Wake-up test

☐ Consider Aborting surgery

☐ Consider Calcium Channel Blocker (topical to cord or iv)

*The checklist assumes baseline anesthetic regimen is 1/3-1/2 MAC of halogenated anesthetic (desflurane) and TIVA (total intravenous anesthesia) with propofol +/- ketamine.

Fig. 4. Checklist for the response to an intraoperative neuromonitoring alert, from Ziewacz and colleagues.[38] BIS, bispectral index; BP, blood pressure; HR, heart rate; I/O, input/output; MAC, minimum alveolar concentration; MAP, mean arterial pressure; MEP, motor evoked

The success and efficacy of the algorithm-designed checklist described earlier should not overpower significant potential pitfalls and drawbacks of checklist use that were identified across specialties and disciplines. It is key to remember that checklists are not designed to substitute training, responsibility, or judgment. Factors like profession, department, and location can vary while the checklist is made for and implemented in specific social and cultural contexts.[39] The bureaucratic nature of checklists leads to resistance by practitioners, which can lead to incomplete penetrance even when mandated. This concept was demonstrated in a study by Calland and colleagues[40] that studied the implementation of a surgical checklist by randomly assigning surgeons to a checklist or no checklist group. The subjective reviews of the cases by surgeons reported less effective communication between the team, whereas video reviews demonstrated significant improvement in explicit communication of roles and responsibility as well as other positive safety-related team behaviors. The factors found in other studies that were successful in implementing checklists, like surgical leaders enthusiastically explaining and demonstrating why checklists can be effective, were the ones that were placed at the top of the algorithm.

Loss of intraoperative monitoring signals represents an event that is conducive to checklist use due to its time-critical nature and multidisciplinary management complexity. It is a stressful situation in which surgical, anesthetic, and technical factors could be the possible causal element. The identification and resolution of the situation requires a rapid and coordinated approach. Other checklists have been implemented like the comprehensive protocol for managing high-risk spine patients at Northwestern by Halpin and colleagues[41] that encompasses the full scope of care of these patients. However, such protocols are less suited for situations requiring a rapid response like in the case of IONM signal change.[41] The neuromonitoring alert checklist developed by Ziewacz and colleagues[38] has been tested to be effective, and has been reported to be brief and straightforward to use. These encouraging results must be tempered by the lack of clinical efficacy data, which would need to be demonstrated by lower neurologic injury rates in a large, multi-center, randomized controlled trial.[42,43]

SUMMARY

Overall literature opinions on use of IOMN is divided. Clark and colleagues demonstrated a correlation between a decrease in intraoperative MEPs and new postoperative neurologic deficits in cervical or cervicothoracic myelopathy cases. The sensitivity and specificity of MEP monitoring as a diagnostic test varies based on risk factors such as patient comorbidities, age, and preoperative neurologic function.[21]

To truly determine the effectiveness of IONM, we recommend the implementation of a standard procedure for neuromonitoring across several sites to gather data. One such checklist could come from Ziewacz and colleagues,[38] who have created an effective checklist for the multidisciplinary response to significant intraoperative neuromonitoring alert in spine surgery. Although the initial implementation of a standardized IONM plan may be complicated, it may also lead to increased interdisciplinary

---

potential; RR, respiration rate; SSEP, somatosensory evoked potential. (*From* Ziewacz, J. E., Berven, S. H., Mummaneni, V. P., Tu, T.-H., Akinbo, O. C., Lyon, R., & Mummaneni, P. V. (2012). The design, development, and implementation of a checklist for intraoperative neuromonitoring changes. *Neurosurgical Focus, 33*(5), E11. https://doi.org/10.3171/2012.9.FO-CUS12263, with permission. (Figure 2 in original)).

cooperation among the surgeons, anesthesiologists, and neuromonitoring technicians of the surgical team and may contribute to further advancements in IONM.

CLINICS CARE POINTS

- Although the usage and cost-benefit analysis of intraoperative monitoring is questioned in simple spinal surgeries, its utility is valuable in high-risk procedures such as spinal deformity and spinal tumor surgeries.

- Usage of combined SSEP and MEP increases the sensitivity and specificity of the IONM for detecting injury.

- More high-quality studies are required to determine the validity of IONM benefits in procedures with low risk of injury.

- For IONM to be helpful, it needs to be performed by practitioners that are skilled at both the technical and interpretative aspects of monitoring.

- The activities of the monitoring team must integrate well with those of the surgical and the anesthesia team. The monitoring team needs to communicate efficiently and effectively in settings of changes in IONM so that both surgical and anesthesia teams be aware of the changes.

DISCLOSURE

This research received no specific grant from any funding agency in the public, commercial, or not-for-profit sectors. The authors have no personal or institutional interest with regard to the authorship and/or publication of this article.

REFERENCES

1. Nasser R, Yadla S, Maltenfort MG, et al. Complications in spine surgery: a review. J Neurosurg Spine 2010;13(2):144–57.
2. Fehlings MG, Brodke DS, Norvell DC, et al. The evidence for intraoperative neurophysiological monitoring in spine surgery: does it make a difference? Spine 2010; 35(9S):S37–46. Available at:https://journals.lww.com/spinejournal/Fulltext/2010/04201/The_Evidence_for_Intraoperative_Neurophysiological.6.aspx.
3. Tamaki T, Kubota S. History of the development of intraoperative spinal cord monitoring. Eur Spine J 2007;16(Suppl 2):S140–6.
4. Park J-H, Hyun S-J. Intraoperative neurophysiological monitoring in spinal surgery. World J Clin Cases 2015;3(9):765–73.
5. Papastefanou SL, Henderson LM, Smith NJ, et al. Surface electrode somatosensory-evoked potentials in spinal surgery: implications for indications and practice. Spine 2000;25(19):2467–72.
6. Jones SC, Fernau R, Woeltjen BL. Use of somatosensory evoked potentials to detect peripheral ischemia and potential injury resulting from positioning of the surgical patient: case reports and discussion. Spine J 2004;4(3):360–2.
7. Shils JL, Sloan TB. Intraoperative neuromonitoring. Int Anesthesiol Clin 2015; 53(1):53–73. Available at: https://journals.lww.com/anesthesiaclinics/Fulltext/2015/05310/Intraoperative_Neuromonitoring.5.aspx.
8. Stecker MM. A review of intraoperative monitoring for spinal surgery. Surg Neurol Int 2012;3(Suppl 3):S174–87.
9. Charalampidis A, Jiang F, Wilson JRF, et al. The Use of intraoperative neurophysiological monitoring in spine surgery. Global Spine J 2020;10(1 Suppl):104S–14S.

10. Bose B, Sestokas AK, Schwartz DM. Neurophysiological monitoring of spinal cord function during instrumented anterior cervical fusion. Spine J Official J 2004;4(2):202–7.
11. Agarwal N, Hamilton DK, Ozpinar A, et al. Intraoperative neurophysiologic monitoring for adult patients undergoing posterior spinal fusion. World Neurosurg 2017;99:267–74.
12. Uribe JS, Vale FL, Dakwar E. Electromyographic monitoring and its anatomical implications in minimally invasive spine surgery. Spine (Phila Pa 1976) 2010; 35(26S):S368–74. Available at: https://journals.lww.com/spinejournal/Fulltext/201 0/12151/Electromyographic_Monitoring_and_Its_Anatomical.14.aspx.
13. Cole T, Veeravagu A, Zhang M, et al. Intraoperative neuromonitoring in single-level spinal procedures: a retrospective propensity score–matched analysis in a national longitudinal database. Spine 2014;39(23):1950–9. Available at: https://journals.lww.com/spinejournal/Fulltext/2014/11010/Intraoperative_Neurom onitoring_in_Single_Level.6.aspx.
14. Chachan S, Bae J. Intraoperative neuromonitoring during thoracic spine surgery BT- minimally invasive thoracic spine surgery. In: Lee S-H, Bae J, Jeon S-H, editors. Minimally Invasive Thoracic Spine Surgery. Singapore: Springer Singapore; 2021. p. 55–8.
15. Biscevic M, Sehic A, Krupic F. Intraoperative neuromonitoring in spine deformity surgery: modalities, advantages, limitations, medicolegal issues – surgeons' views. EFORT Open Rev 2020;5(1):9–16.
16. Roth SG, Lange S, Haller J, et al. A prospective study of the intra- and postoperative efficacy of intraoperative neuromonitoring in spinal cord stimulation. Stereotact Funct Neurosurg 2015;93(5):348–54.
17. Appel S, Biron T, Goldstein K, et al. Effect of intra- and extraoperative factors on the efficacy of intraoperative neuromonitoring during cervical spine surgery. World Neurosurg 2019;123:e646–51.
18. Krause KL, Cheaney B II, Obayashi JT, et al. Intraoperative neuromonitoring for one-level lumbar discectomies is low yield and cost-ineffective. J Clin Neurosci 2020;71:97–100.
19. Huang Z, Chen L, Yang J, et al. Multimodality intraoperative neuromonitoring in severe thoracic deformity posterior vertebral column resection correction. World Neurosurg 2019;127:e416–26.
20. Lall RR, Lall RR, Hauptman JS, et al. Intraoperative neurophysiological monitoring in spine surgery: indications, efficacy, and role of the preoperative checklist. Neurosurg Focus 2012;33(5):E10.
21. Clark AJ, Ziewacz JE, Safaee M, et al. Intraoperative neuromonitoring with MEPs and prediction of postoperative neurological deficits in patients undergoing surgery for cervical and cervicothoracic myelopathy. Neurosurg Focus 2013;35(1):E7.
22. Costa P, Bruno A, Bonzanino M, et al. Somatosensory- and motor-evoked potential monitoring during spine and spinal cord surgery. Spinal Cord 2007;45(1):86–91.
23. Eggspuehler A, Sutter MA, Grob D, et al. Multimodal intraoperative monitoring (MIOM) during cervical spine surgical procedures in 246 patients. Eur Spine J 2007;16(2):209–15.
24. Smith PN, Balzer JR, Khan MH, et al. Intraoperative somatosensory evoked potential monitoring during anterior cervical discectomy and fusion in nonmyelopathic patients—a review of 1,039 cases. Spine J 2007;7(1):83–7.
25. Xu R, Ritzl EK, Sait M, et al. A role for motor and somatosensory evoked potentials during anterior cervical discectomy and fusion for patients without myelopathy: Analysis of 57 consecutive cases. Surg Neurol Int 2011;2:133.

26. Kelleher MO, Tan G, Sarjeant R, et al. Predictive value of intraoperative neuro-physiological monitoring during cervical spine surgery: a prospective analysis of 1055 consecutive patients. J Neurosurg Spine 2008;8(3):215–21.
27. Fan D, Schwartz DM, Vaccaro AR, et al. Intraoperative neurophysiologic detection of iatrogenic C5 nerve root injury during laminectomy for cervical compression myelopathy. Spine 2002;27(22):2499–502.
28. Svensson LG, Crawford ES, Hess KR, et al. Experience with 1509 patients undergoing thoracoabdominal aortic operations. J Vasc Surg 1993;17(2):357–68 [discussion: 368-370].
29. Weinzierl MR, Reinacher P, Gilsbach JM, et al. Combined motor and somatosensory evoked potentials for intraoperative monitoring: intra- and postoperative data in a series of 69 operations. Neurosurg Rev 2007;30(2):109–16 [discussion: 116].
30. Wiedemayer H, Sandalcioglu IE, Armbruster W, et al. False negative findings in intraoperative SEP monitoring: analysis of 658 consecutive neurosurgical cases and review of published reports. J Neurol Neurosurg Psychiatry 2004;75(2):280–6.
31. Wilber RG, Thompson GH, Shaffer JW, et al. Postoperative neurological deficits in segmental spinal instrumentation. A study using spinal cord monitoring. J Bone Joint Surg Am 1984;66(8):1178–87.
32. Traynelis Vincent MD, Abode-Iyamah Kingsley, Leick Katie, Bender Sarah, Greenlee Jeremy. Cervical decompression and reconstruction without intraoperative neurophysiological monitoring. Neurosurgery: Spine 2012;16.
33. Ney JP, van der Goes DN, Watanabe JH. Cost-effectiveness of intraoperative neurophysiological monitoring for spinal surgeries: Beginning steps. Clin Neurophysiol 2012;123(9):1705–7.
34. Devlin VJ, Anderson PA, Schwartz DM, et al. Intraoperative neurophysiologic monitoring: Focus on cervical myelopathy and related issues. Spine J 2006;6(6 Suppl):212S–24S.
35. Fehlings MG, Brodke DS, Norvell DC, et al. The evidence for intraoperative neurophysiological monitoring in spine surgery: does it make a difference? Spine 2010;35(9 Suppl):S37–46.
36. Hilibrand AS, Schwartz DM, Sethuraman V, et al. Comparison of transcranial electric motor and somatosensory evoked potential monitoring during cervical spine surgery. J Bone Joint Surg Am 2004;86(6):1248–53.
37. Lee JY, Hilibrand AS, Lim MR, et al. Characterization of neurophysiologic alerts during anterior cervical spine surgery. Spine 2006;31(17):1916–22.
38. Ziewacz JE, Berven SH, Mummaneni VP, et al. The design, development, and implementation of a checklist for intraoperative neuromonitoring changes. Neurosurg Focus 2012;33(5):E11.
39. Fourcade A, Blache J-L, Grenier C, et al. Barriers to staff adoption of a surgical safety checklist. BMJ Qual Saf 2012;21(3):191–7.
40. Calland JF, Turrentine FE, Guerlain S, et al. The surgical safety checklist: Lessons learned during implementation. Am Surg 2011;77(9):1131–7.
41. Halpin RJ, Sugrue PA, Gould RW, et al. Standardizing care for high-risk patients in spine surgery: The Northwestern high-risk spine protocol. Spine 2010;35(25):2232–8.
42. Degani, A., Wiener, E., & Ames Research Center. (1994). On the design of flight-deck procedures. TECHNICAL PUBLICATION - Government Publication. https://doi.org/10.21949/1403608.
43. Deletis V, Sala F. Intraoperative neurophysiological monitoring of the spinal cord during spinal cord and spine surgery: a review focus on the corticospinal tracts. Clin Neurophysiol 2008;119(2):248–64.

Neurosurgery for the Neurologist: Peripheral Nerve Injury and Compression (What can be Fixed?)

Megan M. Jack, MD, PhD, Brandon W. Smith, MD, Robert J. Spinner, MD*

KEYWORDS

- Peripheral nerve injury • Compressive neuropathies • Peripheral nerve imaging

KEY POINTS

- Neurologists are frequently the gatekeepers to neurosurgeons; as such they should be aware of indications for, types and timing of commonly performed surgical procedures, and expected outcomes of these surgeries.
- Patients with nerve injuries can be treated with a variety of nerve techniques (including neurolysis, nerve repair, nerve grafts, or nerve transfers) and/or soft tissue or bony procedures (such as tendon or free muscle transfer; or bony fusion).
- Patients with persistent or severe symptoms of nerve compression can often benefit from surgical decompression.

INTRODUCTION

The fields of Neurology and Neurosurgery intersect to care for specific patient populations, particularly those with certain pathologies that require surgical intervention for either diagnosis or treatment. Inflammation/vasculitis, tumors, neuropathic pain, trauma, dystonia, stroke, and compression neuropathies are all areas in which neurologists and nerve surgeons work together to treat patients. In this chapter, you will be introduced to the diagnosis and management of peripheral nerve injuries and the management of nerve compression syndromes that can be treated with surgical intervention and achieve favorable/optimal outcomes. Understanding this information will help guide you in evaluating patients, understanding indications for referral, and knowing potential surgical options for patients with peripheral nerve injuries or compressive neuropathies.

Mayo Clinic, Department of Neurologic Surgery, 200 1st Street SW, Rochester, MN 55905, USA
* Corresponding author.
E-mail address: spinner.robert@mayo.edu

Neurol Clin 40 (2022) 283–295
https://doi.org/10.1016/j.ncl.2021.11.001
0733-8619/22/© 2021 Elsevier Inc. All rights reserved.

neurologic.theclinics.com

PERIPHERAL NERVE INJURY

Nerve injury is a potentially devastating and costly problem in our health care system. Nerve injury resulting from trauma or iatrogenic injury can result in a range of symptoms from pain to loss of sensation and complete paralysis of the muscles innervated by the given nerve. Initially, a detailed peripheral nerve baseline examination forms the foundation for which management decisions are made in the future. A few guiding principles based on the anatomic structure of a nerve tend to direct the diagnosis and surgical management of peripheral nerve injuries.

Nerve injuries can occur from various insults, but a unifying treatment principle can be applied to most traumatic nerve injuries. Nerves that demonstrate both electrophysiologic and functional recovery following injury should be treated nonoperatively with watchful waiting. In these instances, patients are likely to make considerable recovery without any surgical intervention, particularly in cases of early functional recovery. On the other hand, for patients requiring surgery, "The Rule of 3's plus 1" is a guiding mantra in treating traumatic injuries (**Fig. 1**). This principle states that a sharp nerve injury should be treated within 3 days, ragged, or contaminated nerve transection should be treated within 3 weeks, blunt nerve injury should be treated within 3 months, and bony or soft tissue reconstruction for chronic injuries or failed intervention should be considered after 1 year. These concepts stem from an understanding of nerve microanatomy and depend on the overall continuity of the nerve structure and its potential for regrowth or repair.

Outcomes following surgical intervention are highly dependent on several factors. Peripheral nerves are known for their different capacities to regenerate following injury. For instance, the proximal ulnar nerve injuries are less likely to achieve a good functional outcome compared with high median or radial nerve injuries; this is directly related to the distance required for regeneration so intrinsic (ie, hand) muscle recovery is much more difficult to achieve than extrinsic (ie, forearm) muscle recovery. In the lower limb sciatic nerve, the tibial division demonstrates better motor and sensory recovery compared with the peroneal division for unknown reasons. More proximal injuries are known to be worse than more distal injuries. Younger patients, especially infants, are known to have better outcomes compared with older patients. Early surgical primary nerve repairs are considered more optimal than later intervention.

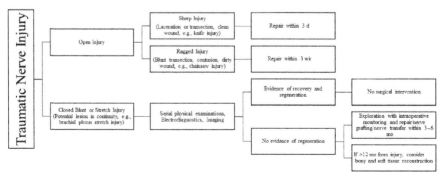

Fig. 1. "The Rule of 3's plus 1" provides guidelines for operating traumatic nerve injuries: a sharp nerve injury within 3 days; a ragged or contaminated nerve transection with 3 weeks; a closed blunt or stretch injury without electrophysiologies and clinical recovery by 3 to 6 months; and a chronic injury without recovery after prior surgery or delayed intervention can be considered for other types of bony or soft tissue reconstruction after 1 year.

Primary nerve repairs generally recover better than nerve grafts. The mechanism of injury ultimately is one the most important factors to guide surgical decision making.

Early Surgical Intervention

As governed by "the rule of 3's plus 1," specific types of traumatic injuries are treated within days, weeks, months, or years following injury. A sharp nerve injury can be sustained after a complete laceration from sharp objects such as razors, blades, or knives. A clean laceration results in the immediate loss of nerve dysfunction. It necessitates reconstruction urgently as a transected nerve has no potential for spontaneous recovery. Without repair, the distal axons will undergo Wallerian degeneration, while the proximal axons will attempt to grow distally. Without distal scaffolding for these axons to grow through, a neuroma of the proximal stump will form that could potentially become painful. The timing of repair for a sharp, clean injury necessitates an urgent referral to a nerve surgeon as this injury should be treated within *3 days*.[1] There are no methods for immediate restoration of nerve function as the distal nerve will continue to undergo Wallerian degeneration no matter how quickly or precisely the nerve is repaired. The axons must cross the gap and grow down the now axonless nerve at a rate of approximately 1 mm per day. A delay in surgical intervention beyond 3 days results in undesirable retraction of the proximal and distal nerve stumps along with scar formation making a direct repair difficult to perform.

Other nerve injuries may occur soon after injury, but the neurologic examination may worsen under observation. Such peripheral nerve injuries may occur related to displaced bones or bone fractures, expanding hematomas, or other growing mass lesions like pseudoaneurysms. Peripheral nerves may become trapped within a joint or within the fracture line of a long bone. Similarly, expanding hematomas following trauma can lead to the compression of the surrounding structures, including nerve (s), resulting in motor and sensory deficits. Typically, in these clinical scenarios, patients often have severe pain often out of proportion to the presumed injury. In the case of acute compression with neurologic deficits, an emergent plan should be made to relieve the offending compression, if possible. These clinical scenarios are important to recognize early to prevent ongoing peripheral nerve injury.

Ragged lacerations are injuries whereby the cut in the nerve is not uniform and/or will contain debris. Injuries such as those that occur with a chain saw are classified as ragged transection injuries. This type of injury is often treated *3 weeks* after injury. Although a ragged laceration has the same distal pathophysiology as a sharp laceration resulting in Wallerian degeneration, excess time before surgical intervention is given to ensure the wound is cleared of infectious material and for the extent of trauma on the nerve ends to be made more apparent. In the ideal scenario, direct end-to-end nerve repair of the proximal and distal nerve stumps is completed, however, this is not always possible. If a small gap exists, the nerves can be freed from the surrounding tissue and their usual anatomic locations to make the ends meet in a tension-free manner. Typically, these injuries require interpositional nerve grafting.

Delayed Surgical Intervention

In contrast to traumatic mechanisms whereby the nerve is known to be completely discontinuous and requires more urgent intervention, other types of injuries, such as blunt or stretch injuries, potentially have the capacity for nerve regeneration if the nerve is in continuity. The degree of nerve injury results in different likelihoods for spontaneous recovery. Some more mild injuries (ie, neuropraxia) resolve in a short period, whereas more severe stretch injuries (ie, neurotmesis) cause nerve damage with no potential for recovery. It is also important to understand that specific nerves are known to recover better than others. In general, lower extremity nerve injuries have significantly poorer outcomes than those in the upper extremity.[2] To determine if the nerve will spontaneously recover without surgery, a longer period of observation is required for these specific injury patterns. These patients should be observed with serial physical examinations and EMG testing to evaluate for signs of early recovery. A recovering nerve should be observed as the natural history of recovery has the capacity to outperform nerve surgery in these cases.

In cases where no clinical and electrophysiologic evidence of recovery is evident by *3 to 6 months*, surgical intervention should occur.[1] Ancillary testing can help guide surgical decision making. Preoperative imaging with either MRI or ultrasound can provide information regarding the length/extent of injury, presence, or absence of neuroma formation, and potential areas of compression distal to the site of injury. Similarly, intraoperative neurophysiologic testing at the time of surgery may help to guide decision making for blunt injuries. Surgical exploration will show the gross extent of injury evidenced by neuroma formation; however, it does not provide information about the damage or lack thereof within the nerve. Nerve action potential (NAP) testing can help to determine if the neuroma has internal fascicular architecture allowing it to conduct nerve signals.[3] If there is an NAP present, external neurolysis by itself is performed as this results in favorable results in over 94% of nerves (1255/1422).[4] If an NAP is not obtained across the lesion, there is low probability for useful recovery; the neuroma can be excised and a repair/reconstruction, completed.

There are different techniques within the surgeon's armamentarium to repair/reconstruct nerves and restore function. Primary surgical repair involves suturing the 2 ends of a nerve together to *reconnect* them. A tension-free repair is imperative; thus, this is only indicated in injuries whereby approximation of the proximal and distal ends can be achieved. Key techniques that help accomplish this are the mobilization of the nerve, positioning the joint in some degree of flexion, and nerve transposition whereby applicable. Some surgeons will even use bony shortening or nerve elongation techniques to facilitate direct end-to-end repair. In cases whereby a primary repair cannot be achieved due to injury to the nerve over an extended distance, nerve grafting is typically used (**Fig. 2**). In this procedure, an expendable sensory donor nerve, such as sural, superficial radial, or lateral or medial antebrachial nerve, is used as an interpositional graft to *bridge* the proximal and distal ends of nerves and serve as a conduit for axons to grow through.

Some nerve injuries have a low likelihood of recovery with direct nerve repair or nerve grafting. Nerve transfers are newer techniques that take advantage of a functioning and expendable distal donor motor nerve, branch, or fascicle to provide innervation closer to the motor end plate. Injuries necessitating long nerve grafts or very proximal injuries tend to have less favorable outcomes. Recovering motor function is a race against time. After a nerve injury, the motor endplate experiences severe degeneration a year after injury. Our goal is that nerve surgery is performed between 3 and 6 months after injury to give time for the axons to begin to grow to their target before this point. However, very proximal lesions make this difficult even with swift intervention due to the distance the axons must regrow to reach their end-organ targets. An alternative strategy of reinnervating a muscle is the use of nerve transfers, that is, to *bypass* the area of injury and use an expendable motor nerve or fascicle from another muscle nearby.[5] This approach is referred to as a motor nerve transfer, and one of the most famous of these is an ulnar fascicular transfer to the biceps motor branch of the musculocutaneous nerve when attempting to restore elbow flexion.[5,6] An important factor in determining suitable surgical candidates for nerve transfers is the muscle that is innervated by the donor nerve or fascicle must have sufficient

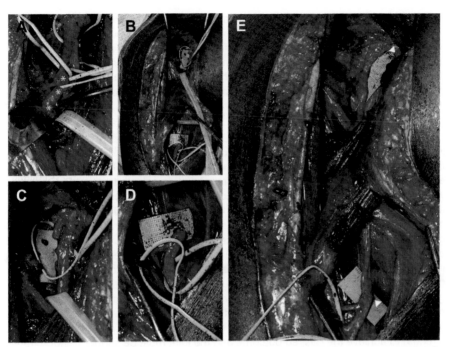

Fig. 2. Infraclavicular brachial plexus exploration of a patient after a traumatic right brachial plexus injury with a neuroma in continuity of the musculocutaneous nerve (*A*, white *asterisk*). Intraoperative electrodiagnostic testing did not demonstrate a NAP across the neuroma. The neuroma was excised (*B*) with the proximal (*C*) and distal (*D*) nerve ends exposed. Sural nerve was harvested and two 13 cm cable grafts were sutured into place (*E, white arrow* heads).

power, generally, strength at least 4/5 on the MRC grading scale. Nerve transfers are best performed within the 3 to 6 month period after nerve injury, but because their distal connections (ie, shortened distance to the muscle end plate) can be considered in cases up to 1 year after injury.

Brachial plexus injuries in both adult and pediatric patients require special consideration with regards to surgical timing and outcomes. Given the proximal location of the brachial plexus and the potential sites for injury, a few more pieces of information are helpful in guiding treatment beyond clinical examination and electrodiagnostic findings. A key point of information in brachial plexus trauma is the injury's location in relationship to the dorsal root ganglion (DRG). A complete preganglionic injury, also known as an avulsion, has no capacity for spontaneous recovery, whereas a postganglionic injury resulting in a neuroma-in continuity may recover. The location of injury in relationship to the DRG also dictates whether the spinal nerve can be used for reconstruction purposes when surgical intervention is deemed necessary. Intraoperative neurophysiology can be used to evaluate the spinal nerves with somatosensory and motor evoked potentials. SSEPs help to evaluate the integrity of the dorsal nerve rootlets and MEPs help to evaluate the ventral rootlets. The use of NAP testing would also be critical in evaluating the postganglionic lesions. The decision making and reconstructive strategies are complex and evolving. In addition to considering a purely anatomic reconstruction scheme, nerve surgeons must determine the priorities for reinnervation. An injury at the level of the proximal brachial plexus in an adult has little hope for restoring useful hand function with standard nerve reconstruction techniques, and in many algorithms, hand restoration is foregone in favor of restoring shoulder and elbow function.[6] An early referral to a peripheral nerve surgeon is key for evaluating brachial plexus injuries as surgical intervention, if warranted, is often attempted at 3 to 6 months following injury. This time frame provides a balance—weighing the risks of unnecessary surgery (in a recovering nerve) with the benefits of operating earlier and operating too late when the trajectory of nerve recovery is more defined.

Late Surgical Intervention

In general, standard techniques of nerve reconstruction typically do not fare well in patients after 1 year from injury. New distal nerve transfers may offer an opportunity to extend this, perhaps even to 18 months from injury in selected cases. Patients that are 1 year or more after the injury can be considered for bony or soft tissue reconstructive techniques to achieve some recovery of function. Bony fusions, while seemingly considered to limit movement, intended to stabilize joints to improve overall functional capacity. For instance, shoulder arthrodesis can improve pain due to instability as well as hand-to-mouth movement after brachial plexus repair by placing the arm in an improved position.[7] Selective wrist fusions and/or thumb arthrodesis are frequently performed. Tendon transfers (whereby a functioning tendon and muscle is moved to give power to a weakened joint) may be considered. For instance, the tibialis posterior tendon can be transferred anteriorly to treat a foot drop from different conditions.[8] Like nerve transfers, the muscle/tendon that is being transferred must have sufficient strength to achieve the desired outcome and the joint must be supple. Tendon transfers are not under the same time restrictions that nerve transfers are and can be performed outside the 1-year time mark. Similarly, free functioning muscle transfer (FFMT) is another alternative technique that primarily is reserved for late-stage surgical reconstruction. This procedure involves harvesting a functioning muscle and transferring a neurovascularized pedicle to restore function. For instance, the gracilis muscle is often used to restore elbow flexion following brachial plexus injury. Other similar procedures are used to achieve elbow extension, finger and wrist extension, and primitive grip. Patients with delayed presentation *beyond 1 year* or failed primary nerve repairs may be appropriate candidates for FFMT.[6]

NERVE COMPRESSION SYNDROMES

Nerves normally pass through anatomic structures such as fascia or ligaments that form a tunnel; however, in pathologic states, these same locations can be sites of nerve compression when either the tunnel is narrowed or the contents within the tunnel are enlarged causing an overall relative reduced space for the nerve. There are classic compression syndromes that are well substantiated and accepted, and then a growing number of entities that are being defined and are more controversial. We will go into detail about the less disputed and more common entities such as carpal tunnel syndrome, cubital tunnel syndrome, peroneal neuropathy, and lateral femoral cutaneous neuropathy. In these syndromes, the clinical description, physical examination findings, electrodiagnostic studies, and imaging each form one leg of a "four-legged table" to support the diagnosis of compression syndrome (ie, the more legs of the table that can be supported, the more stable is the table!). Some of the other more disputed compression symptoms will be mentioned, but we will not go into detail on them as their evidence needs continued development. In these instances, the diagnosis is harder to establish because often one or more of the "legs of the table" are missing to support a definitive diagnosis.

Nerve compressions can result in symptoms ranging from mild pain or sensory changes without motor deficit to complete loss of motor and sensory function in the impacted nerve territory and severe pain. Generally, nerve compression syndromes differ from traumatic injuries in that their onset is often more indolent without a direct relationship to any isolated insult. The workup of suspected compressive mononeuropathy may include investigation for a focal lesion such as a mass (eg, cyst or tumor), especially when it occurs at unusual sites.

Two methodologies to visualize the peripheral nervous system include MRI and ultrasonography. MRI of the peripheral nervous system helps to provide clear delineations between nerves and surrounding tissues. There have been some advancements in this technology including MRI neurography which can demonstrate the underlying fascicular architecture in some cases. MRI in compression neuropathies can also show conformational changes in the nerve at areas of compression. T2 sequencing can aid in demonstrating edema within the nerve and denervated muscle, which is commonly seen in traumatic or compression injuries. Ultrasonography has many advantages including its portability, low cost and its being noninvasive and widely available. Although the resolution of the probes continues to improve, the separation of anatomic structures is less clear to an untrained eye. Ultrasound can be used to examine nerves in continuity in trauma, as well as determine the relative size and shape of the nerve at areas of entrapment.

Carpal Tunnel Syndrome

Median nerve entrapment at the level of the carpal tunnel is the most common nerve entrapment syndrome that we encounter as nerve surgeons. Carpal tunnel syndrome (CTS) tends to affect women more than men and is relatively common in the general population with an estimated prevalence of 1% to 5%. The classic presentation of CTS includes pain/paresthesia in the median nerve territory (radial 3 ½ digits), while sparing the palmar branch. The carpal tunnel itself is composed of a ligamentous roof that passes from the medial to the lateral aspect of the carpal bones, with the carpal bones themselves consisting of the floor. The nerve is not alone in its passage through the tunnel and instead is accompanied by 9 flexor tendons to the volar aspect of the hand. The basic pathophysiology of CTS involves a mismatch in space between the size of the carpal tunnel and the size of the median nerve and tendons that pass through the anatomic space. In cases without adequate space for the nerve to exist freely, the nerve can become compressed. When the syndrome is left to progress, numbness, weakness, and atrophy can occur.

For mild and nonprogressive CTS, a trial of conservative therapy is warranted. Steroid injections at the carpal tunnel and neutral splinting are first-line interventions to decrease the symptomatology and to halt the progression of the disease. In patients with persistent symptoms or progressive moderate and severe CTS, surgical intervention is indicated. There are many methods for decompressing the carpal tunnel and this is an area of ongoing debate. Carpal tunnel decompression is often done through an open incision on the palm with visualization and decompression of the median nerve from the wrist crease to the distal end of the transverse carpal ligament. Relief from symptoms is seen in more than 80% of appropriately selected patients, but sensory and motor symptoms may take up to a year to recover.[9,10] Many factors have been hypothesized to influence the outcomes following carpal tunnel decompression including the duration of symptoms, severity of nerve abnormalities on electrodiagnostic studies, age, and worker's compensation.[2]

In many areas of surgery, including CTS, there has been an increasing trend to perform treatments in less invasive ways. The first attempt at this in CTS was by performing "mini" incisions to decompress the transverse carpal ligament. This procedure then progressed to include endoscopic nerve decompression by using even smaller incisions and an endoscopic camera to perform the decompression. Both open and endoscopic techniques are successful at decompressing the median nerve and relieving symptoms; however, endoscopic surgery allows for earlier return to work, but has higher risk for neural injuries.[11–13] More recent attempts have used ultrasound-guided decompression either with novel bladed instruments or even using a thread to effectively saw the ligament percutaneously.[14–16] Comparative studies will need to be performed to demonstrate the superiority of one technique over the other.

Cubital Tunnel Syndrome

The second most encountered compression syndrome for the neurosurgeon is cubital tunnel syndrome at the elbow (CuTS). In addition to the cubital tunnel itself, other sites of compression for the ulnar nerve near the elbow include the arcade of Struthers, intermuscular septum, retro-condylar groove, and Osbourne's band. Ulnar neuropathy at the elbow caused by these compressive structures can result in sensory changes and pain in the ulnar distribution. More advanced cases can experience motor changes as well as the atrophy of the intrinsic hand muscles innervated by the ulnar nerve.

Mild CuTS can be treated with injections, padding, and activity modifications. Cases that fail conservative therapy or have more severe motor involvement should be considered for surgical intervention. Surgery is most often performed by an open incision and decompression along the various compression points.

The biggest controversy in surgery for CuTS, however, involves debate on in situ decompression versus transposition of the nerve ventral to the medial epicondyle. Different techniques are available, each with personal preferences and biomechanical advantages (including subcutaneous, intramuscular, submuscular transpositions, and medial epicondylectomy). In a large meta-analysis, decompression and transposition had equivalent clinical outcomes; however, transposition of the ulnar nerve was associated with increased risks.[17,18] The risks identified with anterior transposition include ulnar nerve devascularization, increased surgical complexity, and increased complication rates.[2] Because of this, most surgeons will perform the transposition if there are signs of nerve subluxation on physical examination or intraoperatively; some surgeons perform transposition in all cases of CuTS. The outcomes for surgery for CuTS are variable but slightly below that for CTS; however, they are still favorable for patients.[19] It is thought some of the variability is related to the severity of the disorder and the precise surgical technique chosen.[20] Surgery for CuTS is therefore commonly performed to halt the progression of symptoms and provide relief in patients before they become too severe. Akin to CTS, some surgeons are performing ulnar nerve decompression and transposition via an endoscopic approach with differing levels of success.[21,22]

Fibular Tunnel

The most common lower extremity entrapment syndrome that we see is peroneal nerve compression at the fibular neck. The common peroneal nerve is part of the sciatic nerve and travels in the posterior thigh whereby it bifurcates approximately 10 cm proximal to the knee joint. It then travels laterally, staying medial to the biceps femoris tendon and then coursing obliquely, wrapping around the fibular neck to travel underneath the muscles of the lateral compartment through the fibular tunnel whereby the common peroneal nerve divides into the articular, deep, and superficial branches.

Peroneal neuropathy can present as sensory changes in the deep and/or superficial branches of the nerve, or as a foot drop. There are fewer conservative options for peroneal neuropathy with foot drop than other compressive syndromes. Injections, discontinuation of the offending behaviors, and hydrodissection can be attempted; however, decompression is a favored method for the treatment of peroneal neuropathy at the fibular neck.[23] The decompression is a low morbidity, outpatient procedure. The common peroneal nerve is isolated proximal to the fibular head and is neurolysed through the fibular tunnel. The leading edge of the peroneal muscles is often a tight compressive band of fascia, which is then released over the nerve by cutting the fascial band.[24] The peroneal nerve may be resistant to recovery, so it is important to halt the progression of the disease before it becomes too severe. Good outcomes can be seen with peroneal nerve decompression and given the low morbidity nature of the procedure remains a worthwhile and often rewarding option.[25]

Meralgia Paresthetica

The only sensory neuropathy that we will discuss is lateral femoral cutaneous nerve (LFCN) entrapment or meralgia paresthetica, which was one of the earliest nerve entrapments to be described. The LFCN branches off the lumbar plexus and travels in the retroperitoneum before exiting the abdomen below the inguinal ligament generally medial to the anterior superior iliac spine (ASIS). The nerve then travels to innervate the lateral aspect of the thigh. It is important to note there are many variations to this anatomy including the median and lateral position of the nerve with regards to the ASIS and the terminal branching pattern of the LFCN. The pain and paresthesias involve the lateral aspect of the thigh and, although this dermatome is not critical for function, the pain can be quite debilitating.

Weight reduction or avoidance of compressive clothing should be attempted. Some groups advocate for the use of injections for the diagnosis and management of LFCN syndrome; however, many agree that long-term relief from an injection is a rarity. Thus, surgical intervention is advocated for refractory symptoms. Standard treatment includes decompression of the nerve as it passes under the inguinal ligament with transposition. The current area of debate among nerve surgeons is whether a neurectomy should be performed in the management of the meralgia paresthetica. Some advocate for neurolysis alone as the primary surgical intervention, while others regularly perform neurectomy.[26] A recent systematic review and meta-analysis found improved pain relief and lower rates of revision following the neurectomy of the LFCN.[27,28]

Other Controversial Compression Neuropathies

There are some conditions that have a much more controversial standing within the peripheral nerve community. These typically include pain syndromes or other disorders whereby one or more of the diagnostic legs of a table does not support the definitive diagnosis. These compression neuropathies will be briefly discussed along with potential surgical options that are being performed by surgeons with differing frequency and enthusiasm.

There are groups whereby much of their practice consists of surgery for patients with neurogenic thoracic outlet syndrome (nTOS), and there are some that feel this diagnosis is rare. Patients with true TOS have objective evidence of nerve dysfunction on EMG/NCS and account for less than 1% of all cases.[29] By far, most of the cases of TOS, are considered disputed TOS whereby findings on electrodiagnostic testing are absent. Patients with nTOS will present with proximal upper extremity pain, distal paresthesias, and are often exacerbated by activity and overhead positioning. In many suspected cases, physical examination, imaging, and electrodiagnostic testing are often normal. Positive TOS maneuvers are often found in asymptomatic individuals. The diagnostic criteria are vague and vastly vary from institution to institution making selection of appropriate surgical patients difficult.[30] Physiotherapy is the mainstay of treatment of patients with suspected nTOS.[31] In practices that perform surgical intervention, several different approaches are considered. The supraclavicular approach to the brachial plexus to perform a scalenectomy with or without first rib resection is a commonly used technique.[32] Many busy academic nerve surgeons only perform a handful of these cases per year with varying results.[33]

There are also a group of neuropathies including the long thoracic nerve, suprascapular nerve, posterior interosseous nerve at the arcade of Frohse, and anterior interosseous nerve at the tendinous edge of the pronator teres that are considered compression neuropathies by some groups; however, many others feel that these often result from an inflammatory process.[34,35] The inflammatory theory would explain other features, including the associated triggers and the spontaneous resolution seen in many patients, but often not seen in patients with more classic compression neuropathies. For those groups that believe these clinical entities are the result of compression and not inflammation, surgical intervention to decompress the involved nerves at areas of potential compression is completed.[36]

Pain syndromes are also a relatively new field whereby peripheral nerve surgery may have a role. Several pain syndromes including radial tunnel syndrome, pronator (teres) syndrome, piriformis syndrome, and pudendal neuralgia are considered by some to be compressive neuropathies. Spontaneous syndromes may often be attributed to micro-trauma. While surgical outcome studies are more limited for these conditions, initial management should be conservative. Painful diabetic neuropathy has more recently had investigated to determine if lower extremity decompression of the peroneal and tibial nerve branches can improve symptoms.[37,38] As with other controversial compressive neuropathies, the evidence remains insufficient to recommend surgical intervention for painful diabetic neuropathy.[37]

Headache management is an emerging area of nerve surgery. A subset of headache syndromes is considered, by some, to be the result of compression of nerves providing cranial sensory innervation.[39,40] This is an evolving topic and there remains a lack of consensus among nerve surgeons as to the applicability for nerve decompressions or neurectomies in the treatment of nerve-related headache syndromes. Some physicians think patients that have failed standard medical therapy and have had good relief with either nerve blocks or Botox injections should be considered for surgical evaluation.[2] Again, further study is necessary to better understand the implications of available surgical techniques in the treatment of headaches.

SUMMARY

A comprehensive multidisciplinary approach is essential for patients with peripheral nerve disorders. Trauma and compressive neuropathies are 2 very common disorders encountered by both neurologists and neurosurgeons. In many instances, both pathologies have surgical interventions available to patients to improve their symptoms. Thus, it remains imperative when evaluating patients to understanding the timing and indications for referral as well as possible surgical options for patients with peripheral nerve injuries and compressive neuropathies.

CLINICS CARE POINTS

- Successful results can be achieved with peripheral nerve surgery for patients with nerve injuries and compression.

- High-resolution peripheral nerve imaging and electrophysiology are important in the evaluation of patients with peripheral nerve disorders.
- Timely referral can dictate the type of surgery performed and ultimately the surgical results.

REFERENCES

1. Midha R, Grochmal J. Surgery for nerve injury: current and future perspectives. J Neurosurg 2019;130:675–85.
2. Mackinnon SE. Nerve surgery. New York, NY: Thieme Medical Publishers; 2015.
3. Wang H, Spinner R. Intraoperative testing and monitoring during peripheral nerve surgery. Handbook Clin Neurophysiol 2008;8.
4. Kim D, Midha R, Murovic JA. Spinner: Kline & Hudson's nerve injuries - operative results for major nerve injuries, entrapments, and tumors, vol. 2. Saunders Elsevier; 2008.
5. Peters BR, Van Handel AC, Russo SA, et al. Five reliable nerve transfers for the treatment of isolated upper extremity nerve injuries. Plast Reconstr Surg 2021; 147:830e–45e.
6. Maldonado AA, Bishop AT, Spinner RJ, et al. Five operations that give the best results after brachial plexus injury. Plast Reconstr Surg 2017;140:545–56.
7. Carlsen BT, Bishop AT, Shin AY. Late reconstruction for brachial plexus injury. Neurosurg Clin N Am 2009;20:51–64, vi.
8. Krishnamurthy S, Ibrahim M. Tendon transfers in foot drop. Indian J Plast Surg 2019;52:100–8.
9. Hybbinette CH, Mannerfelt L. The carpal tunnel syndrome. A retrospective study of 400 operated patients. Acta Orthop Scand 1975;46:610–20.
10. Phalen GS. The carpal-tunnel syndrome. Clinical evaluation of 598 hands. Clin Orthop Relat Res 1972;83:29–40.
11. Li Y, Luo W, Wu G, et al. Open versus endoscopic carpal tunnel release: a systematic review and meta-analysis of randomized controlled trials. BMC Musculoskelet Disord 2020;21:272.
12. Scholten RJ, Mink van der Molen A, Uitdehaag BM, et al. Surgical treatment options for carpal tunnel syndrome. Cochrane Database Syst Rev 2007;2007: CD003905.
13. Shin EK. Endoscopic versus open carpal tunnel release. Curr Rev Musculoskelet Med 2019;12:509–14.
14. Burnham RS, Loh EY, Rambaransingh B, et al. A controlled trial evaluating the safety and effectiveness of ultrasound-guided looped thread carpal tunnel release. Hand (N Y) 2021;16:73–80.
15. Hebbard P, Thomas P, Fransch SV, et al. Microinvasive carpal tunnel release using a retractable needle-mounted blade. J Ultrasound Med 2020;40(7):1451–8.
16. Wang PH, Wu PT, Jou IM. Ultrasound-guided percutaneous carpal tunnel release: 2-year follow-up of 641 hands. J Hand Surg Eur 2021;46:305–7.
17. Bartels RH, Verhagen WI, van der Wilt GJ, et al. Prospective randomized controlled study comparing simple decompression versus anterior subcutaneous transposition for idiopathic neuropathy of the ulnar nerve at the elbow: part 1. Neurosurgery 2005;56:522–30 [discussion 522–30].
18. Said J, Van Nest D, Foltz C, et al. Ulnar nerve in situ decompression versus transposition for idiopathic cubital tunnel syndrome: an updated meta-analysis. J Hand Microsurg 2019;11:18–27.

19. Giöstad A, Nyman E. Patient characteristics in ulnar nerve compression at the elbow at a tertiary referral hospital and predictive factors for outcomes of simple decompression versus subcutaneous transposition of the ulnar nerve. Biomed Res Int 2019;2019:5302462.
20. Mowlavi A, Andrews K, Lille S, et al. The management of cubital tunnel syndrome: a meta-analysis of clinical studies. Plast Reconstr Surg 2000;106:327–34.
21. Fok MWM, Cobb T, Bain GI. Endoscopic cubital tunnel decompression - Review of the literature. J Orthop Surg (Hong Kong) 2021;29. 2309499020982084.
22. Palmer BA, Hughes TB. Cubital tunnel syndrome. J Hand Surg Am 2010;35: 153–63.
23. Song B, Marathe A, Chi B, et al. Hydrodissection as a therapeutic and diagnostic modality in treating peroneal nerve compression. Proc (Bayl Univ Med Cent) 2020;33:465–6.
24. Morimoto D, Isu T, Kim K, et al. Microsurgical decompression for peroneal nerve entrapment neuropathy. Neurol Med Chir (Tokyo) 2015;55:669–73.
25. Tarabay B, Abdallah Y, Kobaiter-Maarrawi S, et al. Outcome and prognosis of microsurgical decompression in idiopathic severe common fibular nerve entrapment: prospective clinical study. World Neurosurg 2019;126:e281–7.
26. Payne R, Seaman S, Sieg E, et al. Evaluating the evidence: is neurolysis or neurectomy a better treatment for meralgia paresthetica? Acta Neurochir (Wien) 2017;159:931–6.
27. de Ruiter GC, Kloet A. Comparison of effectiveness of different surgical treatments for meralgia paresthetica: results of a prospective observational study and protocol for a randomized controlled trial. Clin Neurol Neurosurg 2015; 134:7–11.
28. Lu VM, Burks SS, Heath RN, et al. Meralgia paresthetica treated by injection, decompression, and neurectomy: a systematic review and meta-analysis of pain and operative outcomes. J Neurosurg 2021;1–11.
29. Jones MR, Prabhakar A, Viswanath O, et al. Thoracic outlet syndrome: a comprehensive review of pathophysiology, diagnosis, and treatment. Pain Ther 2019; 8:5–18.
30. Ruopsa N, Ristolainen L, Vastamäki M, et al. Neurogenic Thoracic outlet syndrome with supraclavicular release: long-term outcome without rib resection. Diagnostics (Basel) 2021;11:450.
31. Balderman J, Abuirqeba AA, Eichaker L, et al. Physical therapy management, surgical treatment, and patient-reported outcomes measures in a prospective observational cohort of patients with neurogenic thoracic outlet syndrome. J Vasc Surg 2019;70:832–41.
32. Hwang JS, Kim J, Kim S, et al. Diagnosis of neurogenic thoracic outlet syndrome based on the clinical status. Ann Vasc Surg 2021;76:454–62.
33. George EL, Arya S, Rothenberg KA, et al. Contemporary practices and complications of surgery for thoracic outlet syndrome in the United States. Ann Vasc Surg 2021;72:147–58.
34. Maldonado AA, Amrami KK, Mauermann ML, et al. Nontraumatic "isolated" posterior interosseous nerve palsy: reinterpretation of electrodiagnostic studies and MRIs. J Plast Reconstr Aesthet Surg 2017;70:159–65.
35. Suematsu N, Hirayama T. Posterior interosseous nerve palsy. J Hand Surg Br 1998;23:104–6.
36. Sigamoney KV, Rashid A, Ng CY. Management of atraumatic posterior interosseous nerve palsy. J Hand Surg Am 2017;42:826–30.

37. Albers JW, Jacobson R. Decompression nerve surgery for diabetic neuropathy: a structured review of published clinical trials. Diabetes Metab Syndr Obes 2018; 11:493–514.
38. Best TJ, Best CA, Best AA, et al. Surgical peripheral nerve decompression for the treatment of painful diabetic neuropathy of the foot - A level 1 pragmatic randomized controlled trial. Diabetes Res Clin Pract 2019;147:149–56.
39. Baldelli I, Mangialardi ML, Salgarello M, et al. Peripheral occipital nerve decompression surgery in migraine headache. Plast Reconstr Surg Glob Open 2020;8: e3019.
40. Lucia Mangialardi M, Baldelli I, Salgarello M, et al. Decompression surgery for frontal migraine headache. Plast Reconstr Surg Glob Open 2020;8:e3084.

Chiari Malformation (Update on Diagnosis and Treatment)

Jared S. Rosenblum, MD[a], I. Jonathan Pomeraniec, MD, MBA[b], John D. Heiss, MD[b],*

KEYWORDS

- Chiari malformation - Diagnosis - Treatment - Syrinx

KEY POINTS

- Chiari Malformation Type I is typically diagnosed by greater than 5 mm of cerebellar tonsillar ectopy below the foramen magnum, typically due to the reduced size of the bony posterior fossa
- Recent investigations have found CMI with a spacious posterior fossa, suggesting that there are additional mechanisms for cerebellar ectopy
- Patient selection and proper choice of surgical intervention are critical for the successful resolution of signs and symptoms of CMI and syringomyelia

INTRODUCTION

History—Initial Observations

Cerebellar ectopy may be acquired, for example, due to mass effect or changes in cerebrospinal fluid pressures, or congenital.[1] Chiari malformations, which are now recognized as a spectrum of congenital anomalies involving the craniocervical junction, vary in age of onset, presenting symptoms, and etiology.[1,2] The cause of these malformations has been long debated. In 1891, Hans Chiari, an Austrian pathologist, elaborated on the relationship between cerebellar ectopy and hydrocephalus.[3,4] In this initial report, Chiari described 3 pathologies, which are now considered Chiari Malformations I through III (CMI–III).

As the title of his article suggested, the unifying theme of these pathologies was the displacement of the cerebellum through the craniocervical junction at the foramen magnum. In Type I (CMI), Chiari observed elongation and ectopia of the cerebellar tonsils and the medial portions of the inferior lobes of the cerebellum, which he described as cone-shaped.[4] Of critical note, Chiari only found Type I cerebellar ectopy in cases

[a] National Institutes of Health, National Cancer Institute, Neuro-Oncology Branch, 37 Convent Drive, MSC 4254, Bethesda, MD, 20892 USA; [b] National Institutes of Health, National Institute of Neurological Disorders and Stroke, Surgical Neurology Branch, 10 Center Drive, Room 3D20, Bethesda, MD, 20892 USA
* Corresponding author.
E-mail address: heissj@ninds.nih.gov

Neurol Clin 40 (2022) 297–307
https://doi.org/10.1016/j.ncl.2021.11.007
0733-8619/22/© 2022 Elsevier Inc. All rights reserved.

neurologic.theclinics.com

Abbreviations	
CM	Chiari malformation
CMI	Chiari malformation, type I
CSF	cerebrospinal fluid
EPAS1	endothelial PAS domain protein 1
HIF	hypoxia-inducible factor
CDE	Common Data Elements

of congenital hydrocephalus, not in cases of acute or late-onset hydrocephalus,[4] suggesting a primary congenital etiology rather than an acquired pathology. In Type II (CMII), Chiari reported greater hindbrain and brainstem displacement through the craniocervical junction associated with a cervicothoracic syrinx, congenital lumbosacral dysraphism, and neural tube defect.[4] Chiari described Type III (CMIII) based on one case of a 5-month-old child with what he called "hydrencephalocele cerebellaris cervicalis," which included spina bifida, an enlarged skull, convergent strabismus, absence of the tentorium, cervical "hydromyelocele" communicating with the fourth ventricle, and complete herniation of the cerebellum into the spinal canal.[4]

While others described cerebellar ectopy in the setting of hydrocephalus before this report, Chiari was the first to investigate the origins of this relationship. In a more extensive cadaveric study several years later (1896), Chiari confirmed the above classification and added a fourth type of malformation (CMIV), which lacked cerebellar displacement through the craniocervical junction due to cerebellar hypoplasia.[3,5] While this spectrum of pathologies was related to hydrocephalus, the severity of the hydrocephalus in this series did not correlate with the extent of the craniospinal malformation, which prompted Chiari to hypothesize another mechanism was responsible for obstruction of the flow of cerebrospinal fluid.[3,5] He proposed that insufficient development of the cranial bones played a critical role in these pathologies. Supporting this hypothesis were observations by both Julius A. Arnold, who in 1894 published a case of cerebellar ectopy and spina bifida without hydrocephalus,[3,6] and John Cleland, who described a similar case with hydrocephalus in 1883.[3,7] These initial descriptions of CMI-IV made by Arnold, Chiari, and Cleland fueled debates and studies surrounding the acquired or congenital nature of cerebellar ectopy in Chiari Malformations and remain the basis of our ongoing investigations, diagnosis, and management.

Section highlights

- Chiari Malformations I–IV are a spectrum of congenital malformations with varied age of onset, presenting symptoms, and etiologies that may be associated with syringomyelia

- The unifying theme of CMI–III is the displacement of the hindbrain through the craniocervical junction

- Chiari and others proposed that insufficient development of the bony posterior fossa played a critical role in cerebellar ectopy in these malformations.

DISCUSSION
Recent Insights—Syringomyelia and Chiari Malformation Type I

Early observations by Chiari and others suggested a shared mechanism of cerebellar ectopy and disorders of cerebrospinal fluid, that is, hydrocephalus and syringomyelia.

Critical animal studies by Dorcus Padget furthered our understanding of the embryologic underpinnings of CMI–IV and the relationship to dysraphism, such as occurs in the more severe Chiari Malformations and Dandy–Walker malformation.[8] Further studies by Miguel Marín-Padilla supported the concept that these malformations—CMI–IV, Dandy–Walker malformations, and various forms of dysraphism—result from varying failures of neuraxial induction of dorsal structures.[9]

The shared embryologic origin of these pathologies, though some nuances are still currently debated,[1,2] provided a rationale for the investigations into the pathophysiologic relationship of cerebellar ectopy and syringomyelia. This original question led Chiari to report his findings. CMI in adults can have a presentation ranging from an asymptomatic MRI incidental finding to signs and symptoms of central myelopathy from syringomyelia, including suspended sensory loss, pain, upper extremity muscle atrophy, and lower extremity spasticity.[1]

Theories on the formation of a syrinx in CMI were proposed, including the "waterhammer" theory proposed by Gardner in the 1950s that postulated obstruction of the outlets of the fourth ventricle, enlarged CSF arterial pressure waves directed into the obex and progressive dilation of the spinal cord central canal.[1,12] Williams' theorized that cranial–spinal pressure dissociation during the Valsalva maneuver caused by the ectopic tonsils obstructing the foramen magnum CSF pathway drove CSF into the obex and spinal cord central canal. Gardner's and Williams' theories required a patent communication of the obex and upper pole of the syrinx to transmit CSF and its pressure.[1] Imaging and postmortem studies did not demonstrate this patent communication in most cases, invalidating these theories.[1] Oldfield and Heiss (current author) led further investigations to elucidate the pathophysiology of syringomyelia in CMI.[1,10,11] Their studies involved CSF pressure measurements, phase-contrast magnetic resonance imaging (PC-MRI) CSF and syrinx flow studies, and intraoperative cardiac-gaited MRI in patients with Chiari I malformation and syringomyelia. The findings of these studies supported a theory in which the flow through the CSF spaces at the foramen magnum was impeded by the ectopic cerebellar tonsils, preventing the normal movement of CSF across the foramen magnum during the cardiac cycle. Instead of CSF, the ectopic cerebellar tonsils descended into the cervical spinal canal during the cardiac systole, acting on the enclosed spinal subarachnoid space, creating enlarged spinal subarachnoid pressure waves, and driving cerebrospinal fluid from the subarachnoid space into the perivascular and extracellular space of the spinal cord, resulting in syrinx formation. After forming the syrinx, these enlarged spinal subarachnoid pressure waves acted on the spinal cord surface, induced movement of syrinx fluid, and expanded the syrinx diameter and length (Fig. 1).[1,11] Surgical intervention involving suboccipital craniectomy, C-1 laminectomy, and duraplasty expanded the CSF space at the foramen magnum and resolved the syrinx. The cerebellar tonsils assumed a regular shape and ascended toward the foramen magnum after the surgical procedure.[11]

CMI in most cases arises because the internal volume of the posterior fossa is inadequate to contain its neural contents and not from a primary maldevelopment of the cerebellum. Treatment of CM1 by surgically enlarging the posterior fossa results in the cerebellar tonsils ascending and assuming a regular shape, supporting this premise. Meticulous morphologic studies by Misao Nishikawa and embryologic studies by Charles Raybaud support the contention that CMI developed from a small posterior fossa. This conclusion has profound implications for the management of CMI because it directs treatment toward enlarging the posterior fossa rather than modifying a congenital brain abnormality.[13,14]

Normal

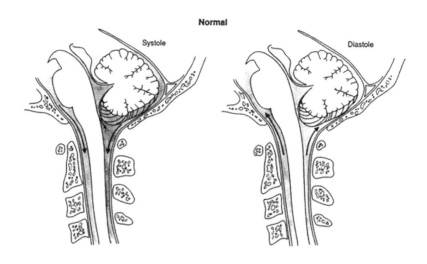

Preoperative

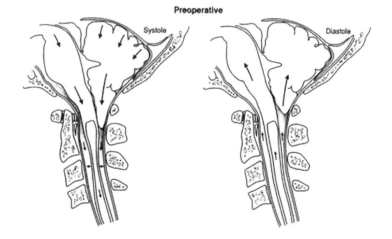

Post Operative

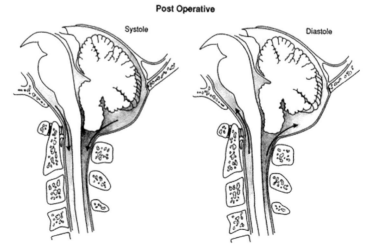

Section Highlights

- Several theories were developed to explain syringomyelia in CMI
- The prevailing theory, supported by physiologic studies in patients with CMI using phase-contrast MRI and ultrasound, proposes that the occlusion of the subarachnoid spaces at foramen magnum leads to the formation of the syrinx cavity by the movement of cerebrospinal fluid through perivascular and extracellular spaces in the spinal cord
- Surgical decompression of the posterior fossa results in return of the cerebellar tonsils to the normal position and resolution of the syrinx, suggesting that, in most cases, cerebellar ectopy is secondary to an abnormally small volume of the bony posterior fossa

Controversies and Ongoing Investigations

Reduced posterior fossa size and crowding of neural structures is not the only cause of tonsillar ectopia in CM1.[1,15] Oldfield described in 2016 CM1 cases for which the cerebellar tonsils extended below the foramen magnum in patients with normal posterior fossa volume.[15] Based on this and other studies, Raybaud recently proposed that these cases of cerebellar ectopy resulted from an overgrowth of the cerebellum.[16] This suggests that any developmental mismatch causing the posterior fossa contents to exceed that of the posterior fossa volume results in cerebellar tonsillar ectopy and CMI.

Studies of syndromes with impaired bone development have further supported the concept that a mismatch between the growth of the bony posterior fossa and its contents may result in cerebellar ectopy. For example, CMI is often a feature of achondroplasia and fibrous dysplasia.[17,18] We recently identified CMI and occult spinal dysraphism in patients with *EPAS1*-gain-of-function syndrome (Pacak–Zhuang syndrome) and the corresponding mouse model.[19] This syndrome, originally described as a syndrome characterized by multiple paragangliomas, somatostatinoma, and polycythemia, is caused by early somatic mosaicism of gain-of-function mutations in *EPAS1*, encoding the protein hypoxia-inducible factor 2α (HIF-2α).[19] Thus, while this syndrome does not represent isolated CMI, it is a sporadic disease that can be studied to understand CMI better. Despite occasional familial occurrences, it is most often sporadic and still has no known genetic cause.[20]

Section highlights

- Recently, cerebellar tonsillar ectopy was described in patients with a spacious posterior fossa, suggesting that reduced posterior fossa size and crowding of neural structures is not the only cause of tonsillar ectopia and CMI
- Tonsillar ectopia can arise in a normal bony posterior fossa if the combined volume of the posterior fossa neural contents and CSF is abnormally large.

Fig. 1. Illustrations showing normal anatomy and flow of CSF in the subarachnoid space at the foramen magnum during the cardiac cycle in a normal healthy volunteer *(upper)*; obstructed flow of CSF in the subarachnoid space at the foramen magnum resulting in the cerebellar tonsils acting as a piston on the cervical subarachnoid space, creating cervical subarachnoid pressure waves that compress the spinal cord from without and propagating syrinx fluid movement *(center)*; and relief of the obstruction of the subarachnoid space at the foramen magnum, eliminating the mechanism of progression of syringomyelia *(lower)*. (*Adapted from* Heiss JD, Patronas N, DeVroom HL, et al. Elucidating the pathophysiology of syringomyelia. J Neurosurg. 1999;91(4):553-562. doi:10.3171/jns.1999.91.4.0553; with permission).

Practical Considerations

Recent investigations into the etiology of Chiari Malformations have practical implications for diagnosing, managing, and treating these pathologies. Historically, the disease of CMI without syringomyelia has been challenging to define. Radiologists diagnose CM1 in symptomatic and asymptomatic individuals with an MRI finding of cerebellar tonsillar ectopy at least 5 mm below the foramen magnum.[16] Further, there is still ongoing debate about the interplay between the extent of cerebellar ectopy and the development of a syrinx. There have been studies that have proposed additional classifications of Chiari Malformations such as CM0 for patients with less than 5 mm of tonsillar ectopia and associated cervical syringomyelia.[2] It has been suggested that these cases arise from neural and CSF pathway crowding within the foramen magnum and diminished flow of cerebrospinal fluid through the subarachnoid spaces. This proposal, which agrees with the theory outlined above, raises the question of the best treatment of such patients.

While we now recognize that congenital Chiari Malformations broadly belong to a class of pathologies with a shared embryologic origin, ongoing imaging and physiologic studies continue to propose more nuanced definitions to reflect 2 primary considerations. First, if these pathologies have a common source, why are some more limited than others, for example, CMI than CMII? Second, what is the best intervention in cases of CMI without syringomyelia and atypical clinical symptoms? From the studies discussed, the most practical implication is that the diagnosis of CMI and the decision to intervene to resolve CM1 symptoms or syringomyelia should not be based on cerebellar ectopy alone but the evidence of the diminished flow of cerebrospinal fluid across the craniocervical junction assessed by phase-contrast magnetic resonance imaging.[1,2] The aim of intervention thus should be the restoration of CSF flow across the craniocervical junction. While this was demonstrated in previous studies, this outcome has only recently been compared among the various surgical interventions for CM1.

Section highlights

- Observations of cervical syringomyelia, a crowed posterior fossa, but less than 5 mm of tonsillar ectopia, that is, CM0, support diminished flow of CSF as the critical mechanism for syrinx formation.

- Phase-contrast MRI demonstrates constricted and obstructed CSF pathways in CM0 and in patients with a crowded posterior fossa, CM1 symptoms, but no tonsillar herniation or syringomyelia.

Controversies of Management

With our understanding of the natural history and etiologies of CMI evolving, management remains complex. We recently elaborated the history, importance of patient selection, and rationales for surgical treatments in symptomatic CMI with or without syringomyelia.[21] The early surgical management of these patients by McConnell and Parker only involved a posterior fossa decompression.[22] Later, several authors described craniocervical decompression in the treatment of CMI.[23,24] On recognizing that syringomyelia was associated with CMI, Gardner at Cleveland Clinic aimed to eliminate the postulated "water-hammer" pulsation by removing the bone from the posterior aspect of the foramen magnum, opening the fourth ventricle, and plugging the obex, which Levy later found could permanently damage the hypoglossal and vagal nuclei.[25–27] After these early procedures, several surgical procedures have been advocated, including extradural craniocervical decompression alone or with the following additional steps: scoring the dura, opening the dura, dissecting the arachnoid, exploring the fourth ventricle, and shrinking cerebellar tonsils, all with subsequent dural repair (duraplasty).[21] These various procedures have similar outcomes in the medical literature.[21] Recently, some investigators have advocated performing less invasive interventions such as posterior fossa decompression alone or with dural scoring.[28–32]

As we previously elaborated, surgical intervention in CMI should provide enough enlargement of the subarachnoid space at the foramen magnum to relieve tonsillar impaction and reverse the signs and symptoms of CMI.[21] The extent of expansion of the CSF spaces is more often reported in pediatric than adult studies.[21] As investigations into the surgical management of CMI in both adults and children continue to search for the optimal intervention, standardization of patient selection, reporting, and measurements is required. The recent development of Common Data Elements for use in research regarding CMI by the National Institute of Neurologic Disorders and Stroke at NIH represents a significant advancement for investigations to determine the best or most effective treatments, interventions, and management for patients with CMI.[33] This standardization of terminology and methods for studies, including case report forms, outcome measure recommendations, and data definitions assembled by a group of 30 experts, will serve to guide investigations regarding CMI.[33] These guidelines are available on the NINDS CDE website (https://www.commondataelements.ninds.nih.gov/Chiari%20I%20Malformation).

After the release of the Common Data Elements for CMI in 2016, several studies have evaluated surgical interventions for CMI. A single institutional study of 177 patients (97 with syringomyelia) assessed the effect of posterior fossa decompression (150 with opening the dura and intra-arachnoidal dissection; 135 with reduction of the cerebellar tonsils) on the postoperative resolution of signs and symptoms and size of the posterior fossa cisterns and syrinx.[34] This study found that clinical improvement was strongly correlated with enlargement of the subarachnoid cisterns, which also strongly correlated with a reduction in the syrinx cavity.[34]

Several recent studies have investigated the success of these varied interventions in resolving specific pathologies associated with CMI. The Park-Reeves Syringomyelia Research Consortium recently evaluated whether extradural decompression of the posterior fossa alone or with duraplasty is superior at halting the progression of scoliosis in CMI.[35] This large multicenter retrospective and prospective study of 1257 pediatric patients with CMI, as defined by cerebellar tonsillar descent greater than 5 mm below foramen magnum with an associated syrinx of greater than 3 mm in axial width, found that there was no difference in the occurrence of surgical correction of scoliosis between groups having undergone extradural decompression alone (n = 51) or with duraplasty (n = 346).[35] However, patients treated with duraplasty were less likely to have curve progression; further, older age at the time of surgery and more significant preoperative curves were more strongly associated with subsequent fusion.[35] The same group also evaluated complication rates with different grafts used for duraplasty within the 6-month postoperative period. They found higher rates of pseudomeningocele and meningitis in the group receiving nonautologous grafts (n = 422), which included bovine pericardium, bovine collagen, synthetic, and human cadaveric allograft, than in the group receiving autografts (n = 359).[36]

Cases of CMI with syringomyelia and complex pathology of the craniovertebral junction may require occipital-cervical fusion and ventral decompression as adjuncts to posterior fossa decompression.[37,38] In another multicenter retrospective study by the Park-Reeves Syringomyelia Research Consortium, 12 of 637 patients who underwent posterior fossa decompression alone (n = 132) or with duraplasty (n = 505) subsequently required occipital-cervical fusion, 4 of which also needed ventral decompression.[37] Of note, these patients had platybasia, Klippel–Feil syndrome, and/or basilar invagination.[37]

These recent studies highlight the need for continued investigation into the proper and optimal surgical management of CMI. The recent advances in the understanding of the pathogenesis of CMI may also impact our practical management regarding patient selection for surgery. Further, the recent development of Common Data Elements for CMI will fundamentally change future investigations.

Section highlights

- There is still on-going debate regarding the optimal surgical intervention for the resolution of symptoms and syrinx in CMI
- Available options include posterior fossa decompression alone or with dural scoring, intraarachnoidal dissection, exploration of the fourth ventricle, and/or reduction of the cerebellar tonsils
- Recent studies have supported less invasive interventions such as posterior fossa decompression alone in selected cases of CM1 without syringomyelia.
- The Common Data Elements for CMI developed by NINDS at NIH provide the framework for continued investigations in CMI

SUMMARY

Congenital Chiari Malformations range in complexity from cerebellar tonsillar ectopy to complex neuraxial malformations with long-debated etiologies. Fundamental anatomic, physiologic, and embryologic studies over the past 50 years have deepened our understanding of the original question asked in early reports by Chiari: what is the relationship between tonsillar ectopy and syringomyelia or hydrocephalus? We are now better able to classify Chiari Malformations and make more informed decisions regarding surgical intervention based on our better understanding of the pathophysiology of these malformations. Continued investigations into the pathogenesis of Chiari Malformations through recently discovered sporadic diseases with associated Chiari Malformation pathologies will continue to inform our understanding of Chiari Malformations. Further, there remain practical questions in more nuanced presentations of CMI that warrant further investigation.

CLINICS CARE POINTS

- Chiari Malformation Type I (CMI) is typically defined by cerebellar tonsillar ectopy of at least 5 mm below the foramen magnum. The bony posterior fossa volume is small in most cases.
- Syringomyelia in CM1 arises from the cerebellar tonsils impeding normal CSF flow across the foramen magnum during the cardiac cycle. Surgical relief of the obstruction to CSF flow results in syrinx resolution.
- There are many options for surgical intervention, including posterior fossa decompression alone and with dural scoring, intraarachnoidal dissection, exploration of the fourth ventricle, or reduction of the cerebellar tonsils. Their success in resolving syringomyelia depends on their ability to permanently establish a patent subarachnoid space at the foramen magnum.

- Some cases of CMI have a spacious posterior fossa, suggesting that a reduced bony posterior fossa may not be the only mechanism for cerebellar ectopy. These patients have less constricted CSF pathways and are less likely to have an associated syrinx.
- The recent development of the Common Data Elements for CMI provides a framework for continued investigation into CM1 pathogenesis, pathophysiology, and optimal surgical management.

DISCLOSURE

The authors have nothing to disclose.

ACKNOWLEDGMENTS

The authors acknowledge support from the Intramural Research Program at the National Cancer Institute (J.R.) and the National Institute of Neurological Disorders and Stroke (I.J.P. and J.H.) at the NIH, United States.

REFERENCES

1. Oldfield EH. Pathogenesis of Chiari I-Pathophysiology of syringomyelia: implications for therapy: a summary of 3 decades of clinical research. Neurosurgery 2017;64(CN_Suppl_1):66–77.
2. Hiremath SB, Fitsori A, Boto J, et al. The perplexity surrounding chiari malformations—are we any wiser now? AJNR Am J Neuroradiol 2020;41(11):1975–81.
3. Koehler PJ. Chiari's description of cerebellar ectopy (1891): With a summary of Cleland's and Arnold's contributions and some early observations on neural-tube defects. J Neurosurg 1991;75:823–6.
4. Chiari H. Concerning alterations in the cerebellum resulting from cerebral hydrocephalus. Pediatr Neurosci 1891;13:3–8.
5. Chiari H. Uber Veranderungen des Kleinhirns, des Pons und der Medulla Oblongata infolge von kongenitaler Hy- drocephalie des Grosshirns. Denkschr der Kais Akad Wiss Wien math-naturw 1896;63:71–116.
6. Arnold J. Myelocyste, transposition von Gewebskeimen und Sympodie. Zieglers Beitr Pathol Anal 1894;16:1–28.
7. Cleland J. Contribution to the study of spina bifida, encephalocele, and anencephalus. J Anat Physiol 1883;17:257–92.
8. Padget DH. Development of so-called dysraphism; with embryologic evidence of clinical Arnold-Chiari and Dandy-Walker malformations. Johns Hopkins Med J 1972;130(3):127–65.
9. Marín-Padilla M. Cephalic axial skeletal-neural dysraphic disorders: embryology and pathology. Can J Neurol Sci 1991;18(2):153–69.
10. Buell TJ, Heiss JD, Oldfield EH. Pathogenesis and Cerebrospinal Fluid Hydrodynamics of the Chiari I Malformation. Neurosurg Clin N Am 2015;26(4):495–9.
11. Heiss JD, Patronas N, DeVroom HL, et al. Elucidating the pathophysiology of syringomyelia. J Neurosurg 1999;91(4):553–62.
12. Gardner WJ, Angel J. The mechanism of syringomyelia and its surgical correction. Clin Neurosurg 1958;6:131–40.
13. Raybaud C, Jallo GI. Chapter 2: Chiari I deformity in children: etiopathogenesis and radiologic diagnosis. In: Manto M, Huisman TAGM, editors. Handbook of clinical neurologyVol 155, 3rd series. Edinburgh (U.K): Elsevier; 2018. p. 25–48.

14. Nishikawa M, Sakamoto H, Hakuba A, et al. Pathogenesis of Chiari malformation: a morphometric study of the posterior cranial fossa. J Neurosurg 1997; 86:40–7.

15. Taylor DG, Mastorakos P, Jane JA, et al. Two distinct populations of Chiari I malformation based on presence or absence of posterior fossa crowdedness on magnetic resonance imaging. J Neurosurg 2016;126(6):1–7.

16. Raybaud C, Jallo GI. Chiari I deformity in children: etiopathogenesis and radiologic diagnosis. Handb Clin Neurol 2018;155:25–48.

17. Pan KS, Heiss JD, Brown SM, et al. Chiari I malformation and basilar invagination in fibrous dysplasia: prevalence, mechanisms, and clinical implications. J Bone Miner Res 2018;33(11):1990–8.

18. Urbizu A, Khan TN, Ashley-Koch AE. Genetic dissection of Chiari malformation type I using endophenotypes and stratification. J. Rare Dis. Res. Treat, 2 (2), 2017, 35-42 Available at: www.rarediseasesjournal.com. December 23, 2021

19. Rosenblum JS, Cappadona AJ, Argersinger DP, et al. Neuraxial Dysraphism in EPAS1-Associated Syndrome due to Improper Mesenchymal Transition. Neurol Genet 2020;6(3):e414.

20. Kniffin CL, McKusick VA. OMIM-online mendelian inheritance in man: Chiari malformation type, I. Available at: https://www.omim.org/entry/118420#title. July 27, 2021.

21. Mastorakos P, Heiss JD. Chapter 38: treatment of the adult Chiari I Malformation. In: Tubbs RS, Turgut M, Oakes W J, editors. The Chiari malformations. Cham, Switzerland: Springer Nature Switzerland AG; 2020. p. 443–57.

22. McConnell AA, Parker HL. A deformity of the hindbrain associated with internal hydrocephalus. Its relation to the Arnold-Chiari malformation. Brain 1938;61: 415–29.

23. Adams RD, Schatzki R, Scovill WB. The Arnold- Chiari malformation. Diagnosis, demonstration by intraspinal Lipiodol and successful surgical treatment. N Engl J Med 1941;225:125–31.

24. Bucy PC, Lichtenstein BW. Arnold-Chiari deformity in an adult without obvious cause. J Neurosurg 1945;2:245–50.

25. Gardner WJ, Goodall RJ. The surgical treatment of Arnold-Chiari malformation in adults; an explanation of its mechanism and importance of encephalography in diagnosis. J Neurosurg 1950;7(3):199–206.

26. Levy WJ, Mason L, Hahn JF. Chiari malformation presenting in adults: a surgical experience in 127 cases. Neurosurgery 1983;12(4):377–90.

27. Pillay PK. Thecoperitoneal shunting for syringomy- elia. J Neurosurg 1991;75(5): 835–6.

28. Chauvet D, Carpentier A, George B. Dura splitting decompression in Chiari type 1 malformation: clinical experience and radiological findings. Neurosurg Rev 2009;32(4):465–70.

29. Durham SR, Fjeld-Olenec K. Comparison of posterior fossa decompression with and without duraplasty for the surgical treatment of Chiari malformation Type I in pediatric patients: a meta-analysis. J Neurosurg Pediatr 2008;2(1):42–9.

30. Isu T, Sasaki H, Takamura H, et al. Foramen magnum decompression with removal of the outer layer of the dura as treatment for syringomyelia occurring with Chiari I malformation. Neurosurgery 1993;33(5):844–9 [discussion: 9-50].

31. Kotil K, Ton T, Tari R, et al. Delamination technique together with longitudinal incisions for treatment of Chiari I/syringomyelia complex: a prospective clinical study. Cerebrospinal Fluid Res 2009;6:7.

32. Romero FR, Pereira CAdB. Suboccipital craniectomy with or without duraplasty: what is the best choice in patients with Chiari type 1 malformation? Arq Neuropsiquiatr 2010;68(4):623–6.
33. Luciano MG, Batzdorf U, Kula RW, et al. Chiari I Malformation Common Data Element Working Group. Development of Common Data Elements for Use in Chiari Malformation Type I Clinical Research: An NIH/NINDS Project. Neurosurgery 2019;85(6):854–60.
34. Batzdorf U, McArthur DL, Bentson JR. Surgical treatment of Chiari malformation with and without syringomyelia: experience with 177 adult patients. J Neurosurg 2013;118(2):232–42.
35. Sadler B, Skidmore A, Gewirtz J, et al. Extradural decompression versus duraplasty in Chiari malformation type I with syrinx: outcomes on scoliosis from the Park-Reeves Syringomyelia Research Consortium. J Neurosurg Pediatr 2021;1–9. https://doi.org/10.3171/2020.12.PEDS20552.
36. Yahanda AT, Adelson PD, Akbari SHA, et al. Dural augmentation approaches and complication rates after posterior fossa decompression for Chiari I malformation and syringomyelia: a Park-Reeves Syringomyelia Research Consortium study. J Neurosurg Pediatr 2021;1–10.
37. CreveCoeur TS, Yahanda AT, Maher CO, et al. Occipital-cervical fusion and ventral decompression in the surgical management of Chiari-1 Malformation and Syringomyelia: analysis of data from the Park-Reeves Syringomyelia Research Consortium. Neurosurgery 2021;88(2):332–41.
38. Hale AT, Adelson PD, Albert GW, et al, Park-Reeves Syringomyelia Research Consortium Investigators. Factors associated with syrinx size in pediatric patients treated for Chiari malformation type I and syringomyelia: a study from the Park-Reeves Syringomyelia Research Consortium. J Neurosurg Pediatr 2020;1–11. https://doi.org/10.3171/2020.1.PEDS19493.

Current State of the Art in Endovascular Stroke Treatment

David Dornbos III, MD[a], Adam S. Arthur, MD, MPH[b],*

KEYWORDS

- Thrombectomy • Acute ischemic stroke • Balloon-guide catheter • Endovascular

KEY POINTS

- Given robust clinical trials, thrombectomy for large vessel occlusion ischemic stroke is well indicated for up to 24 hours following onset
- New device development of balloon-guide catheters, more navigable aspiration catheters, and small distal catheters is opening up more patients to the procedure
- Ongoing trials are evaluating thrombectomy for large core infarcts, distal occlusions, and first-line aspiration

INTRODUCTION

With an incidence of nearly 800,000 strokes per year within the United States, stroke has become a leading cause of death and disability.[1] The socioeconomic impact of acute ischemic stroke (AIS) is substantial, costing the United States health care system an estimated $46 billion annually.[2] This underscores the need for improved stroke prevention through lifestyle and risk factor modification, enhanced stroke care delivery, technological advancements, and improved stroke recovery and rehabilitation.

Once arterial occlusion and decreased cerebral perfusion occur, the race commences to restore reperfusion before ischemic penumbra can progress to completed infarct. A perfusion deficit and lack of oxygen delivery to brain parenchyma results in loss of ATP synthesis and irreversible neuronal death within minutes. However, the rate of permanent ischemic change is highly variable, ranging from less than 35,000 to greater than 27 million neurons per minute.[3] Despite a proximal arterial occlusion, accessory perfusion of brain tissue from collateral vessels can maintain adequate oxygen levels to avoid cell death, and the degree of collateralization produces the wide range of ischemic progression observed in these patients. The utility of adequate hydration, oxygen

[a] Department of Neurosurgery, University of Kentucky College of Medicine, 780 Rose St, Lexington, KY 40508, USA; [b] Department of Neurosurgery, Semmes-Murphey Clinic, University of Tennessee Health Science Center, Memphis, Tennessee, USA
* Corresponding author. 6325 Humphreys Blvd, Memphis, TN 38120
E-mail address: aarthur@semmes-murphey.com

Neurol Clin 40 (2022) 309–319
https://doi.org/10.1016/j.ncl.2021.11.008
0733-8619/22/© 2022 Elsevier Inc. All rights reserved.
neurologic.theclinics.com

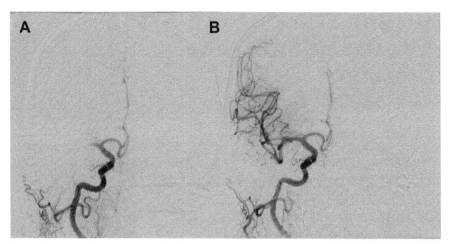

Fig. 1. Emergent large vessel occlusion (ELVO). (*A*) Digital subtraction angiography (PA projection) depicting a right M1 occlusion in the setting of AIS. (*B*) Following aspiration thrombectomy, full recanalization of the right MCA territory was achieved.

supplementation, and avoidance of hypotension are key factors to enhance collateral blood flow to penumbral regions before endovascular intervention in patients with an emergent large vessel occlusion (ELVO) (**Fig. 1**). While these maneuvers can decrease the risk of permanent ischemia, restoration of normal perfusion is ultimately needed.

Intravenous tissue plasminogen activator (TPA) has been the standard of care for patients presenting within 4.5 hours for nearly 3 decades.[4] While TPA has been shown to increase long-term functional independence, the recanalization efficacy of TPA is quite poor, particularly in the setting of ELVO, only restoring vessel patency in 30% to 40% of cases.[5–7] For this reason, endovascular treatment of acute ischemic stroke has become standard of care in patients with ELVO.

DISCUSSION
Efficacy of mechanical thrombectomy

Early clinical trials
While initial clinical trials found no benefit for mechanical thrombectomy in combination with IV TPA in the setting of AIS,[8–10] further device development and improved patient selection resulted in a significant clinical benefit for patients undergoing thrombectomy.[11–15] While inclusion criteria between these initial trials varied slightly (**Table 1**), they established that patients greater than 18 years of age with a good premorbid functional status (modified Rankin scale [mRS] <2), absence of a large completed infarct, and treated within 6 hours of stroke onset were able to achieve functional independence with greater frequency than those treated without endovascular thrombectomy. These trials precipitated an explosion in device development, enhanced imaging modalities and software, and adjunctive treatments for ischemic stroke.

Expanding the time window
While time to thrombectomy is a major indicator for patient outcomes, neuronal loss experienced during this time is not a linear relationship, but rather a stepwise or sudden decline when autoregulatory reserve and collateral support begin to fail. Based on

Table 1
Major clinical trials establishing the role of mechanical thrombectomy in large vessel occlusion ischemic stroke

Trial	MR Clean	Escape	SWIFT Prime	EXTEND-IA	Revascat
Age (years)	> 18	> 18	18–80	≥ 18	18–85
Prestroke morbidity	None	Barthel score ≥ 90	mRS ≤ 1	mRS ≤ 1	mRS ≤ 1
Coagulopathy	Excluded	Included	Excluded	Excluded	Excluded
Vessel	Anterior circulation	ICA/MCA	ICA/M1	Anterior circulation	ICA/M1
NIHSS	> 2	> 5	8–29	None	≥ 6
IV TPA	Not required	Not required	Required	Required	Not Required
ASPECTS	None	≥ 6	≥ 6	None	≥ 7
Time	6 h to initiation of IAT	12 h to randomization	6 h to groin	6 h to groin	8 h to groin

this assumption, 2 trials (DAWN and DEFUSE 3) were formed to evaluate the potential benefit of thrombectomy in patients beyond 6 hours from stroke onset with good collaterals and the absence of a large core infarct.[16,17] Both trials used automated CT perfusion (**Fig. 2**) imaging to identify patients with a relatively small ischemic core and large penumbral region presenting greater than 6 hours from stroke onset. DEFUSE 3 evaluated patients within 16 hours of known stroke onset, an ischemic core less than 70 cc, and a penumbra:core ratio of 1.8 or greater,[17] whereas DAWN included patients within 24 hours from stroke onset and stratified penumbra and core sizes based on patient age.[16]

Both studies identified a significant shift in functional outcomes toward independence (mRS ≤2) in patients who underwent intervention. Patients treated with thrombectomy in combination with medical therapy were nearly 3-fold more likely to achieve a good outcome when compared with patients undergoing medical treatment alone.[17] This finding was so profound that the number needed to treat to effectively shift one patient from a poor to a good functional outcome was only between 2 and 3.6.[18] Further, there was no difference in symptomatic ICH or mortality between the 2 groups. These trials not only established an expanded cohort of patients with ischemic stroke that benefit from thrombectomy but also shifted the paradigm from a "time-based" approach to a "tissue-based" approach, wherein time as stroke onset is of lesser importance compared with the volume of penumbra and ischemic core. Following these trials, the standard of care for patients with AIS presenting with an ELVO within 24 hours in the absence of a large core infarct dictates proceeding with thrombectomy. Given the profound treatment effect, further investigations have sought to identify patients excluded from these trials that may still achieve benefit from mechanical thrombectomy.

Controversies and current trials

Medium and distal vessel occlusions
Initial trials limited the inclusion of patients to those presenting with more proximal large vessel occlusions, typically of the intracranial internal carotid artery (ICA) or the M1 segment of the middle cerebral artery (MCA). While these trials did not include

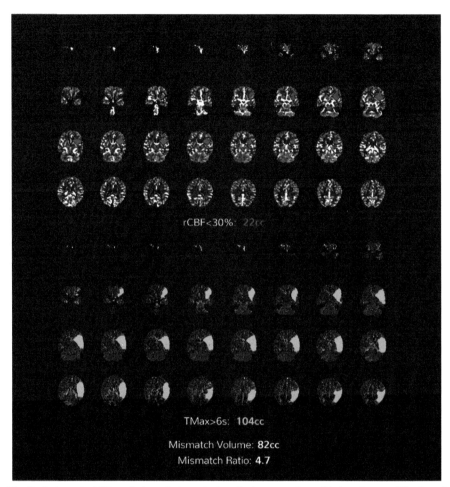

rCBF<30%: 22cc

TMax>6s: **104cc**

Mismatch Volume: **82cc**
Mismatch Ratio: **4.7**

Fig. 2. Automated CT perfusion. Automated perfusion mapping of ischemic core (22 cc) and penumbral tissue (104 cc) provides rapid and efficient estimation of the core infarct and potentially salvageable brain tissue.

medium and distal vessel occlusions, iterative catheter and device development over the past several years have made thrombectomy for these occlusions relatively safe and effective. Several recent meta-analyses have identified that patients presenting with M2 occlusions that undergo thrombectomy obtain high recanalization rates and experience improved clinical outcomes, particularly for occlusion of the dominant M2 division (**Fig. 3**).[19,20] Occlusions of the anterior cerebral artery (ACA) and M3 segment of the MCA are less well characterized, although account for approximately one-third of AIS and are often associated with poor outcome. Further, intravenous fibrinolytics are only effective in one-third to half of the patients presenting with medium and distal vessel occlusions.[21]

Smaller, single-center studies evaluating the use of endovascular thrombectomy for the treatment of medium and distal vessel occlusions have identified high rates of revascularization (83% and higher) and low risk of symptomatic intracranial hemorrhage (<5%).[22,23] With this early experience and the highly efficacious nature of

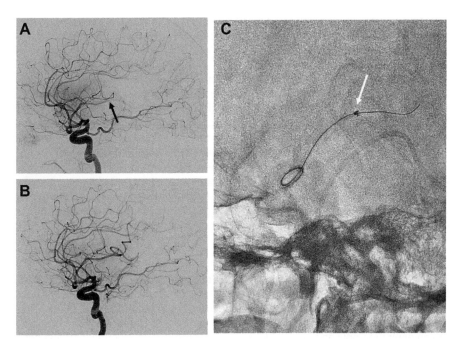

Fig. 3. Medium vessel occlusion. (*A*) Digital subtraction angiography (lateral projection) depicting a distal occlusion (*black arrow*) of a dominant M2 branch of the left MCA. (*B*) Following aspiration thrombectomy, full recanalization of the left MCA territory was achieved. (*C*) Smaller, more navigable aspiration catheters (062-inch, *white arrow*) are better equipped to allow access to distal occlusion.

thrombectomy for ELVO, recent 2019 American Stroke Association guidelines identify endovascular intervention for medium vessel occlusion as a reasonable option (class IIb recommendation) for these patients.[24] Based on these early clinical series and enhanced catheter development, endovascular treatment of distal and medium vessel occlusions is likely to be safe and effective, needing further clinical investigation and randomized trials.

Large core infarct

Early studies predominantly excluded patients based on the size of preprocedural infarct size with Alberta Stroke Program Early Computed Tomography Score (AS-PECTS) of 6 as a typical threshold for a large infarct. Despite this, several studies have evaluated the utility of mechanical thrombectomy in patients presenting with larger infarcts. Patient with low initial ASPECTS ≤6 do appear to get a clinical benefit from reperfusion with a 2-fold improvement in functional outcomes, decreased mortality, and no increase in symptomatic intracranial hemorrhage.[25] As the ASPECTS continues to decrease (≤4), however, this benefit seems to diminish and loses significance. Nonetheless, while the effect is certainly less powerful than in patients with more favorable ASPECTS, successful recanalization is a strong predictor of good outcome in patients with AIS presenting with a large ischemic core.[26]

Using endovascular thrombectomy to save penumbra regions adjacent to a large infarct may also have a secondary advantage of preventing malignant cerebral edema and subsequent craniectomy. Decompressive hemicraniectomy clearly prevents brain herniation and reduces mortality in the setting of a malignant infarction, but the quality of life following this procedure remains controversial.[27-29] With the increased utilization of mechanical thrombectomy, nationwide trends in decompressive hemicraniectomy have noticeably decreased,[30] in part due to endovascular intervention in the setting of larger infarctions.

Further studies to evaluate the utility and clinical benefit of endovascular intervention for ELVO in the setting of a large volume stroke are certainly needed and are ongoing. SELECT 2 is an ongoing randomized controlled trial evaluating the safety and efficacy of endovascular thrombectomy for ELVO (ICA and M1 occlusions) compared with best medical therapy for patients with AIS presenting with large core infarcts within 24 hours of stroke onset.[31] A large infarct in SELECT 2 is defined as ASPECTS 3 to 5 on noncontrast head CT or a stroke of $\geq$50 mL on MRI or CT perfusion. Similarly, TENSION is an ongoing European randomized controlled trial evaluating the efficacy of thrombectomy compared with best medical management in patients presenting within 12 hours of stroke onset and a large infarct, defined as ASPECTS of 3 to 5.[32] These trials will provide clarity to what seems to be a promising additional patient population for endovascular thrombectomy.

Aspiration v stent retriever

The initial trials establishing the clinical benefit of endovascular thrombectomy all utilized stent retrievers in combination with aspiration catheters. While effective in establishing recanalization, dragging a stent retriever across the endothelial surface has been shown to lead to greater endothelial disruption and damage when compared with an aspiration only approach.[33] Early single-center studies found a first-line aspiration-only approach to be highly efficacious with a favorable safety profile and conferring significant cost savings compared with the utilization of stent retrievers as a first-line treatment strategy.[34,35] A follow-up prospective randomized controlled trial (ASTER) failed to show improved angiographic outcomes with a direct aspiration first pass technique, but did identify similar clinical results when compared with a stent retriever first-line approach.[36]

COMPASS was a multicenter randomized open-label noninferiority trial designed to assess clinical functional outcomes in patients treated with direct aspiration first pass than stent retriever first line for the treatment of AIS secondary to ELVO within 6 hours of stroke onset.[37] Good functional outcomes (mRS $\leq$2) were seen, indicating that an aspiration first-line approach to thrombectomy to be noninferior to stent retriever first line. Further, there was no difference between the 2 treatment modalities in the assessed safety outcomes, mortality, or intracranial hemorrhage. While outcomes have remained equivalent, direct aspiration has been shown to be a faster and more cost-effective modality when compared with a first-line stent-retriever approach.[34,35] While this remains a debated topic among neurointerventionalists, there are data to support either modality as a first-line treatment.

Catheter and device development

Balloon-guide catheters

As numerous studies have established the efficacy of endovascular treatment of AIS, further technological advancements have focused on ways to expedite treatment and make thrombectomy a more safe and efficacious procedure. The introduction of balloon guide catheters for use in mechanical thrombectomy came about to improve efficacy and decrease the risk of emboli to new territories (ENT). Utilizing a balloon on the primary guide catheter arrests anterograde flow, limiting blood flow working against clot retrieval. Depending on the location of the thrombus, collateral vascular supply may provide additional reversal of flow with the balloon inflated and aspiration applied.

Numerous studies have found significant benefits for the adjunctive use of balloon-guide catheters in AIS.[38,39] While balloon-guide catheters do add to procedural times and their impact on first-pass effect has been mixed,[40] their use has been shown to decrease the rate of ENT and improve rates of angiographic revascularization. Most importantly, the use of balloon-guide catheters has been independently associated with better clinical outcomes in both long-term functional independence and mortality. Recent balloon-guide development has substantially improved navigability with the introduction of the Walrus (Q'Apel Medical, Fremont, California), BOBBY (MicroVention Inc., Aliso Viejo, California), and BOSS (Marblehead Medical, LLC, Rochester, Minnesota) balloon-guide catheters. As balloon-guide catheter development continues to enhance the ease of use and access in tortuous vasculature, their use in the clinical setting will certainly become more widespread and ubiquitous.

Iterative device development

The first-pass effect, defined as complete revascularization and reperfusion on the first attempt, has been identified as a significant contributor to successful endovascular treatment and long-term clinical outcomes. Numerous technological advancements have been developed to enhance the first-pass effect, including the development of larger bore catheters with improved navigability in the intracranial circulation. Recent publications have found the use of large-bore catheters to be independently associated with improved first-pass effect and better rates of revascularization.[41] Numerous 071, 072, and 074-inch aspiration catheters have been developed with enhanced glide and navigation technology to improve access with these larger catheters.

Given that surface area is directly proportional to suction force, larger aspiration catheters provide an increased suction capacity on the clot interface and theoretically improved aspiration success. Recently, the Trac Star 088 (Imperative Care Inc., Campbell, California) and the Millipede 088 (Perfuze Ltd, Gateway, Ireland) catheters have also been introduced as a means to access the intracranial circulation with 088-inch diameter aspiration catheters to improve the success rates of primary aspiration.[42,43] To maximize surface area and thrombus-catheter interface, beveled-tip aspiration catheters have also been developed, showing promise to further improve revascularization rates and clinical outcomes.[44]

Because potential benefit exists with thrombectomy for medium and distal vessel occlusions, newer generation aspiration catheters have also been developed to target these lesions. Numerous small diameter catheters (035-inch to 054-inch) have been developed to target distal occlusions of M3 segment MCA and A3 segment ACA occlusions. Additionally, new stent retrievers are also being developed to allow safe and efficacious treatment of distal occlusion. Recently, a new generation stent retriever (Tigertriever, Rapid Medical, Yokneam, Israel) has been shown to safely treat distal occlusions with a diameter of only 0.5 to 2 mm.[23,45] Future generations of devices and catheters will continue to focus on enhancing first-pass effect, decreasing ENT, and facilitating navigation and access of tortuous anatomy and more distal vasculature.

Transradial access

The use of transradial access has been shown to have a significantly improved safety profile in the cardiac literature compared with traditional transfemoral access.[46] While early experience in the neurointerventional literature has shown promise,[47] additional procedural time in certain neurointerventional procedures has limited its broad use and application for thrombectomy. Despite this, numerous centers have adopted a radial-first approach with thrombectomy in the absence of prohibitive anatomic factors with good results. In the setting of thrombectomy for ELVO in AIS, radial access has been shown to have equivalent door-to-procedure times, procedural length, first-pass effectiveness, and revascularization rates.[48,49] Importantly, transradial access for thrombectomy was found to have a superior access-site complication profile when compared with transfemoral access.[49] Other studies, however, have found trans-femoral access to be associated with improved revascularization, fewer passes, and better overall outcomes, potentially due to higher use of balloon-guide catheters from this approach.[50] Further studies, improved practitioner experience, and radial-specific catheters will be needed to determine the viability of this approach moving forward.

Future directions

Device and catheter development will continue to move endovascular stroke care forward, but perhaps the biggest area of enhanced patient outcomes will come from the improved delivery of care to the patient. The rise of stroke certification led to a tiered delivery system, akin to that of the tiered levels of trauma care. Much debate has arisen in terms of whether patients should be brought to a nearby primary stroke center before transfer to a comprehensive stroke center (drip and ship) or simply brought immediately to a comprehensive stroke center. There are theoretic benefits to both with early time to TPA in the drip-and-ship model but with early time to endovascular intervention with the latter model.[51] More recently, a third model for which the interventional team is mobile and able to transfer the entire treatment team to individual hospitals within a network was found to have improved revascularization times and short term outcomes.[52] While all of these models are likely needed to serve different communities and geographic areas, improvements in the delivery of endovascular care to patients is certainly ongoing.

SUMMARY

Mechanical thrombectomy has been shown to be a powerful and highly effective procedure that improves clinical outcomes in patients with AIS with ELVO. Further studies are identifying additional patients that may benefit from this procedure, including patients with large infarcts and occlusions of medium and distal intracranial vessels. As iterative catheter and device development continues, the safety and efficacy of mechanical thrombectomy will continue to improve and benefit future patients with stroke.

CLINICS CARE POINTS

1. Mechanical thrombectomy has been shown to be highly efficacious for patients with AIS with an ELVO
2. Development of balloon-guide catheters, large bore aspiration catheters, smaller devices, and improved navigability is allowing this procedure to be delivered in a safer and more efficacious manner
3. Trials assessing the utility of thrombectomy in patients with large infarcts and distal occlusions are ongoing

REFERENCES

1. Koton S, Rexrode KM. Trends in stroke incidence in the United States: Will women overtake men? Neurology 2017;89(10):982–3.

2. Virani SS, Alonso A, Benjamin EJ, et al. Heart disease and stroke Statistics-2020 Update: a Report from the American Heart Association. Circulation 2020;141(9): e139–596.

3. Desai SM, Rocha M, Jovin TG, et al. High Variability in Neuronal Loss. Stroke 2019;50(1):34–7.

4. National Institute of Neurological, D. and P.A.S.S.G. Stroke rt. Tissue plasminogen activator for acute ischemic stroke. N Engl J Med 1995;333(24):1581–7.

5. Demchuk AM, Burgin WS, Christou I, et al. Thrombolysis in brain ischemia (TIBI) transcranial Doppler flow grades predict clinical severity, early recovery, and mortality in patients treated with intravenous tissue plasminogen activator. Stroke 2001;32(1):89–93.

6. Muchada M, Rodriguez-Luna D, Pagola J, et al. Impact of time to treatment on tissue-type plasminogen activator-induced recanalization in acute ischemic stroke. Stroke 2014;45(9):2734–8.

7. Molina CA, Montaner J, Arenillas JF, et al. Differential pattern of tissue plasminogen activator-induced proximal middle cerebral artery recanalization among stroke subtypes. Stroke 2004;35(2):486–90.

8. Broderick JP, Palesch YY, Demchuk AM, et al. Endovascular therapy after intravenous t-PA versus t-PA alone for stroke. N Engl J Med 2013;368(10):893–903.

9. Ciccone A, Valvassori L, Nichelatti M, et al. Endovascular treatment for acute ischemic stroke. N Engl J Med 2013;368(10):904–13.

10. Kidwell CS, Jahan R, Gorbein J, et al. A trial of imaging selection and endovascular treatment for ischemic stroke. N Engl J Med 2013;368(10):914–23.

11. Berkhemer OA, Fransen PS, Beumer D, et al. A randomized trial of intraarterial treatment for acute ischemic stroke. N Engl J Med 2015;372(1):11–20.

12. Campbell BC, Micthell PJ, Kleing TJ, et al. Endovascular therapy for ischemic stroke with perfusion-imaging selection. N Engl J Med 2015;372(11):1009–18.

13. Goyal M, Demchuk AM, Menon BK, et al. Randomized assessment of rapid endovascular treatment of ischemic stroke. N Engl J Med 2015;372(11):1019–30.

14. Jovin TG, Chamorro A, Cobo E, et al. Thrombectomy within 8 hours after symptom onset in ischemic stroke. N Engl J Med 2015;372(24):2296–306.

15. Saver JL, Goyal M, Bonafe A, et al. Stent-retriever thrombectomy after intravenous t-PA vs. t-PA alone in stroke. N Engl J Med 2015;372(24):2285–95.

16. Nogueira RG, Jadhav AP, Haussen DC, et al. Thrombectomy 6 to 24 hours after stroke with a Mismatch between Deficit and Infarct. N Engl J Med 2018;378(1): 11–21.

17. Albers GW, Marks MP, Kemp S, et al. Thrombectomy for stroke at 6 to 16 hours with selection by perfusion imaging. N Engl J Med 2018;378(8):708–18.

18. Martinez-Gutierrez JC, Leslie-Mazwi T, Chandra KL, et al. Number needed to treat: a primer for neurointerventionalists. Interv Neuroradiol 2019;25(6):613–8.

19. Saber H, Narayanan S, Palla M, et al. Mechanical thrombectomy for acute ischemic stroke with occlusion of the M2 segment of the middle cerebral artery: a meta-analysis. J Neurointerv Surg 2018;10(7):620–4.

20. Menon BK, Hill MD, Davalos A, et al. Efficacy of endovascular thrombectomy in patients with M2 segment middle cerebral artery occlusions: meta-analysis of data from the HERMES Collaboration. J Neurointerv Surg 2019;11(11):1065–9.

21. Saver JL, Chapot R, Agid R, et al. Thrombectomy for distal, medium vessel occlusions: a Consensus Statement on Present Knowledge and Promising Directions. Stroke 2020;51(9):2872–84.

22. Grossberg JA, Rebello LC, Haussen DC, et al. Beyond large vessel occlusion Strokes: distal occlusion thrombectomy. Stroke 2018;49(7):1662–8.

23. Rikhtegar R, Mosimann PJ, Weber R, et al. Effectiveness of very low profile thrombectomy device in primary distal medium vessel occlusion, as rescue therapy after incomplete proximal recanalization or following iatrogenic thromboembolic events. J Neurointerv Surg 2021.

24. Powers WJ, Rabinstein AA, Ackerson T, et al. Guidelines for the early management of patients with acute ischemic stroke: 2019 Update to the 2018 Guidelines for the early management of acute ischemic stroke: a Guideline for Healthcare Professionals from the American Heart Association/American stroke Association. Stroke 2019;50(12):e344–418.

25. Desilles JP, Consoli A, Redjem H, et al. Successful reperfusion with mechanical thrombectomy is associated with Reduced Disability and mortality in patients with Pretreatment Diffusion-Weighted imaging-Alberta stroke Program early Computed Tomography Score </=6. Stroke 2017;48(4):963–9.

26. Panni P, Gory B, Xie Y, et al. Acute stroke with large ischemic Core treated by thrombectomy. Stroke 2019;50(5):1164–71.

27. Hofmeijer J, Kappelle LJ, Algra A, et al. Surgical decompression for space-occupying cerebral infarction (the Hemicraniectomy after Middle Cerebral Artery infarction with Life-threatening Edema Trial [HAMLET]): a multicentre, open, randomised trial. Lancet Neurol 2009;8(4):326–33.

28. Juttler E, Schwab S, Schmiedek P, et al. Decompressive Surgery for the treatment of malignant infarction of the middle cerebral artery (DESTINY): a randomized, controlled trial. Stroke 2007;38(9):2518–25.

29. Vahedi K, Vicaut E, Mateo J, et al. Sequential-design, multicenter, randomized, controlled trial of early decompressive craniectomy in malignant middle cerebral artery infarction (DECIMAL Trial). Stroke 2007;38(9):2506–17.

30. Rumalla K, Ottenhausen M, Kan P, et al. Recent Nationwide impact of mechanical thrombectomy on decompressive Hemicraniectomy for acute ischemic stroke. Stroke 2019;50(8):2133–9.

31. Sarraj A, Hassan AE, Abraham M, et al. EXPRESS: a randomized controlled trial to Optimize Patientas selection for endovascular treatment in acute ischemic stroke (SELECT2): study Protocol. Int J Stroke 2021. 17474930211035032.

32. Bendszus M, Bonekamp S, Berge E, et al. A randomized controlled trial to test efficacy and safety of thrombectomy in stroke with extended lesion and extended time window. Int J Stroke 2019;14(1):87–93.

33. Peschillo S, Diana F, Berge J, et al. A comparison of acute vascular damage caused by ADAPT versus a stent retriever device after thrombectomy in acute ischemic stroke: a histological and ultrastructural study in an animal model. J Neurointerv Surg 2017;9(8):743–9.

34. Turk AS, Frei D, Fiorella D, et al. ADAPT FAST study: a direct aspiration first pass technique for acute stroke thrombectomy. J Neurointerv Surg 2014;6(4):260–4.

35. Turk AS, Spiotta A, Frei D, et al. Initial clinical experience with the ADAPT technique: a direct aspiration first pass technique for stroke thrombectomy. J Neurointerv Surg 2014;6(3):231–7.

36. Lapergue B, Blanc R, Gory B, et al. Effect of endovascular contact aspiration vs stent retriever on Revascularization in patients with acute ischemic stroke and large vessel occlusion: the ASTER randomized clinical trial. JAMA 2017;318(5):443–52.

37. Turk AS 3rd, Siddiqui A, Fifi JT, et al. Aspiration thrombectomy versus stent retriever thrombectomy as first-line approach for large vessel occlusion (COMPASS): a multicentre, randomised, open label, blinded outcome, non-inferiority trial. Lancet 2019;393(10175):998–1008.

38. Baek JH, Kim BM, Kang DH, et al. Balloon guide catheter is Beneficial in endo-vascular treatment Regardless of mechanical recanalization Modality. Stroke 2019;50(6):1490–6.
39. Nguyen TN, Castonguay AC, Noguiera RG, et al. Effect of balloon guide catheter on clinical outcomes and reperfusion in Trevo thrombectomy. J Neurointerv Surg 2019;11(9):861–5.
40. Bourcier R, Marnat G, Labreuche J, et al. Balloon guide catheter is not Superior to Conventional guide catheter when stent retriever and contact aspiration are com-bined for stroke treatment. Neurosurgery 2020;88(1):E83–90.
41. Perez-Garcia C, Maegerlein C, Rosati S, et al. Impact of aspiration catheter size on first-pass effect in the combined use of contact aspiration and stent retriever technique. Stroke Vasc Neurol 2021;6(4):553–60.
42. Nogueira RG, Mohammaden MH, Al-Bayati AR, et al. Preliminary experience with 088 large bore intracranial catheters during stroke thrombectomy. Interv Neuro-radiol 2021;27(3):427–33.
43. Fitzgerald S, Ryan D, Thornton J, et al. Preclinical evaluation of Millipede 088 intracranial aspiration catheter in cadaver and in vitro thrombectomy models. J Neurointerv Surg 2021;13(5):447–52.
44. Vargas J, Blalock J, Venkatraman A, et al. Efficacy of beveled tip aspiration cath-eter in mechanical thrombectomy for acute ischemic stroke. J Neurointerv Surg 2021;13(9):823–6.
45. Gruber P, Diepers M, von Hessling A, et al. Mechanical thrombectomy using the new Tigertriever in acute ischemic stroke patients - a Swiss prospective multi-center study. Interv Neuroradiol 2020;26(5):598–601.
46. Valgimigli M, Frigoli E, Leonardi S, et al. Radial versus femoral access and biva-lirudin versus unfractionated heparin in invasively managed patients with acute coronary syndrome (MATRIX): final 1-year results of a multicentre, randomised controlled trial. Lancet 2018;392(10150):835–48.
47. Li Y, Chen SH, Spiotta AM, et al. Lower complication rates associated with trans-radial versus transfemoral flow diverting stent placement. J Neurointerv Surg 2021;13(1):91–5.
48. Sur S, Snelling B, Khandelwal P, et al. Transradial approach for mechanical thrombectomy in anterior circulation large-vessel occlusion. Neurosurg Focus 2017;42(4):E13.
49. Munich SA, Vakharia K, McPheeters MJ, et al. Transition to transradial access for mechanical thrombectomy-Lessons Learned and comparison to transfemoral ac-cess in a Single-Center case series. Oper Neurosurg (Hagerstown) 2020;19(6): 701–7.
50. Siddiqui AH, Waqas M, Neumaier J, et al. Radial first or patient first: a case series and meta-analysis of transradial versus transfemoral access for acute ischemic stroke intervention. J Neurointerv Surg 2021;13(8):687–92.
51. Wei D, Oxley TJ, Nistal DA, et al. Mobile Interventional stroke Teams Lead to Faster treatment Times for thrombectomy in large vessel occlusion. Stroke 2017;48(12):3295–300.
52. Morey JR, Oxley TJ, Wei D, et al. Mobile Interventional stroke Team model Im-proves early outcomes in large vessel occlusion stroke: the NYC MIST trial. Stroke 2020;51(12):3495–503.

Decompressive Craniectomy for Stroke: Who, When, and How

Gregory J. Cannarsa, MD[a],*, J. Marc Simard, MD, PhD[a,b,c]

KEYWORDS

- Decompressive craniectomy • Large hemispheric infarct • Malignant cerebral edema
- Ischemic stroke • Glibenclamide

KEY POINTS

- In patients up to 60 years of age, decompressive craniectomy for large hemispheric infarction (LHI) reduces mortality and improves the rate of good functional outcome when performed up to 48 hours after the onset of stroke.
- In patients more than 60 years of age, decompressive craniectomy for LHI reduces mortality but the likelihood of poor functional outcome is higher than in younger patients.
- The data on decompressive craniectomy more than 48 hours after stroke onset are limited but suggest that it does not carry the same benefit as earlier intervention.
- Early imaging studies, including MRI and CT perfusion, can help determine which patients with LHI are likely to benefit from early decompressive craniectomy.
- Decompressive craniectomy, although a commonly used procedure, has many associated risks and complications, and necessitates a second surgical intervention – cranioplasty.

INTRODUCTION

Large vessel occlusion ischemic stroke, or large hemispheric infarction (LHI), accounts for 24% to 38% of all acute ischemic stroke.[1] LHI of the anterior circulation has an incidence of 20 per 100,000 persons per year.[2] LHI comprises a minority of all strokes, but is responsible for up to 96% of poststroke mortality; unfortunately,

Funding: This article was not funded. JMS is supported by grants from the Department of Veterans Affairs (I01BX002889), the Department of Defense (SCI170199), the National Heart, Lung and Blood Institute (R01HL082517), and the NINDS (R01NS060801; R01NS102589; R01NS105633).[50]

[a] Department of Neurosurgery, University of Maryland Medical Center, 22 S Greene Street, S12D, Baltimore, MD 21201, USA; [b] Department of Pathology, University of Maryland Medical Center, 22 S Greene Street, S12D, Baltimore, MD 21201, USA; [c] Department of Physiology, University of Maryland Medical Center, 22 S Greene Street, S12D, Baltimore, MD 21201, USA
* Corresponding author.
E-mail address: gcannarsa@som.umaryland.edu

Neurol Clin 40 (2022) 321–336
https://doi.org/10.1016/j.ncl.2021.11.009
0733-8619/22/© 2021 Elsevier Inc. All rights reserved.
neurologic.theclinics.com

only a minority of patients with large vessel occlusion are eligible for first-line recanalization treatments, including recombinant tissue plasminogen activator (rtPA) and endovascular thrombectomy.[1] A major contributor to the morbidity and mortality following LHI is malignant cerebral edema (MCE). MCE is highly morbid, and is associated with up to 75% to 95% mortality with medical management alone.[3] With an aging population around the world, LHI will continue to increase in prevalence, further burdening the health care systems of the world.

Here, we summarize the major trials of decompressive craniectomy for MCE, including the surgical indications and contraindications, the operative procedure of decompressive craniectomy, as well as possible complications. Additionally, the latest research on the utility of imaging modalities, alternative surgical techniques, and potential medical treatments for MCE are reviewed.

The nature of the Problem

Until the early 2000s, there was little consensus regarding the best treatment of LHI. Studies of small single-center cohorts had suggested that surgical intervention in the form of decompressive craniectomy for MCE might be beneficial.[4,5] Three randomized controlled trials, DECIMAL, DESTINY, and HAMLET, conducted in Germany, France, and the Netherlands, respectively, were undertaken in the 2000s to evaluate the efficacy of decompressive craniectomy compared with intensive medical management for MCE.[6–8] Subsequent pooled analyses of those trials as well as several other randomized trials have shown convincingly that early (<48 hours) surgical intervention in the form of large decompressive craniectomy with duraplasty significantly improves both overall survival (number needed to treat [NNT] = 2) and survival with a good functional outcome (modified Rankin Scale (mRS) $\leq$ 3, NNT = 4).[9] As this initial analysis was published in 2007, further trials have confirmed these initial findings.[10] Additionally, imaging and clinical scoring systems have been developed that help to identify patients that may benefit from decompressive craniectomy before they deteriorate clinically. Also, standardized medical management protocols have been developed for LHI. Other evidence, though of lower grade, has given insight into which patients may achieve the best outcomes from decompressive craniectomy, and when surgical intervention may be futile.

Evidence Favoring Decompressive Craniectomy for Malignant Cerebral Edema

Decompressive craniectomy for MCE has been investigated in several randomized controlled trials, and their results are summarized in **Table 1**. A recent meta-analysis that examined 6 of the 7 trials listed in **Table 1** and also included data from the unpublished DEMITUR trial affirmed that decompressive craniectomy for MCE within 48 hours is associated with a significant increase in good functional outcome.[10] A systematic review that examined outcomes for several years following decompressive craniectomy found lasting benefit, and found that most of the patients would again choose to undergo surgery, even with the benefit of hindsight.[11]

Decompressive craniectomy for MCE is effective, but the question of which patients benefit most is still unclear. Additionally, although the literature reports that "early" (defined as <48 hours after stroke onset) decompressive craniectomy is associated with improvements in outcome, there still is uncertainty at individual institutions regarding the best timing to perform surgery. In the following, we address the main considerations for deciding whether a patient is eligible for and would benefit from decompressive craniectomy.

Table 1
Summary data of the major randomized, controlled trials of decompressive craniectomy compared with medical management

	Decimal[6]	Destiny[7]	Slezins et al[13]	Zhao et al[50]	Hamlet[8]	Destiny II[12]	HeADDFIRST[17]
Year Published	2007	2007	2012	2012	2014	2014	2014
Patients (n)	38	32	28	47	64	112	24
Age Range (years)	18–55	18–60	49–81	29–80	18–60	61–82	18–75
Timing to Surgery (hours)	≤30	12–36	<48	<48	≤96	<48	≤96
Surgical vs Medical mRS 0–3 at last follow-up (% of patients)	15 vs 0	47 vs 27	45 vs 0	25 vs 0	25 vs 25	6 vs 5	29 vs 30
Surgical vs Medical mortality at last follow-up (% of patients)	25 vs 78	18 vs 53	55 vs 92	16.7 vs 69.6	22 vs 59	43 vs 76	36 vs 40

Age in Decision-Making for Decompressive Craniectomy

One of the first major criticisms of the early pooled analysis of the major trials was that patients over 60 years were excluded. To address the age question, DESTINY II, a randomized, controlled trial of decompressive craniectomy in patients greater than 60 years, was initiated. DESTINY II found that decompressive craniectomy was effective in lowering mortality in patients greater than 60 years, with a median age of 70 years.[12] However, as only 6% of patients in the surgical group achieved an mRS score of 3, with no patients achieving an mRS of 0 to 2, the question remains as to whether decompressive craniectomy offers meaningful benefit in patients older than 60 years. In line with the DESTINY II findings, a retrospective review of decompressive craniectomy in 131 patients found a significant mortality benefit regardless of whether patients were age 70 years or greater, but did not find a significant association of surgical intervention with good functional outcome.[3]

In contrast to the published DESTINY II trial, the unpublished DEMITUR trial (data reported in a recent meta-analysis for which the authors were able to obtain the unpublished data) had highly favorable outcomes for decompressive craniectomy in patients more than 60 years, with up to 66% of patients obtaining a favorable outcome.[10] The meta-analysis that included these data showed that age greater than 60 years did not significantly change the benefit of decompressive craniectomy. Importantly, the authors noted that the use of unpublished data should be viewed with caution. Another trial of 28 patients published in 2012 found a mortality benefit for decompressive craniectomy in all patients, but found that there were no survivors more than 60 years old in the surgical group.[13] In line with these findings, DECAP, a prospective, single-center observational study of 40 patients who fit the DESTINY II criteria found a trend toward higher rates of death and severe disability compared with patients with DESTINY II (77.5% vs 59%, $P = .077$).[14] The authors expressed surprise with their findings, as their cohort was significantly younger than the comparable DESTINY II cohort (64 vs 70 years, $P < .001$). They advised that patients' families should be counseled regarding the high likelihood of death or severe disability following decompressive craniectomy. As to the question of quality of life after decompressive craniectomy, especially in older patients, a systematic review of patients found that quality of life in those more than 60 years tended to be lower.[11] Given the above findings, it is recommended that for patients older than 60 years, a discussion regarding the low likelihood of a good functional outcome following decompressive craniectomy should be had with the patient, if possible, and with the patient's family, to explicitly clarify goals of care.

THE ROLE OF THE HISTORY AND PHYSICAL EXAM

Patients who present with LHI generally have comorbidities and a past medical history that can affect both their eligibility for decompressive craniectomy as well as their overall prognosis. It should be noted that the major trials of decompressive craniectomy all had strict inclusion and exclusion criteria, especially with regards to medical history. The major trials for decompressive craniectomy excluded all patients with an mRS ≥2, any patient with contraindications to anesthesia, life expectancy less than 3 years, other serious illness that could affect outcome, and noncorrectable coagulopathy.[10] In practice, decompressive craniectomy can be potentially be performed despite most of these conditions, although the risks of surgery may be higher.

The National Institutes of Health Stroke Scale (NIHSS) has been an important inclusion criterion in past trials, and retrospective data indicate that it can predict which patients will likely develop MCE. All randomized trials to date have enrolled patients with an NIHSS greater than 15 with dominant hemisphere LHI, and NIHSS greater than 14 with nondominant hemisphere LHI. Affirming these criteria, an NIHSS greater than 13.5 was found to be highly sensitive and specific for MCE in a series of 95 patients.[15] A systematic review and meta-analysis examining predictors of MCE after LHI found younger age and higher NIHSS to be significantly associated with MCE.[16] With an MRI demonstrating a large volume infarction, a clinical examination with NIHSS greater than 22 at 24 hours predicts a high likelihood of developing MCE.

TIMING OF INTERVENTION

As with the age criterion, the data on the timing of intervention for decompressive craniectomy are heterogeneous and are strongly anchored to the initial 48-h threshold used as the inclusion criterion in most of the major trials with the exceptions of HAMLET and HeADDFIRST.[8,17] To reiterate, meta-analyses of the major randomized, controlled trials reported to date support the efficacy of decompressive craniectomy within 48 hours.[10,18] However, due to the small number of patients reported who have undergone decompressive craniectomy beyond 48 hours, the data on later surgery are unclear. A recent meta-analysis focusing on the timing of decompressive craniectomy concluded that the outcome of patients who underwent decompressive craniectomy after 48 hours was not worse compared with those operated before 48 hours.[19] The authors noted that most studies, both prospective and retrospective, have been limited due to small sample sizes. An earlier, larger analysis of 1301 decompressive craniectomy patients from the Nationwide Inpatient Sample Database found an association between later surgery (>72 hours) and increased mortality, and likelihood of discharge to institutional facility, suggesting decompressive craniectomy after 72 hours may be less beneficial.[20]

HeADDFIRST, a randomized trial conducted in 2014 with a randomization period of up to 96 hours, approached the enrollment of patients differently than previous trials; they registered patients who fit inclusion criteria similar to prior major trials but only randomized patients who fit further criteria including radiographic evidence of edema and shift as well as neurologic decline.[17] Importantly, no patient in the registered, but nonrandomized group died, suggesting that adding imaging and clinical deterioration criteria to inclusion criteria might avoid the performance of decompressive craniectomy in those patients who otherwise may not develop MCE (**Fig. 1**). Additionally, even though the average time to randomization in HeADDFIRST was significantly longer than previous major trials, overall mortality was not affected, suggesting later surgical intervention may be noninferior.

IMAGING

Initial imaging of large vessel occlusion ischemic stroke patients consists initially of a head CT without contrast as well as a CT angiogram of the brain. With the advent of rapid CT perfusion intended to help select patients presenting in a delayed fashion for endovascular treatment, more imaging data are available to predict which patients may develop MCE necessitating decompressive craniectomy. Previous trials have used a CT infarct threshold of at least 50% of MCA territory.[10] This volume determination has been confirmed in a meta-analysis of imaging factors associated with the development of MCE, with an expected dramatic increase in the likelihood of MCE with larger volumes of MCA territory infarction.[16]

Noncontrast head CT also informs whether other major vascular territories are affected, including the anterior cerebral artery (ACA) and posterior cerebral artery (PCA) territories. A recent retrospective review of 137 decompressive craniectomy patients found the involvement of other vascular territories to be significant in predicting poor functional outcome, and that simple volume alone was not predictive of outcome.[21] Patients with complete MCA infarctions with a total volume similar to patients with subtotal MCA infarctions plus infarction of either the ACA or PCA territory had significantly better outcomes, suggesting that the distribution of the infarct is more important than the total volume.

Advances in CT angiography and perfusion studies are allowing for improved prediction in those patients who are likely to require decompressive craniectomy. A recent study focusing on the CTA ASPECTS showed that a score ≤5 was a relatively specific threshold to predict the development of MCE (sensitivity 46%; specificity

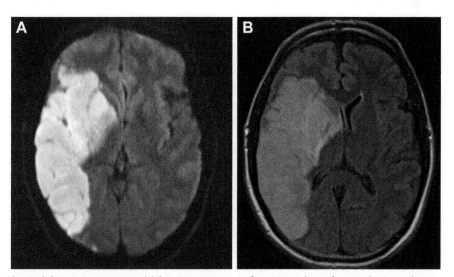

Fig. 1. (*A*) DWI Sequence and (*B*) FLAIR sequence of an MRI 5 days after stroke ictus demonstrating a large, hemispheric infarct without any significant swelling or midline shift.

97%; positive predictive value 78%; negative predictive value 65%).[22] Along with CT angiography, CT perfusion is improving the ability to identify patients at risk for MCE; multiple parameters, including time-to-peak and cerebral blood flow, show robust ability to aid in edema prediction.[15,23] Affirming the value of CT perfusion, a series analyzing CT perfusion than noncontrast head CT found higher predictive ability with perfusion CT.[24]

Multiple randomized trials have used DWI infarct volume on early MRI for patient selection. The DWI threshold in the major trials has been greater than 145 cc.[10] Multiple retrospective studies have analyzed radiologic predictors of MCE on MRI and found that DWI infarct volume greater than 82 cc before 6 hours after stroke ictus to have high specificity (98%) for development of MCE.[25] Additional studies have confirmed DWI as well as perfusion-weighted imaging to be predictive of MCE.[26] To help control for cerebral atrophy, one study found that measuring and accounting for the hemi-intercaudate distance, a proxy of cerebral atrophy, significantly improves the predictive value of MRI DWI size.[27]

THERAPEUTIC OPTIONS

Medical management for MCE has evolved during the era of trials of decompressive craniectomy, with general guidelines summarized in prior literature.[28] The early trials had recommended medical management guidelines to all participating centers but did not require strict adherence. In contrast, HeADDFIRST, which was the first major trial with a standardized medical management protocol (SMMP) and a formal adherence agreement among all investigators, had a mortality rate at 180 days of only 40% in the medical group, which compared favorably with their surgical mortality of 36%.[17] The authors posit that their SMMP may have played a role in the relatively low mortality in their medical cohort.

DECOMPRESSIVE CRANIECTOMY: SURGICAL TECHNIQUE

After medical management for MCE has been exhausted, and with adherence to previously discussed surgical criteria, both inclusion and exclusion criteria, the indications, risks, and goals of decompressive craniectomy should be honestly discussed with the patient and family before obtaining surgical consent. In the operating room, the patient is intubated, undergoes large-bore IV access, which may include a central line, and has placement of an arterial line for continuous blood pressure monitoring. The patient's head is secured using a Mayfield (Integra Life Sciences) skull clamp. The patient is positioned with a gel bump under the shoulder and the head is positioned so that the lateral aspect is uppermost. The hair is usually shaved to expedite cleansing and surgical preparation of the site, although there is no evidence that shaving is necessary to reduce infection.[29]

The midline of the head is marked, and a large "question mark" shaped incision is marked from the rostral hairline near the middle forehead to the zygoma (**Fig. 2**). After sterile draping, the skin is infiltrated with local anesthetic. The incision is developed with the application of Raney hemostatic clips to the scalp edges. The temporalis muscle is incised using a Bovie electrocautery. The scalp together with the underlying temporalis muscle is dissected from the skull using periosteal elevators, widely exposing the skull. Multiple burr holes are placed along the margins of the planned craniectomy. The size of the craniectomy is planned to be at least 15 cm from anterior to posterior and 12 cm from inferior to superior, as there are retrospective data and physiologic data supporting improved outcomes from a larger craniectomy.[30] Following the completion of the burr holes, the dura with periosteum is dissected

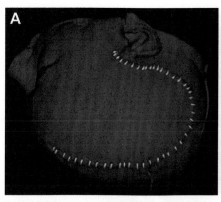
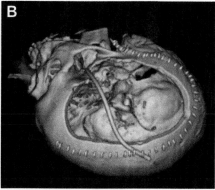

Fig. 2. (*A*) 3D reconstruction of a head CT performed postoperatively after decompressive craniectomy. The white staples demonstrate the shape of the incision, an inverted, reverse question mark. (*B*) 3D reconstruction of the same patient's head CT demonstrating the craniectomy defect underneath incision. The white tubing in the center of the defect is the subgaleal drain.

from the bone. A craniotomy saw is used to cut the intervening bone between the burr holes. The sphenoid wing is not cut using craniotomy due to its width and depth. The bone flap is typically elevated at this stage with careful fracture of the tip of the sphenoid wing, at which point the bone flap can be removed, revealing the underlying dura (**Fig. 3**). The wound is irrigated to remove blood and bone dust.

An expansile duraplasty is performed. The dura can be opened in several different patterns: a "C-shaped incision," a stellate opening, or with parallel linear dural incisions, as shown in **Fig. 4**. Duraplasty is then performed using either a graft that can be sutured to the existing dura, as shown in **Fig. 5**, or using dural substitutes that function as "on-lay" grafts not requiring sutures. Following the completion of the duraplasty, a layer of SEPRAFILM (Baxter) may be placed on the dura to reduce the development of adhesions between the dura and scalp, to facilitate later cranioplasty. A subgaleal drain is placed inside the wound and the scalp is closed in 2 layers with absorbable sutures for the galea and either staples or sutures for the skin. A postoperative head CT is obtained and demonstrates the extent of decompression (**Fig. 6**).

The bone flap can be stored in a bone bank freezer or it can be placed subcutaneously in the abdomen of the patient, to be replaced later at the time of cranioplasty. There is no significant difference in complications between the 2 methods of storage of the bone flap.[31,32]

SURGICAL ALTERNATIVES TO DECOMPRESSIVE CRANIECTOMY

There are surgical alternatives to decompressive craniectomy, although, to date, no alternative has been subjected to a randomized controlled trial. In addition to decompressive craniectomy, "strokectomy," or the removal of infarcted brain to further decompress the viable brain, has been performed in small, retrospective series without significant complications.[33,34] A larger retrospective series of 101 decompressive craniectomy patients found that 20 patients went on to require resection of infarcted brain due to persistent increased midline shift and/or unilateral nonreactive pupil, suggesting strokectomy may be necessary for a subset of LHI patients.[35] Another retrospective series of 59 patients who underwent decompressive craniectomy alone found that continued effacement of the basal cisterns, as well as continued

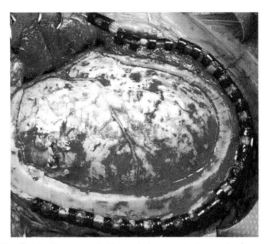

Fig. 3. The operative field after completion of the craniectomy, before opening the dura.

compression of the lateral ventricles on postoperative imaging, was significantly associated with a poor functional outcome, suggesting that decompressive craniectomy alone may sometimes be inadequate and that strokectomy may improve outcome by lowering ICP and mass effect.[36]

Strokectomy alone without decompressive craniectomy has been trialed in small series. A series of 15 patients who underwent a small craniotomy with temporal lobectomy and aggressive CSF drainage showed outcomes comparable to series with decompressive craniectomy.[37] Another small case series of 4 strokectomy patients versus 20 decompressive craniectomy patients showed a trend toward better outcomes with strokectomy, suggesting noninferiority.[38] Lastly, a retrospective review of 68 patients compared strokectomy to decompressive craniectomy alone and to decompressive craniectomy with strokectomy, and found no significant difference

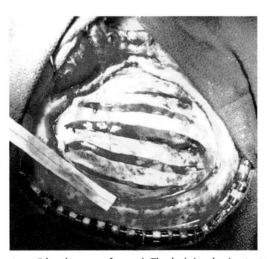

Fig. 4. A "strip durotomy" has been performed. The bulging brain stretches and separates the strips of dura, allowing the brain to herniate without being strangulated at the bony edges (the cotton strip is ½ inch wide).

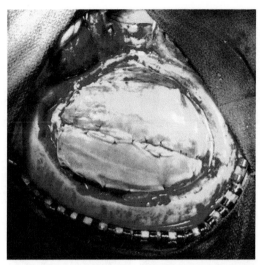

Fig. 5. A dural substitute has been sutured in, completing the duraplasty.

in outcomes, suggesting strokectomy may be noninferior to decompressive craniectomy.[39] At this time, further prospective data are needed to determine if strokectomy is a safe, viable alternative to decompressive craniectomy.

COMPLICATIONS OF DECOMPRESSIVE CRANIECTOMY

Decompressive craniectomy along with ensuing cranioplasty is associated with numerous complications. These complications have been summarized previously in a comprehensive systematic review and can be broadly categorized into hemorrhagic, infectious, and CSF disturbance-related complications.[40]

Hemorrhage after craniectomy or cranioplasty has been reported in up to 20.7% of patients and can occur in the parenchyma in the form of hemorrhagic transformation, the subdural space, as well as the epidural space. Several retrospective series of decompressive craniectomy found that hemorrhagic transformation rates ranged from 29% to 59% but without apparent significant impact on outcome (**Fig. 7**).[41]

Infectious complications after craniectomy, as with hemorrhagic complications, can occur in multiple compartments leading to meningitis/ventriculitis, cerebral abscess, subdural empyema, as well as epidural abscesses and superficial skin infections due to the long length of the incision and devascularization of the scalp flap. Infectious complications specifically after decompressive craniectomy for stroke have been reported to be the highest among all indications for craniectomy at 13.7%.[40]

CSF disturbances after decompressive craniectomy are often delayed and include hydrocephalus, hygroma formation, and the syndrome of the trephined. Of all the indications for craniectomy, those patients who underwent craniectomy for MCE had the highest reported rate of hydrocephalus postoperatively, at 25.5%, and a subset of patients will require permanent CSF diversion, most commonly in the form of a ventriculoperitoneal shunt (**Fig. 8**).[40] Additionally, subdural hygroma has been found in up to 12.5% of patient postoperatively. Once the initial edema is resolved, over the longer term, patients are at risk for the syndrome of the trephined, also known as "sinking flap" syndrome or paradoxic herniation, when the brain shifts to the side contralateral to the craniectomy (**Fig. 9**A).[42] Importantly, the only lasting treatment of these disturbances is the replacement of the bone flap (cranioplasty) (see **Fig. 9**B).

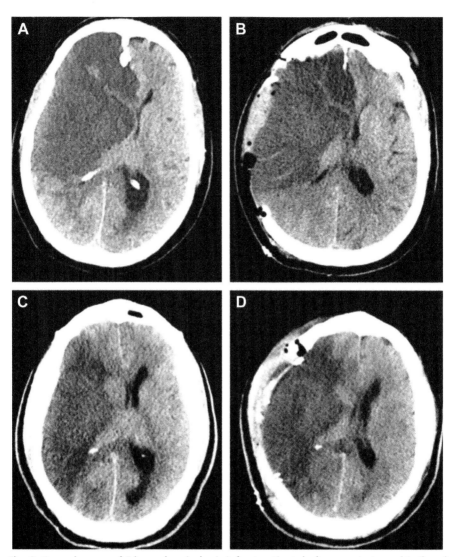

Fig. 6. Example cases of 2 large, hemispheric infarct patients before craniectomy (*A, C*) and after craniectomy (*B, D*). Midline shift in both cases has improved, though some shift still persists.

Another serious complication of craniectomy and cranioplasty is seizures leading to potential epilepsy. A retrospective review of 36 patients found that 19 of 24 patients who survived the acute period went on to have multiple seizures with the development of epilepsy.[43]

While not the focus of this review, it should be noted that the decision to perform decompressive craniectomy implies that the patient will require another surgery, cranioplasty, at a later date. The above-mentioned systematic review also details the numerous complications of cranioplasty, which are not insignificant. Ultimately, these complications and their respective rates are important for an educated and informed discussion with any patient and their family who may require a decompressive craniectomy.

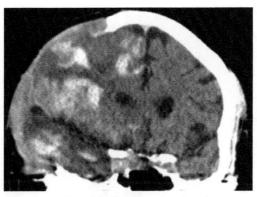

Fig. 7. Hemorrhagic transformation of ischemic stroke after decompressive craniectomy.

FUTURE DIRECTIONS

While surgical decompression in the form of decompressive craniectomy or other surgical intervention has been shown to be effective, the search for medical treatment options for MCE is ongoing. The only pharmaceutical to enter randomized clinical trials for the treatment of MCE is intravenous glibenclamide (glyburide), a sulfonylurea initially approved for use in diabetes, but with basic and clinical data supporting an inhibitory effect on the formation of cerebral edema through inhibition of the SUR1-TRPM4 ion transporter.[44,45] Glibenclamide for the treatment of MCE is currently in a phase III trial, the CHARM trial, to assess for efficacy in improving good functional outcomes in patients at risk for MCE after LHI.[46] The phase II trial evaluating glibenclamide for MCE after LHI, GAMES-RP, was not significant for its primary outcome, but did show a significant reduction in midline shift, with subsequent post hoc analysis showing that

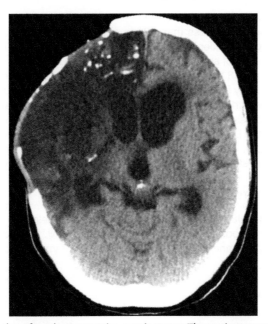

Fig. 8. Hydrocephalus after decompressive craniectomy. The patient required a ventriculo-peritoneal shunt after the cranioplasty due to persistent hydrocephalus.

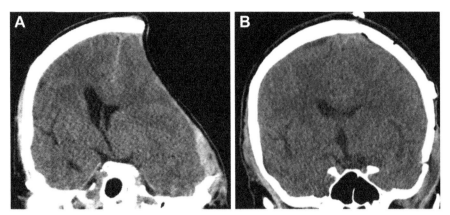

Fig. 9. (*A*) Paradoxic herniation after decompressive craniectomy with (*B*) near-immediate resolution of herniation postoperatively after cranioplasty.

glibenclamide was significantly associated with lower net lesional water uptake compared with placebo.[47,48] Importantly, while there was no difference in the rate of decompressive craniectomy between the glibenclamide and placebo groups, the glibenclamide group had significantly lower rates of neurologic decline (increases in NIHSS) compared with placebo. Other compounds including aquaporin inhibitors have shown promise in basic, preclinical models, but have not yet been trialed in humans.[49]

SUMMARY

Decompressive craniectomy for LHI reduces mortality and improves good functional outcomes when performed less than 48 hours after onset of stroke in patients less than 60 years of age. In patients over 60 years with LHI, the data support a decrease in mortality but the rate of severe disability is higher than in younger patients. Decompressive craniectomy 48 hours after stroke onset does not carry the same benefit as early intervention. Early imaging studies including MRI and CT perfusion can be used to help determine which patients with large vessel occlusion stroke are likely to benefit from early decompressive craniectomy. Decompressive craniectomy is a commonly performed procedure but has many associated risks and complications, as does subsequent cranioplasty. The development of medical therapeutic options for MCE is ongoing, with the most promising candidate, glibenclamide, currently in phase III trials.

DECLARATION OF INTEREST

J.M. Simard holds a US patent (7,285,574), "A novel non-selective cation channel in neural cells and methods for treating brain swelling." J.M. Simard is a member of the Board of Directors and holds shares in Remedy Pharmaceuticals and is a paid consultant for Biogen.

CLINICS CARE POINTS

- Multiple randomized, controlled trials support the efficacy of early decompressive craniectomy in the treatment of malignant cerebral edema after ischemic stroke.

- Early imaging studies including MRI and CT perfusion, when combined with clinical exam findings, can help to identify those patients most likely to require decompressive craniectomy.
- The only pharmaceutical treatment of malignant cerebral edema that has been examined in randomized clinical trials is glibenclamide, with basic and clinical evidence suggesting it may be effective in reducing the severity of MCE.

DISCLOSURE

Dr G. Cannarsa: No disclosures. Dr J.M. Simard: holds a US patent (7,285,574), "A novel non-selective cation channel in neural cells and methods for treating brain swelling." J.M. Simard is a member of the Board of Directors and holds shares in Remedy Pharmaceuticals and is a paid consultant for Biogen.

REFERENCES

1. Malhotra K, Gornbein J, Saver JL. Ischemic strokes due to large-vessel occlusions contribute disproportionately to stroke-related dependence and death: a review. Front Neurol 2017;8(NOV). https://doi.org/10.3389/FNEUR.2017.00651.
2. Rai AT, Seldon AE, Boo S, et al. A population-based incidence of acute large vessel occlusions and thrombectomy eligible patients indicates significant potential for growth of endovascular stroke therapy in the USA. J Neurointerv Surg 2017;9(8):722–6.
3. Yu JW, Choi J-H, Kim D-H, et al. Outcome following decompressive craniectomy for malignant middle cerebral artery infarction in patients older than 70 years old. J Cerebrovasc Endovasc Neurosurg 2012;14(2):65.
4. Koh MS, Goh KYC, Tung MYY, et al. Is decompressive craniectomy for acute cerebral infarction of any benefit? Surg Neurol 2000;53(3):225–30.
5. Kilincer C, Asil T, Utku U, et al. Factors affecting the outcome of decompressive craniectomy for large hemispheric infarctions: a prospective cohort study. Acta Neurochir (Wien) 2005;147(3):587–94.
6. Vahedi K, Vicaut E, Mateo J, et al. Sequential-design, multicenter, randomized, controlled trial of early decompressive craniectomy in malignant middle cerebral artery infarction (DECIMAL Trial). Stroke 2007;38(9):2506–17.
7. Jüttler E, Schwab S, Schmiedek P, et al. Decompressive surgery for the treatment of malignant infarction of the middle cerebral artery (DESTINY): a randomized, controlled trial. Stroke 2007;38(9):2518–25.
8. Hofmeijer J, Kappelle LJ, Algra A, et al. Surgical decompression for space-occupying cerebral infarction (the Hemicraniectomy After Middle Cerebral Artery infarction with Life-threatening Edema Trial [HAMLET]): a multicentre, open, randomised trial. Lancet Neurol 2009;8(4):326–33.
9. Vahedi K, Hofmeijer J, Juettler E, et al. Early decompressive surgery in malignant infarction of the middle cerebral artery: a pooled analysis of three randomised controlled trials. Lancet Neurol 2007;6(3):215–22.
10. Reinink H, Jüttler E, Hacke W, et al. Surgical decompression for space-occupying hemispheric infarction: a systematic review and individual patient meta-analysis of randomized clinical trials. JAMA Neurol 2021;78(2):208–16.
11. van Middelaar T, Nederkoorn PJ, van der Worp HB, et al. Quality of life after surgical decompression for space-occupying middle cerebral artery infarction: systematic review. Int J Stroke 2015;10(2):170–6.

12. Jüttler E, Unterberg A, Woitzik J, et al. Hemicraniectomy in older patients with extensive middle-cerebral-artery stroke. N Engl J Med 2014;370(12):1091–100.
13. Slezins J, Keris V, Bricis R, et al. Preliminary results of randomized controlled study on decompressive craniectomy in treatment of malignant middle cerebral artery stroke. Med 2012;48(10):521–4.
14. Rahmig J, Wöpking S, Jüttler E, et al. Decompressive hemicraniectomy in elderly patients with space-occupying infarction (decap): a prospective observational study. Neurocrit Care 2019;31(1):97–106.
15. Lee CL, Kandasamy R, Mohammad Raffiq MAB. Computed tomography perfusion in detecting malignant middle cerebral artery infarct. Surg Neurol Int 2019; 10:159.
16. Wu S, Yuan R, Wang Y, et al. Early prediction of malignant brain edema after ischemic stroke: a systematic review and meta-analysis. Stroke 2018;49(12): 2918–27.
17. Frank JI, Schumm LP, Wroblewski K, et al. Hemicraniectomy and durotomy upon deterioration from infarction-related swelling trial: randomized pilot clinical trial. Stroke 2014;45(3):781–7.
18. Lu XC, Huang BS, Zheng JY, et al. Decompressive craniectomy for the treatment of malignant infarction of the middle cerebral artery. Sci Rep 2014;4:7070.
19. Goedemans T, Verbaan D, Coert BA, et al. Outcome after decompressive craniectomy for middle cerebral artery infarction: timing of the intervention. Clin Neurosurg 2020;86(3):E318–25.
20. Dasenbrock HH, Robertson FC, Vaitkevicius H, et al. Timing of decompressive hemicraniectomy for stroke: a nationwide inpatient sample analysis. Stroke 2017;48(3):704–11.
21. Kamran S, Akhtar N, Salam A, et al. CT pattern of Infarct location and not infarct volume determines outcome after decompressive hemicraniectomy for malignant middle cerebral artery stroke. Sci Rep 2019;9(1). https://doi.org/10.1038/s41598-019-53556-w.
22. Davoli A, Motta C, Koch G, et al. Pretreatment predictors of malignant evolution in patients with ischemic stroke undergoing mechanical thrombectomy. J Neurointerv Surg 2018;10(4):340–4.
23. Dittrich R, Kloska SP, Fischer T, et al. Accuracy of perfusion-CT inpredicting malignant middle cerebral artery brain infarction. J Neurol 2008;255(6):896–902.
24. Lee SJ, Lee KH, Na DG, et al. Multiphasic helical computed tomography predicts subsequent development of severe brain edema in acute ischemic stroke. Arch Neurol 2004;61(4):505–9.
25. Thomalla G, Hartmann F, Juettler E, et al. Prediction of malignant middle cerebral artery infarction by magnetic resonance imaging within 6 hours of symptom onset: a prospective multicenter observational study. Ann Neurol 2010;68(4): 435–45.
26. Tracol C, Vannier S, Hurel C, et al. Predictors of malignant middle cerebral artery infarction after mechanical thrombectomy. Rev Neurol (Paris) 2020;176(7–8): 619–25.
27. Beck C, Kruetzelmann A, Forkert ND, et al. A simple brain atrophy measure improves the prediction of malignant middle cerebral artery infarction by acute DWI lesion volume. J Neurol 2014;261(6):1097–103.
28. Bevers MB, Kimberly WT. Critical care management of acute ischemic stroke. Curr Treat Options Cardiovasc Med 2017;19(6). https://doi.org/10.1007/s11936-017-0542-6.

29. Broekman MLD, Van Beijnum J, Peul WC, et al. Neurosurgery and shaving: What's the evidence? A review. J Neurosurg 2011;115(4):670–8.

30. Flechsenhar J, Woitzik J, Zweckberger K, et al. Hemicraniectomy in the management of space-occupying ischemic stroke. J Clin Neurosci 2013;20(1):6–12.

31. Rosinski CL, Chaker AN, Zakrzewski J, et al. Autologous bone cranioplasty: a retrospective comparative analysis of frozen and subcutaneous bone flap storage methods. World Neurosurg 2019;131:e312–20.

32. Mirabet V, García D, Yagüe N, et al. The storage of skull bone flaps for autologous cranioplasty: literature review. Cell Tissue Bank; 2021. https://doi.org/10.1007/s10561-020-09897-2.

33. Lee SC, Wang YC, Huang YC, et al. Decompressive surgery for malignant middle cerebral artery syndrome. J Clin Neurosci 2013;20(1):49–52.

34. Schwake M, Schipmann S, Möther M, et al. Second-look strokectomy of cerebral infarction areas in patients with severe herniation. J Neurosurg 2020;132(1):1–9.

35. Kürten S, Munoz C, Beseoglu K, et al. Decompressive hemicraniectomy for malignant middle cerebral artery infarction including patients with additional involvement of the anterior and/or posterior cerebral artery territory—outcome analysis and definition of prognostic factors. Acta Neurochir (Wien) 2018;160(1):83–9.

36. Fatima N, Razzaq S, El Beltagi A, et al. Decompressive craniectomy: a preliminary study of comparative radiographic characteristics predicting outcome in malignant ischemic stroke. World Neurosurg 2020;133:e267–74.

37. Tartara F, Colombo EV, Bongetta D, et al. Strokectomy and extensive cisternal csf drain for acute management of malignant middle cerebral artery infarction: technical note and case series. Front Neurol 2019;10(SEP):1017.

38. Moughal S, Trippier S, AL-Mousa A, et al. Strokectomy for malignant middle cerebral artery infarction: experience and meta-analysis of current evidence. J Neurol 2020. https://doi.org/10.1007/s00415-020-10358-9.

39. Kostov DB, Singleton RH, Panczykowski D, et al. Decompressive hemicraniectomy, strokectomy, or both in the treatment of malignant middle cerebral artery syndrome. World Neurosurg 2012;78(5):480–6.

40. Kurland DB, Khaladj-Ghom A, Stokum JA, et al. Complications associated with decompressive craniectomy: a systematic review. Neurocrit Care 2015;23(2):292–304.

41. Al-Jehani H, Petrecca K, Martel P, et al. Decompressive craniectomy for ischemic stroke: effect of hemorrhagic transformation on outcome. J Stroke Cerebrovasc Dis 2016;25(9):2177–83.

42. Akins PT, Guppy KH. Sinking skin flaps, paradoxical herniation, and external brain tamponade: a review of decompressive craniectomy management. Neurocrit Care 2008;9(2):269–76.

43. Brondani R, Garcia De Almeida A, Abrahim Cherubini P, et al. High risk of seizures and epilepsy after decompressive hemicraniectomy for malignant middle cerebral artery stroke. Cerebrovasc Dis Extra 2017;7(1):51–61.

44. Sheth KN, Taylor Kimberly W, Elm JJ, et al. Exploratory analysis of glyburide as a novel therapy for preventing brain swelling. Neurocrit Care 2014;21(1):43–51.

45. Pergakis M, Badjatia N, Chaturvedi S, et al. BIIB093 (IV glibenclamide): an investigational compound for the prevention and treatment of severe cerebral edema. Expert Opin Investig Drugs 2019;28(12):1031–40.

46. Phase 3 study to evaluate the efficacy and safety of intravenous BIIB093 (Glibenclamide) for severe cerebral edema following large hemispheric infarction - Full Text View - ClinicalTrials.gov. Available at: https://clinicaltrials.gov/ct2/show/NCT02864953. June 21, 2021.

47. Kimberly WT, Bevers MB, Von Kummer R, et al. Effect of IV glyburide on adjudicated edema endpoints in the GAMES-RP Trial. Neurology 2018;91(23):E2163–9.
48. Sheth KN, Elm JJ, Molyneaux BJ, et al. Safety and efficacy of intravenous glyburide on brain swelling after large hemispheric infarction (GAMES-RP): a randomised, double-blind, placebo-controlled phase 2 trial. Lancet Neurol 2016; 15(11):1160–9.
49. Yao Y, Zhang Y, Liao X, et al. Potential therapies for cerebral edema after ischemic stroke: a mini review. Front Aging Neurosci 2021;12. https://doi.org/10.3389/fnagi.2020.618819.
50. Zhao J, Su YY, Zhang Y, et al. Decompressive hemicraniectomy in malignant middle cerebral artery infarct: a randomized controlled trial enrolling patients up to 80 years old. Neurocrit Care 2012;17(2):161–71.

Surgical Indications and Options for Hypertensive Hemorrhages

Kelsey M. Bowman, MD, Azam S. Ahmed, MD*

KEYWORDS

- Intracerebral hemorrhage • Hypertensive hemorrhage • Surgery
- Endoscopic surgery

KEY POINTS

- Medical management continues to be the mainstay of treatment for spontaneous hypertensive intracerebral hemorrhage.
- Treatment goals include admission to a neurosurgical intensive care unit, aggressive blood pressure control, reversal of anticoagulation, and control of intracranial pressure.
- Surgical intervention can be lifesaving in patients with midline shift, elevated intracranial pressure, and/or depressed Glasgow Coma Score.
- Surgical intervention has not been shown to definitively improve functional outcomes in these patients.
- Endoscopic and minimally invasive techniques for hematoma evacuation have been proposed and have been technically successful in early studies, but their superiority to open procedures has not been established.

INTRODUCTION AND BACKGROUND

Spontaneous intracerebral hemorrhage (SICH) is the second most common type of stroke, accounting for approximately 15% of all strokes.[1,2] It is, nevertheless, the largest cause of stroke mortality. The case fatality rate is high, with 40% mortality at 1 month and 54% at 1 year.[2] Patients who survive have significant morbidity, with only 12% to 39% obtaining functional independence.[2]

SICH is usually caused by rupture of small, penetrating arteries, secondary to hypertensive changes or amyloid angiopathy. Long-standing hypertension can result in degeneration of the media and smooth muscle of small arteries/arterioles and formation of microaneurysms.[2–4] This pathology is the most common identified in nonlobar ICH. Common locations for hypertensive ICH, in descending order of frequency, include the basal ganglia (putamen most commonly), thalamus, pons, cerebellum,

Department of Neurological Surgery, University of Wisconsin, 600 Highland Avenue, K4/850, CSC-8660, Madison, Wisconsin 53792, USA
* Corresponding author.
E-mail address: azam.ahmed@neurosurgery.wisc.edu

Neurol Clin 40 (2022) 337–353
https://doi.org/10.1016/j.ncl.2021.12.001
0733-8619/22/© 2022 Elsevier Inc. All rights reserved.

and lobar. Lobar ICH, in contrast, is more frequently associated with the deposition of amyloid protein within the walls of the arteries within the cortex, a phenomenon known as cerebral amyloid angiopathy.

The ICH score was developed as a simple prognostic tool for outcome stratification in ICH (**Table 1**).[5] The 6-point scale can be used to predict mortality. Factors known to be associated with poor outcomes include large hematoma size or hematoma expansion, intraventricular hemorrhage, infratentorial location, and increased age. Patients with a hematoma volume greater than 60 mL and a Glasgow Coma Score (GCS) less than 8 have a greater than 90% predicted 30-day mortality.[5]

DISCUSSION
Medical Management

Intensive care unit admission
Medical management is the mainstay of treatment for SICH. Patients should be admitted expeditiously to a neurosurgical intensive care unit or transferred immediately to a hospital that can provide this level of care[6] (**Box 1**). Studies demonstrate that admission to a specialized neurosurgical intensive care unit or stroke unit results in decreased overall mortality when compared with a general intensive care unit.[7] Additionally, a prolonged time in the emergency department before admission is associated with poorer outcomes at hospital discharge.[8]

Table 1 ICH score	
Category	**Points**
GCS	
3–4	2
5–12	1
13–15	0
Volume	
>30 cm³	1
<30 cm³	0
IVH	
Yes	1
No	0
Location	
Infratentorial	1
Supratentorial	0
Age	
≥80	1
<80	0
Total Score	Mortality
0	0%
1	13%
2	26%
3	72%
4	97%
5–6	100%

Box 1

American Heart Association/American Stroke Association Recommendation

- "Initial monitoring and management of ICH patients should take place in an intensive care unit or dedicated stroke unit with physician and nursing neuroscience acute care expertise (Class I; Level of Evidence B)."[6]

Blood pressure control

Hypertension is common in patients with ICH, both as the etiology of the hemorrhage and as an autoregulatory response to elevated ICPs caused by the hemorrhage. Intensive blood pressure (BP) management is one of the most important aspects of treatment (**Box 2**). A retrospective study of 1760 patients with ICH showed that elevated systolic and diastolic pressures were associated with increased death and disability.[9] Another study by Rodriguez-Luna and colleagues[10] demonstrated an increased risk of hematoma growth and early neurologic deterioration in patients with a higher proportion of systolic BP readings of greater than 180 mm Hg.

There had been concern that rapid correction of BP would cause worse systemic outcomes and increased perihematomal infarct; however, the INTERACT2 and ICH ADAPT studies demonstrated the safety and efficacy of intensive BP management. In 2013, the INTERACT2 trial randomized 2794 patients to intensive BP management (target systolic B of <140 mm Hg within 1 hour) versus standard management (target systolic BP of <180 mm Hg). Patients in the intensive group had improved functional outcomes compared with controls (odds ratio [OR], 0.87; 95% confidenceinterval [CI], 0.77–1.0; $P = .04$), with no significant increase in the number of adverse events reported.[11] The ICH ADAPT trial in 2013 randomized 75 patients to intensive BP management (systolic BP goal of <150 mm Hg) versus standard management to determine whether intensive management precipitated cerebral infarction.[12] There was no difference between the perihematomal cerebral blood flow in the 2 groups, suggesting that BP reduction does not increase the risk of ischemic stroke.

More recently, a randomized study of 1000 patients (ATACH-2) failed to show a benefit of aggressive BP management when compared with standard treatment with regards to death or disability (relative risk [RR] 1.04; 95% CI, 0.85–1.27).[13] Additionally, the intensive treatment group had a higher rate of adverse renal events (9.0% vs 4.0%; $P = .002$). However, the percentage of patients with primary treatment failure was higher in the intensive group, which may have led to a dampened apparent treatment effect. Interestingly, a recent systematic review which included both the INTERACT2 and ATACH-2 trials, did show a benefit of aggressive BP management with a decreased rate of 90-day death or disability (adjusted OR, 1.12; 95% CI; 1.0–1.26 per 10 mm Hg) and hematoma expansion (adjusted OR, 1.16; 95% CI, 1.02–1.32).

Box 2

American Heart Association/American Stroke Association Recommendations

- "For ICH patients presenting with [systolic BP] between 150 and 220 mm Hg and without contraindication to acute BP treatment, acute lowering of [systolic BP] to 140 mm Hg is safe (Class I; Level of Evidence A) and can be effective for improving functional outcome (Class IIa; Level of Evidence B)."

- "For ICH patients presenting with [a systolic BP] greater than 220 mm Hg, it may be reasonable to consider aggressive reduction of BP with a continuous intravenous infusion and frequent BP monitoring (Class IIb; Level of Evidence C)."[6]

Reversal of anticoagulation

The increasing use of oral anticoagulation has resulted in an increased number of hemorrhages in patients taking these medications. Immediate reversal of these agents is of utmost importance once an ICH is identified (**Box 3**). There are well-established data supporting the use of intravenous vitamin K plus prothrombin complex concentration (PCC) for reversal of warfarin. The administration of PCC leads to rapid reversal of anticoagulation, with normalization of the international normalized ratio (INR) seen within minutes.[14] In 2013, a large, randomized controlled trial (RCT) found that PCC had a higher likelihood of normalizing the INR (INR < 1.3) within 30 minutes when compared with fresh frozen plasma (62.2% vs 9.6%) in patients taking warfarin.[15]

Fewer data are available regarding the reversal of the direct oral anticoagulants, which include the direct Xa inhibitors (apixaban and rivaroxaban). Studies suggest that PCC may be effective at obtaining hemostasis[16] in patients taking these medications. More recently, the US Food and Drug Administration approved the first specific reversal agent for anti-Xa inhibitors, andexanet alfa, a variant of factor Xa that binds to Xa with high affinity, preventing its anticoagulant activity.[17]

Although it is widely accepted that these anticoagulants should be reversed immediately, the picture is less clear with antiplatelet therapy. Studies suggest that patients taking antiplatelet medications have a slightly increased risk of early hematoma expansion and death. Despite this finding, the PATCH trial, an RCT of 190 patients with SICH on antiplatelet therapy, does not support the use of platelet transfusions, with the risk of death or dependence higher in the group that received platelet transfusions compared with standard care.[18]

Control of intracranial pressure

The final component of medical management of ICH is control of ICP (**Box 4**). Most of the data for ICP management are extrapolated from the traumatic brain injury guidelines. The mainstays of treatment include hypertonic and hyperosmolar therapy, head of bed elevation, and sedation.[19] Additionally, an external ventricular drain (EVD) or intraparenchymal pressure monitor should be placed for monitoring if the GCS is less than 8.[19] Steroids should be avoided, based on the results of a randomized trial

---

Box 3
American Heart Association/American Stroke Association Recommendations

- "Patients with ICH whose INR is elevated because of VKA [vitamin K agonist] should have their VKA withheld, receive therapy to replace vitamin K–dependent factors and correct the INR, and receive intravenous vitamin K (Class I; Level of Evidence C). PCCs may have fewer complications and correct the INR more rapidly than FFP [fresh frozen plasma] and might be considered over FFP (Class IIb; Level of Evidence B). rFVIIa [recombinant factor VIIa] does not replace all clotting factors, and although the INR may be lowered, clotting may not be restored in vivo; therefore, rFVIIa is not recommended for VKA reversal in ICH (Class III; Level of Evidence C)."

- "For patients with ICH who are taking dabigatran, rivaroxaban, or apixaban, treatment with FEIBA [factor eight inhibitor bypassing activity], other PCCs, or rFVIIa might be considered on an individual basis. Activated charcoal might be used if the most recent dose of dabigatran, apixaban, or rivaroxaban was taken less than 2 hours earlier. Hemodialysis might be considered for dabigatran (Class IIb; Level of Evidence C)."

- "Protamine sulfate may be considered to reverse heparin in patients with acute ICH (Class IIb; Level of Evidence C)."

- "The usefulness of platelet transfusions in ICH patients with a history of antiplatelet use is uncertain (Class IIb; Level of Evidence C)."[6]

Box 4
American Heart Association/American Stroke Association Recommendations

- "Ventricular drainage as treatment for hydrocephalus is reasonable, especially in patients with decreased level of consciousness (Class IIa; Level of Evidence B)."

- "Patients with a GCS score of ≤8, those with clinical evidence of transtentorial herniation, or those with significant IVH or hydrocephalus might be considered for ICP monitoring and treatment. A [cranial perfusion pressure] of 50 to 70 mm Hg may be reasonable to maintain depending on the status of cerebral autoregulation (Class IIb; Level of Evidence C)."

- "Corticosteroids should not be administered for treatment of elevated ICP in ICH (Class III; Level of Evidence B)."[6]

---

of 93 patients with SICH that demonstrated no change in mortality and an increased rate of complications in patients taking dexamethasone.[20]

Surgical Management

Surgical treatment options

The role of surgery for patients with SICH remains controversial. In theory, surgical intervention should provide clinical benefit by decreasing mass effect, preventing hematoma expansion, and decreasing the ICP, and, therefore, the increasing cerebral perfusion pressures and decreasing the toxic/inflammatory damage caused on the brain.[21] Nevertheless, RCTs have yet to establish a convincing benefit for surgical intervention. Furthermore, the ideal surgical technique has not been proven, with options including craniotomy for hematoma evacuation, decompressive craniectomy (DC), and endoscopic and other minimally invasive procedures for hematoma evacuation.

Open surgery. Open craniotomy for hematoma evacuation is the most used and most studied surgical approach (**Fig. 1**). However, RCTs evaluating the efficacy of this intervention have had mixed results (**Box 5**). One of the earliest clinical trials was performed by Juvela and colleagues in 1989.[22] Fifty-two patients with supratentorial ICH who presented with depressed consciousness or severe neurologic deficit were randomized to either immediate surgical intervention or medical management. There was no difference in mortality or in functional outcomes between the 2 groups. On subgroup analysis, patients with a GCS of 7 to 10 before randomization had lower overall mortality with surgery ($P = .048$). However, all patients who survived were severely disabled. Similarly, Batjer and colleagues[23] randomized 21 patients with hypertensive putaminal hemorrhages to best medical management, medical management plus ICP monitoring, or surgical evacuation. Overall, 71% died or remained comatose at 6 months. Only 19% were functionally independent, and none returned to their prehemorrhage baseline. These outcomes were no different across the 3 groups studied.

The STICH trials[24,25] are 2 of the largest randomized controlled studies investigating the difference in mortality and neurologic outcomes between surgical and conservative management. The original STITCH trial randomized 1033 patients with supratentorial SICH to surgery within 24 hours versus conservative management. The primary end point was a favorable outcome on the Glasgow Outcome Scale at 6 months, dichotomized based on prognosis. There was no significant difference in outcomes between the 2 groups.[24] There were 118 patients (24%) in the conservative group and 122 patients (26%) in the surgical group who had a favorable outcome (OR, 0.89; 95% CI, 0.66–1.19; $P = .414$). Mortality was 37% and 36% in the conservative and surgical groups, respectively (OR, 0.95; 95% CI, 0.73–1.23; $P = .707$). Subgroup

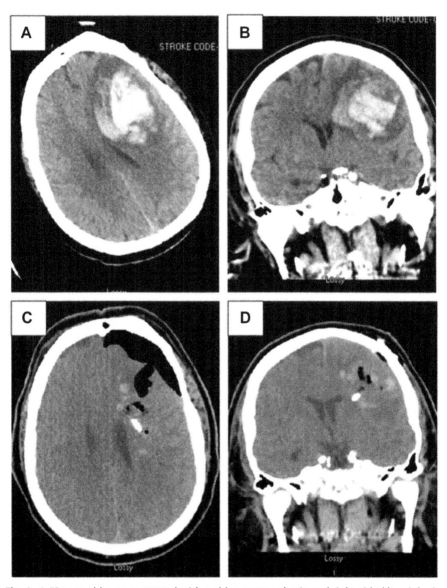

Fig. 1. A 53-year-old man presented with sudden onset aphasia and right-sided hemiplegia. A computed tomography scan showed a 5 × 5 × 7-cm left frontal ICH. He subsequently underwent craniotomy for open surgical hematoma resection. Preoperative axial (*A*) and coronal (*B*) and postoperative axial (*C*) and coronal (*D*) noncontrast computed tomography scans are shown.

analysis suggested that a subset of patients with superficial lobar hemorrhages and a favorable GCS may benefit from surgical intervention. Therefore, STITCH II was designed.[25]

STITCH II randomized 601 patients to surgery or conservative management. To qualify, patients had to be conscious (GCS of >8) and have a superficial lobar

---

Box 5
American Heart Association/American Stroke Association Recommendations

- "For most patients with supratentorial ICH, the usefulness of surgery is not well established (Class IIb; Level of Evidence A)."

- "A policy of early hematoma evacuation is not clearly beneficial compared with hematoma evacuation when patients deteriorate (Class IIb; Level of Evidence A)."

- "Supratentorial hematoma evacuation in deteriorating patients might be considered as a life-saving measure (Class IIb; Level of Evidence C)."[6]

---

hemorrhage measuring 10 to 100 mm^3 within 1 cm of the cortical surface. There was no significant difference in functional outcomes between the groups, with an unfavorable outcome observed in 59% of patients in the conservative group and 62% in the surgical group (OR, 0.86; 95% CI, 0.62–1.20; $P = .367$). There was, however, a nonsignificant, but potentially relevant, survival benefit in the surgical group (24% vs 18%; $P = .095$). It is important to note, however, that there was high crossover to the surgical group, potentially skewing the results, because if there were no crossover, the rate of death and poor outcomes may have been higher in the conservative group.

In contrast with the prior studies, Pantazis and colleagues[26] did show a morbidity benefit to surgery. There were 108 patients with an ICH of greater than 30 mL and a focal neurologic deficit or alteration of consciousness who were randomized to conservative treatment or craniotomy. Patients randomized to the surgical group were more likely to have a favorable neurologic outcome, defined as a Glasgow Outcome Scale of greater than 3 at 12 months (33% vs 9%; $P = .002$). Interestingly, there was no difference in mortality. On subgroup analysis, patients with a GCS of less than 8 or a hematoma volume of greater than 80 mL did not show benefit from surgical intervention with respect to either morbidity or mortality.

Additional open surgical considerations include DC with or without hematoma evacuation. Several studies have addressed this method, again, without convincing results. In general, studies suggest a possible survival benefit in patients undergoing DC with little or no effect on neurologic outcomes (**Box 6**). Patients who may benefit from this intervention include those with large hematomas with significant mass effect or midline shift, a low GCS (≤ 8), and/or refractory elevated ICPs.

One of the earliest series of DC for SICH was reported by Dierssen and colleagues[27] in 1983. They described 73 consecutive patients who underwent DC with hematoma evacuation and compared their outcomes with historical controls. Patients with acute ICH who underwent DC had a lower reported mortality (32% vs 70%; $P = .005$). There were, however, no differences in morbidity. Fung and colleagues[28] investigated the role of DC without hematoma evacuation in 12 patients with large (median volume, 61.3 mL) supratentorial ICH and a lower GCS (median, GCS 8). Compared with matched controls, there was lower mortality in the surgical group (3 patients vs 8

Box 6
American Heart Association/American Stroke Association Recommendation

- "DC with or without hematoma evacuation might reduce mortality for patients with supratentorial ICH who are in a coma, have large hematomas with significant midline shift, or have elevated ICP refractory to medical management (Class IIb; Level of Evidence C)."[6]

patients). An RCT of 40 randomized patients with supratentorial SICH to undergo hematoma evacuation alone or hematoma evacuation plus DC.[29] Overall, there were no significant differences in outcomes between the 2 groups. However, on subgroup analysis, patients with a preoperative GCS of 6 to 12 were more likely to have a good outcome if they underwent DC ($P < .05$).

Endoscopic or minimally invasive surgery. More recently, it has been proposed that endoscopic and other minimally invasive techniques for hematoma evacuation could improve surgical outcomes by causing less surgical disruption to the healthy brain (**Fig. 2; Box 7**). The first RCT looking at this was performed by Auer and colleagues in 1989.[30] One hundred patients with supratentorial SICH were randomized to endoscopic hematoma evacuation or medical management. In patients with subcortical hematomas, there was a lower mortality in the surgical group (30% vs 70%; $P < .05$). Additionally, patients in this subgroup had a higher percentage of good outcomes with surgery (40% vs 25%; $P < .05$). Outcomes were not improved in patients who were stuporous or comatose preoperatively. When stratified by hematoma size, patients with a hematoma size of less than 50 mL had better functional outcomes with surgery when compared with medical management, but a similar mortality. In contrast, in patients with hematomas of greater than 50 mL, surgery showed a mortality benefit, but no difference in neurologic outcomes.

Vespa and colleagues[31] conducted an RCT of 20 patients with a primary ICH of greater than 20 mL who were randomized to computed tomography scan-guided endoscopic hematoma evacuation or medical management. Hematoma evacuation was successful in all cases, with an average decreased of 68%. When compared with historical controls, those who underwent surgery had a trend toward good neurologic outcomes (42.9% vs 23.7%; $P = .19$). A more recent meta-analysis of 3 RCTs comparing endoscopic hematoma evacuation to conventional craniotomy[32] showed no difference in mortality between the 2 groups (RR, 0.58; 95% CI, 0.26–1.29; $P = .18$). However, there was a lower reported complication rate with endoscopic evacuation (RR, 0.37; 95% CI, 0.28–0.49; $P < .001$).

The Penumbra Apollo system (Penumbra Inc, Almeda, CA), an aspiration–irrigation system, is a new device that has promise as an adjunct in endoscopic evacuation. A retrospective analysis of 29 patients who underwent endoscopic evacuation using the Apollo system showed a significant decrease in hematoma volume postoperatively ($P < .001$).[33] Additionally, both the complication and mortality rate were low (6.9% and 13.8%, respectively), suggesting that the device is both safe and effective. The INVEST study, a prospective, multicenter RCT, is currently ongoing to compare the safety and efficacy of endoscopic surgery with the Apollo system to best medical management.[34] The SCUBA technique (Stereotactic ICH Underwater Blood Aspiration) has been proposed as a way to improve on the standard use of the Apollo device.[35] After standard hematoma aspiration with Apollo, the hematoma cavity is then filled with saline, which allows for exploration of the fluid-filled cavity under direct visualization and makes for greater ease of identifying bleeding and achievement of hemostasis. Early experience with this technique in 47 patients was reported by Kellner and colleagues,[35] with an average evacuation of 88.2%. Active bleeding was identified in 23 cases (48.9%), which was stopped with irrigation in 5 cases and electrocautery in the remaining 18. Ongoing investigation of this technique is necessary to determine its efficacy compared with more traditional methods.

The SICHPA trial introduced a new technique for minimally invasive surgical (MIS) evacuation—the placement of a catheter into the hematoma cavity followed by administration of a thrombolytic agent.[36] Seventy-one patients were randomized into a

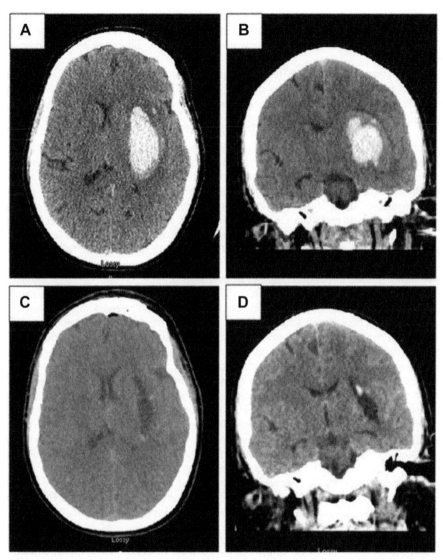

Fig. 2. A 53-year-old hypertensive woman presented with a GCS of 12, right-sided hemiplegia, and a 3.0 × 4.0 × 4.5-cm left basal ganglia ICH. She underwent endoscopic hematoma evacuation. She is now 2 years out from surgery and is independently ambulatory with a cane. Preoperative axial (A) and coronal (B) and postoperative axial (C) and coronal (D) noncontrast computed tomography scans are shown.

Box 7
American Heart Association/American Stroke Association Recommendation

- "The effectiveness of minimally invasive clot evacuation with stereotactic or endoscopic aspiration with or without thrombolytic usage is uncertain (Class IIb; Level of Evidence B)."[6]

surgical or medical group, and outcomes including mortality and functional outcomes were assessed. Despite a significantly larger decrease in hematoma volume after 7 days in the surgical group, there was no significant difference in morbidity or mortality.

Several years later, the MISTIE trials expanded on the results of SICHPA using a similar technique.[37–40] Following a detailed protocol, a cannula was inserted through a burr hole and the hematoma was aspirated. The cannula was then replaced with a catheter, through which tissue plasminogen activator (tPA) was administered postoperatively every 8 hours, until the residual hematoma was less than 15 mL, symptomatic hemorrhage occurred, or the maximum of 9 doses of tPA were administered.[38] In the original MISTIE trial, 96 patients were randomized to surgery or medical management. There were more patients in the surgical group with a good outcome, defined as a modified Rankin score (mRS) of less than 4 at 180 days (33% vs 21%). This difference was nearly significant after correcting for differences in baseline severity between the groups ($P = .05$). There was no difference in 30-day mortality ($P = .542$), symptomatic bleeding ($P = .226$), or infection ($P = .438$) rates. There was, however, an increase in asymptomatic bleeding in the surgery group (22% vs 7%; $P = .051$). Not only was the hematoma volume decreased with surgery, the perihematomal edema volume was decreased as well, with a graded effect of amount of clot removal on edema reduction ($P < .001$).[40]

Subsequently, a larger phase III RCT (MISTIE III) was designed to better evaluate functional outcomes.[37,39] The investigators randomized 506 patients with supratentorial SICH with a hematoma volume of greater than 30 mL. A favorable outcome (mRS of 0–3 at 12 months) was achieved in 45% of patients in the surgical group and 41% in the medical group (adjusted risk difference 4%; 95% CI, –4 to 12; $P = .33$). Secondary analyses showed improved functional outcomes for patients in whom the surgical aim (postoperative hematoma volume of <15 mL) was achieved (adjusted risk difference, 10.5%; 95% CI, 1–20; $P = .03$). There was a nonsignificant trend toward lower 30-day mortality in the surgical group (15% vs 9%; $P = .07$). Interestingly, further analysis of the MISTIE III and STITCH II data suggests that surgical performance may play a role in outcomes.[41] A postoperative ICH volume of less than 28.8 mL in MISTIE III and less than 30.0 mL in STITCH II was associated with increased probability of an mRS of 0 to 3 at 180 days ($P = .01$ and .003, respectively).[41]

Despite mixed results from individual trials, several large meta-analyses have shown more promising results. A Cochrane review published in 2008 included 10 RCTs and 2059 total patients.[42] Both open and MIS techniques were included. Based on the review, surgery was significantly associated with a decreased risk of being dead or dependent at the final follow-up (OR, 0.71; 95% CI, 0.58–0.88; $P = .001$). A large meta-analysis was published in 2012 involving 1955 patients who were randomized to undergo MIS hematoma evacuation or medical management.[43] Both the primary and secondary outcomes of death or dependence or death alone, respectively, showed a significant decrease in the MIS group (OR, 0.54 [$P < .0001$] and OR, 0.53 [$P < .00001$]). Most recently, in 2020, Li and colleagues[44] performed a meta-analysis to compare the safety and efficacy of different surgical techniques to medical management. They found that endoscopic surgery, MIS combined with either urokinase or recombinant tPA (rtPA), and craniotomy were all associated with higher survival rates than standard medical care. Additionally, all 4 surgical interventions decreased the number of surviving patients with severe disability. Among the 4 surgical interventions, endoscopic surgery was the most favorable, with the lowest mortality rates and lowest proportion of patients with severe disability, as well as the lowest risk of rebleeding. Multiple randomized clinical trials are ongoing, including ENRICH, MIND, and EVACUATE, with estimated completion dates in the next several years.[45]

SPECIAL CONSIDERATIONS
Cerebellar Hemorrhage

An infratentorial location is an independent predictor of a poor outcome, regardless of hematoma volume.[5] Infratentorial hemorrhages can cause hydrocephalus by compression of the fourth ventricle and can lead to brainstem compression and/or herniation and, therefore, may be life-threatening at a much smaller size than their supratentorial equivalents. Because of this factor, surgical intervention is regarded as the standard of care for patients with posterior fossa ICH associated with neurologic deterioration, hydrocephalus, or overt brainstem compression (**Box 8**). There have been several nonrandomized studies that suggest that surgical intervention should be performed when the hemorrhage is greater than 3 cm or when these criteria are met. RCTs for cerebellar hemorrhage are challenging; it is clear that surgical and medical management are not equivalent, so high-level data are lacking. Additionally, EVD placement alone without decompression should not be performed.[6]

Kuramatsu and colleagues[46] performed an individual patient data meta-analysis of 578 patients with cerebellar ICH to evaluate functional outcome and survival in patients treated with surgical evacuation versus conservative treatment. Surgical intervention was not significantly related to better functional outcome (30.9% vs 35.5%; OR, 0.94; 95% CI, 0.81–1.09). Patients who underwent surgical intervention, however, did have a higher likelihood of survival (78.3% vs 61.2%; OR, 1.25; 95% CI, 1.07–1.45).

Kobayashi and colleagues[47] suggested a new criterion to guide management that incorporated the patient's GCS and hematoma size. Based on their series of 101 consecutive patients, they proposed dividing patients into 3 categories—(1) patients with a GCS of 14 to 15 and a hematoma size of less than 40 mm, (2) patients with a GCS of less than 14 or a hematoma greater than 40 mm, and (3) patients whose brainstem reflexes were already lost or whose general condition was poor. Patients in the first group are suitable for conservative management, those in the second group should undergo suboccipital craniectomy with hematoma evacuation, and those in the third group should not receive intensive therapy at all. Using these criteria, the authors reported no mortality in group 1, suggesting this may be a reasonable criteria to stratify patients preoperatively.

Data on MIS techniques for posterior fossa hemorrhage are even more limited; however, the outcomes of a small cohort of patients treated with MIS hematoma evacuation was reported in 2019.[48] In this series of 6 patients, MIS techniques were shown to be technically successful, with a median hematoma evacuation of 97.5%, although 1 patient did require reoperation with craniectomy. Mortality and morbidity rates were similar to those reported previously.

Intraventricular Hemorrhage

Intraventricular hemorrhage occurs in approximately 45% of ICH cases. It is independently associated with a poor outcome, increasing the mortality rate of ICH from 20% to 51%.[49,50] Most IVH is secondary to the extension of the ICH into the ventricular

---

Box 8
American Heart Association/American Stroke Association Recommendations

- "Patients with cerebellar hemorrhage who are deteriorating neurologically or who have brainstem compression and/or hydrocephalus from ventricular obstruction should undergo surgical removal of the hemorrhage as soon as possible (Class I; Level of Evidence B). Initial treatment of these patients with ventricular drainage rather than surgical evacuation is not recommended (Class III; Level of Evidence C)."[6]

system, most commonly from the thalamus or basal ganglia.[50] Standard treatment of IVH includes placement of an EVD; however, EVD placement alone is often ineffective because blood within the ventricles can obstruct drainage of the cerebrospinal fluid (**Box 9**).[6] Therefore, studies have been designed to investigate the efficacy of the intrathecal administration of thrombolytic agents.

In 2011, a meta-analysis of several small studies did suggest a benefit to the use of intrathecal thrombolytics.[51] There were 316 patients with spontaneous IVH who were treated with an EVD alone versus EVD plus intraventricular thrombolytic therapy. There was a significant decrease in mortality from 47% to 23% in the group treated with fibrinolysis (OR, 0.32; 95% CI, 0.19–0.52) with no difference in complications.

Later that year, the largest trial to date of intraventricular tPA, the CLEAR-IVH trial, was published.[52,53] Forty-eight patients were randomized to receive intraventricular rtPA or placebo. The preliminary data suggested that the administration of rtPA in patients with spontaneous IVH was safe, without an increased risk of ventriculitis or death in the rtPA group, although there was a nonsignificant trend toward increased bleeding. The use of rtPA was also effective, with a higher rate of blood clot resolution (18% per day vs 8% per day; $P < .001$). Because of the slightly higher rebleeding rate in the rtPA group, a dose-finding study was then undertaken to determine if lower doses would be as effective in clot lysis.[53] This study randomized an additional 16 patients (for a total for 64 patients) to receive 3 different doses of rtPA. The study again confirmed that rtPA accelerates the resolution of IVH, and with a dose-dependent relationship.

In a follow-up study (CLEAR III), 500 patients with SICH with IVH were randomized to treatment with EVD alone versus EVD plus intrathecal tPA (1 mg every 8 hours, up to 12 doses) and their functional outcome at 180 days was assessed, with a good outcome defined as an mRS of less than 4.[54] There was no difference in the number of patients who achieved a good outcome (48% vs 45%; RR, 1.06; 95% CI, 0.88–1.28; $P = .554$). There was a mortality benefit in the tPA arm (18% vs 29%; HR 0.6; 95% CI, 0.51–0.86; $P = .006$); however, this resulted in a higher proportion of patients with an mRS of 5 ($P = .005$). There was no significant difference in bleeding between the 2 groups. A secondary analysis did reveal a significant relationship between the volume of clot remaining in the ventricles and an mRS of less than 4 (OR, 0.96; 95% CI, 0.95–0.97; $P < .0001$).

Additional studies have begun to investigate the efficacy of endoscopic evacuation of IVH given the lack of success with the prior techniques. Two small, retrospective series suggest a potential benefit to endoscopic evacuation of IVH.[55,56] Basaldella and colleagues[55] compared the outcomes of 48 patients who underwent endoscopic IVH evacuation with 48 controls who only underwent EVD placement. Although functional outcomes, as measured by the mRS, were no different between the 2 groups, there was a lesser likelihood of shunt placement in those treated with endoscopic surgery (17% vs 50%). A similar retrospective series compared clinical outcomes in 42 patients, with more promising results.[56] The hematoma clearance rate was higher in

---

Box 9
American Heart Association/American Stroke Association Recommendations

- "Although intraventricular administration of rtPA in IVH appears to have a fairly low complication rate, the efficacy and safety of this treatment are uncertain (Class IIb; Level of Evidence B)."
- "The efficacy of endoscopic treatment of IVH is uncertain (Class IIb; Level of Evidence B)."[6]

those patients treated with endoscopic surgery (71% vs 49%; $P < .05$). Additionally, those patients in the endoscopic surgery group had better functional outcomes on the Glasgow Outcome Scale (3.83 vs 2.75; $P < .05$) and a shorter hospitalization time (12.67 days vs 17.33 days; $P < .05$). Because of the early promise of endoscopic evacuation of IVH, there is currently a large, multicenter, RCT underway to further investigate the benefits of this technique.[57]

SUMMARY

SICH remains a debilitating problem facing neurosurgeons, with high levels of morbidity and mortality. Although large strides in outcomes have been made with regard to ischemic stroke, similar improvements have not been seen with ICH. Efforts to discover an effective surgical intervention have been met with mixed results, and no clearly superior method has been defined. The results of early endoscopic trials, including those using the Apollo system, have shown promise, but additional trials are needed to fully elucidate their efficacy. Given the significant burden of morbidity and mortality associated with ICH, ongoing clinical research efforts should be dedicated to addressing this problem.

CLINICS CARE POINTS

- For most patients with supratentorial ICH, the functional benefit of surgical evacuation is not well established, but surgery may be lifesaving for patients with a moderately depressed GCS or with delayed neurologic deterioration.

- There is no apparent difference in outcomes between patients who were operated on upfront versus those who underwent intervention at time of neurologic deterioration.

- Early data suggest that MIS evacuation is effective, but how it performs compared with conventional surgery remains unclear.

- DC may decrease mortality in patients with low GCS, large hematomas with a midline shift, and in patients with refractory elevated ICPs.

- Surgery should be performed urgently in patients with cerebellar hemorrhages with hydrocephalus, brainstem compression, or declining neurologic examination results.

DISCLOSURE

The authors have nothing to disclose.

REFERENCES

1. Johnson CO, Nguyen M, Roth GA, et al. Global, regional, and national burden of stroke, 1990–2016: a systematic analysis for the Global Burden of Disease Study 2016. Lancet Neurol 2019;18(5):439–58.
2. An SJ, Kim TJ, Yoon BW. Epidemiology, risk factors, and clinical features of intracerebral hemorrhage: an update. J Stroke 2017;19(1):3–10.
3. Qureshi AI, Tuhrim S, Broderick JP, et al. Spontaneous intracerebral hemorrhage. N Engl J Med 2001;344(19):1450–60.
4. Xi G, Keep RF, Hoff JT. Mechanisms of brain injury after intracerebral haemorrhage. Lancet Neurol 2006;5(1):53–63.
5. Hemphill JC, Bonovich DC, Besmertis L, et al. The ICH score: a simple, reliable grading scale for intracerebral hemorrhage. Stroke 2001;32(4):891–7.
6. Hemphill JC, Greenberg SM, Anderson CS, et al. Guidelines for the management of spontaneous intracerebral hemorrhage: a guideline for healthcare

professionals From the American Heart Association/American Stroke Association. Stroke 2015;46(7):2032–60.

7. Diringer MN, Edwards DF. Admission to a neurologic/neurosurgical intensive care unit is associated with reduced mortality rate after intracerebral hemorrhage. Crit Care Med 2001;29(3):635–40.

8. Rincon F, Mayer SA, Rivolta J, et al. Impact of delayed transfer of critically ill stroke patients from the emergency department to the neuro-ICU. Neurocrit Care 2010;13(1):75–81.

9. Zhang Y, Reilly KH, Tong W, et al. Blood pressure and clinical outcome among patients with acute stroke in Inner Mongolia, China. J Hypertens 2008;26(7): 1446–52.

10. Rodriguez-Luna D, Piñeiro S, Rubiera M, et al. Impact of blood pressure changes and course on hematoma growth in acute intracerebral hemorrhage. Eur J Neurol 2013;20(9):1277–83.

11. Anderson CS, Heeley E, Huang Y, et al. Rapid blood-pressure lowering in patients with acute intracerebral hemorrhage. N Engl J Med 2013;368(25):2355–65.

12. Butcher KS, Jeerakathil T, Hill M, et al. The intracerebral hemorrhage acutely decreasing arterial pressure trial. Stroke 2013;44(3):620–6.

13. Qureshi AI, Palesch YY, Barsan WG, et al. Intensive blood-pressure lowering in patients with acute cerebral hemorrhage. N Engl J Med 2016;375(11):1033–43.

14. Pabinger I, Brenner B, Kalina U, et al. Prothrombin complex concentrate (Beriplex ˢ P/N) for emergency anticoagulation reversal: a prospective multinational clinical trial. J Thromb Haemost 2008;6(4):622–31.

15. Sarode R, Milling TJ, Refaai MA, et al. Efficacy and safety of a 4-factor prothrombin complex concentrate in patients on vitamin K antagonists presenting with major bleeding: a randomized, plasma-controlled, phase IIIb study. Circulation 2013;128(11):1234–43.

16. Frontera JA, Lewin JJ III, Rabinstein AA, et al. Guideline for reversal of antithrombotics in intracranial hemorrhage: a statement for healthcare professionals from the Neurocritical Care Society and Society of Critical Care Medicine. Neurocrit Care 2016;24(1):6–46.

17. Momin JH, Candidate P, Hughes GJ. Andexanet Alfa (Andexxa®) for the Reversal of Direct Oral Anticoagulants. P T 2019;44(9):530–49.

18. Baharoglu MI, Cordonnier C, Salman RAS, et al. Platelet transfusion versus standard care after acute stroke due to spontaneous cerebral haemorrhage associated with antiplatelet therapy (PATCH): a randomised, open-label, phase 3 trial. Lancet 2016;387(10038):2605–13.

19. Carney N, Totten AM, O'Reilly C, et al. Guidelines for the Management of Severe Traumatic Brain Injury, Fourth edition. Neurosurgery 2017;80(1):6–15.

20. Poungvarin N, Bhoopat W, Viriyavejakul A, et al. Effects of dexamethasone in primary supratentorial intracerebral hemorrhage. N Engl J Med 1987;316(20): 1229–33.

21. de Oliveira Manoel AL. Surgery for spontaneous intracerebral hemorrhage. Crit Care Lond Engl 2020;24(1):45.

22. Juvela S, Heiskanen O, Poranen A, et al. The treatment of spontaneous intracerebral hemorrhage. A prospective randomized trial of surgical and conservative treatment. J Neurosurg 1989;70(5):755–8.

23. Batjer HH, Reisch JS, Allen BC, et al. Failure of surgery to improve outcome in hypertensive putaminal hemorrhage. A prospective randomized trial. Arch Neurol 1990;47(10):1103–6.

24. Mendelow A, Gregson B, Fernandes H, et al. Early surgery versus initial conservative treatment in patients with spontaneous supratentorial intracerebral haematomas in the International Surgical Trial in Intracerebral Haemorrhage (STICH): a randomised trial. Lancet 2005;365(9457):387–97.
25. Mendelow AD, Gregson BA, Rowan EN, et al. Early surgery versus initial conservative treatment in patients with spontaneous supratentorial lobar intracerebral haematomas (STICH II): a randomised trial. Lancet 2013;382(9890):397–408.
26. Pantazis G, Tsitsopoulos P, Mihas C, et al. Early surgical treatment vs conservative management for spontaneous supratentorial intracerebral hematomas: a prospective randomized study. Surg Neurol 2006;66(5):492–501 [discussion: 501-502].
27. Dierssen G, Carda R, Coca JM. The influence of large decompressive craniectomy on the outcome of surgical treatment in spontaneous intracerebral haematomas. Acta Neurochir (Wien) 1983;69(1–2):53–60.
28. Fung C, Murek M, Z'Graggen WJ, et al. Decompressive hemicraniectomy in patients with supratentorial intracerebral hemorrhage. Stroke 2012;43(12):3207–11.
29. Moussa WMM, Khedr W. Decompressive craniectomy and expansive duraplasty with evacuation of hypertensive intracerebral hematoma, a randomized controlled trial. Neurosurg Rev 2017;40(1):115–27.
30. Auer LM, Deinsberger W, Niederkorn K, et al. Endoscopic surgery versus medical treatment for spontaneous intracerebral hematoma: a randomized study. J Neurosurg 1989;70(4):530–5.
31. Vespa P, Hanley D, Betz J, et al. ICES (intraoperative stereotactic computed tomography-guided endoscopic surgery) for brain hemorrhage: a multicenter randomized controlled trial. Stroke 2016;47(11):2749–55.
32. Zhao XH, Zhang SZ, Feng J, et al. Efficacy of neuroendoscopic surgery versus craniotomy for supratentorial hypertensive intracerebral hemorrhage: a meta-analysis of randomized controlled trials. Brain Behav 2019;9(12):e01471.
33. Spiotta AM, Fiorella D, Vargas J, et al. Initial multicenter technical experience with the apollo device for minimally invasive intracerebral hematoma evacuation. Oper Neurosurg 2015;11(2):243–51.
34. Fiorella D, Arthur AS, Mocco JD. 305 The INVEST Trial: a randomized, controlled trial to investigate the safety and efficacy of image-guided minimally invasive endoscopic surgery with apollo vs best medical management for supratentorial intracerebral hemorrhage. Neurosurgery 2016;63:187.
35. Kellner CP, Chartrain AG, Nistal DA, et al. The Stereotactic Intracerebral Hemorrhage Underwater Blood Aspiration (SCUBA) technique for minimally invasive endoscopic intracerebral hemorrhage evacuation. J Neurointerventional Surg 2018;10(8):771–6.
36. Teernstra OPM, Evers SMaA, Lodder J, et al. Stereotactic treatment of intracerebral hematoma by means of a plasminogen activator: a multicenter randomized controlled trial (SICHPA). Stroke 2003;34(4):968–74.
37. Ziai WC, McBee N, Lane K, et al. A randomized 500-subject open-label phase 3 clinical trial of minimally invasive surgery plus alteplase in intracerebral hemorrhage evacuation (MISTIE III). Int J Stroke Off J Int Stroke Soc 2019;14(5):548–54.
38. Hanley DF, Thompson RE, Muschelli J, et al. Safety and efficacy of minimally invasive surgery plus alteplase in intracerebral haemorrhage evacuation (MISTIE): a randomised, controlled, open-label, phase 2 trial. Lancet Neurol 2016;15(12):1228–37.
39. Hanley DF, Thompson RE, Rosenblum M, et al. Efficacy and safety of minimally invasive surgery with thrombolysis in intracerebral haemorrhage evacuation

(MISTIE III): a randomised, controlled, open-label, blinded endpoint phase 3 trial. Lancet 2019;393(10175):1021–32.

40. Mould WA, Carhuapoma JR, Muschelli J, et al. Minimally invasive surgery plus recombinant tissue-type plasminogen activator for intracerebral hemorrhage evacuation decreases perihematomal edema. Stroke 2013;44(3):627–34.

41. Polster SP, Carrión-Penagos J, Lyne SB, et al. Intracerebral hemorrhage volume reduction and timing of intervention versus functional benefit and survival in the MISTIE III and STICH Trials. Neurosurgery 2021;88(5):961–70.

42. Prasad K, Mendelow AD, Gregson B. Surgery for primary supratentorial intracerebral haemorrhage. Cochrane Database Syst Rev 2008. https://doi.org/10.1002/14651858.CD000200.pub2.

43. Zhou X, Chen J, Li Q, et al. Minimally invasive surgery for spontaneous supratentorial intracerebral hemorrhage: a meta-analysis of randomized controlled trials. Stroke 2012;43(11):2923–30.

44. Li M, Mu F, Su D, et al. Different surgical interventions for patients with spontaneous supratentorial intracranial hemorrhage: a network meta-analysis. Clin Neurol Neurosurg 2020;188:105617.

45. Kobata H, Ikeda N. Recent updates in neurosurgical interventions for spontaneous intracerebral hemorrhage: minimally invasive surgery to improve surgical performance. Front Neurol 2021;12:703189.

46. Kuramatsu JB, Biffi A, Gerner ST, et al. Association of surgical hematoma evacuation vs conservative treatment with functional outcome in patients with cerebellar intracerebral hemorrhage. JAMA 2019;322(14):1392.

47. Kobayashi S, Sato A, Kageyama Y, et al. Treatment of hypertensive cerebellar hemorrhage–surgical or conservative management? Neurosurgery 1994;34(2): 246–50 [discussion: 250-251].

48. Khattar NK, Fortuny EM, Wessell AP, et al. Minimally invasive surgery for spontaneous cerebellar hemorrhage: a multicenter study. World Neurosurg 2019;129: e35–9.

49. Gaberel T, Magheru C, Emery E. Management of non-traumatic intraventricular hemorrhage. Neurosurg Rev 2012;35(4):485–95.

50. Hallevi H, Albright KC, Aronowski J, et al. Intraventricular hemorrhage: anatomic relationships and clinical implications. Neurology 2008;70(11):848–52.

51. Gaberel T, Magheru C, Parienti JJ, et al. Intraventricular fibrinolysis versus external ventricular drainage alone in intraventricular hemorrhage: a meta-analysis. Stroke 2011;42(10):2776–81.

52. Naff N, Williams MA, Keyl PM, et al. Low-dose recombinant tissue-type plasminogen activator enhances clot resolution in brain hemorrhage: the intraventricular hemorrhage thrombolysis trial. Stroke 2011;42(11):3009–16.

53. Webb AJS, Ullman NL, Mann S, et al. Resolution of intraventricular hemorrhage varies by ventricular region and dose of intraventricular thrombolytic: The Clot Lysis: Evaluating Accelerated Resolution of IVH (CLEAR IVH) Program. Stroke 2012;43(6):1666–8.

54. Hanley DF, Lane K, McBee N, et al. Thrombolytic removal of intraventricular haemorrhage in treatment of severe stroke: results of the randomised, multicentre, multiregion, placebo-controlled CLEAR III trial. Lancet 2017;389(10069):603–11.

55. Basaldella L, Marton E, Fiorindi A, et al. External ventricular drainage alone versus endoscopic surgery for severe intraventricular hemorrhage: a comparative retrospective analysis on outcome and shunt dependency. Neurosurg Focus 2012;32(4):E4.

56. Song P, Duan FL, Cai Q, et al. Endoscopic surgery versus external ventricular drainage surgery for severe intraventricular hemorrhage. Curr Med Sci 2018; 38(5):880–7.
57. Zhu J, Tang C, Cong Z, et al. Endoscopic intraventricular hematoma evacuation surgery versus external ventricular drainage for the treatment of patients with moderate to severe intraventricular hemorrhage: a multicenter, randomized, controlled trial. Trials 2020;21(1):640.

Closed-Loop Brain Stimulation and Paradigm Shifts in Epilepsy Surgery

R. Mark Richardson, MD, PhD

KEYWORDS

- Epilepsy surgery • Responsive neurostimulation • Closed-loop
- Deep brain stimulation • Stereo-electroencephalography • Local field potentials
- Seizure network

KEY POINTS

- Epilepsy surgery is underutilized.
- Responsive neurostimulation is Food and Drug Administration approved for focal epilepsy and is highly efficacious.
- Strategies and goals for diagnostic intracranial monitoring surgery have expanded.
- The role of the thalamus in different epilepsies is emerging.
- Generalized epilepsy may be treated effectively with intracranial neuromodulation.

INTRODUCTION

Epilepsy is the fourth most common neurologic disorder. In 2015, the Centers for Disease Control and Prevention estimated that there are at least 3.4 million people with epilepsy in the United States.[1] The cost to society of not optimizing the clinical care of these individuals is quite high. The annual direct medical cost of epilepsy in the United States is estimated to be at least $14 billion in today's dollars,[2] although that number excludes most of the cost burden, such as community service costs and indirect costs from losses in quality of life and productivity. Moreover, costs for individuals with drug-resistant epilepsy (DRE) are as many as 10 times greater than for those whose seizures are prevented by medication.[3]

Thirty percent to 40% of patients with epilepsy have DRE and therefore are surgical candidates.[4] Despite its potential to cure some types of epilepsy, surgery remains a vastly underutilized treatment, with only a small minority of candidates receiving surgical treatments. For example, the 2003 joint position paper from the American Academy of Neurology, American Association of Neurological Surgeons, and the American

Department of Neurosurgery, Massachusetts General Hospital, Harvard Medical School, 55 Fruit Street, Boston, MA 02114, USA
E-mail address: mark.richardson@mgh.harvard.edu

Neurol Clin 40 (2022) 355–373
https://doi.org/10.1016/j.ncl.2021.12.002   **neurologic.theclinics.com**
0733-8619/22/© 2022 The Author. Published by Elsevier Inc. This is an open access article under the
CC BY-NC-ND license (http://creativecommons.org/licenses/by-nc-nd/4.0/).

Epilepsy Society estimated that less than 3% of surgical candidates receive surgery, assuming 4000 epilepsy surgeries performed per year out of 150,000 potential surgical candidates.[5] Subsequent studies have demonstrated no change in epilepsy surgery utilization.[6–8] Moreover, the average time from diagnosis to surgery for a medically refractory patient is reported to be around 18 years, in data from both before and after the joint position paper's recommendation that the patient with DRE should be referred to a comprehensive epilepsy center. DRE is defined as the failure of only 2 appropriately considered medications.[9] Alarmingly, contrary to these guidelines, more than 75% of patients with DRE are not referred to an epilepsy specialist.[10] One of every 10,000 newly diagnosed people with epilepsy will die of sudden unexpected death in epilepsy (SUDEP),[10] but sadly the SUDEP rate is 90-fold higher in those with DRE.[10] Thus, underutilization of epilepsy surgery is a public health crisis that requires proactive intervention.

Traditional resective epilepsy surgery can be curative in many cases but is often viewed incorrectly as dangerous.[9] Surprisingly, 60% to 75% of neurologists are not aligned with epilepsy specialists on best referral practices, with obstacles to referral including knowledge deficits regarding the definition of DRE, existing practice guidelines, indications and timing for epilepsy surgery referral, and understanding the numerous types of epilepsies that are amenable to surgery.[11] It may be helpful that several advances have become mainstream over the last decade that increase surgical options for patients with focal epilepsy, while being minimally invasive. These options include intracranial neuromodulation devices that can record from the brain, providing highly useful chronic and patient-specific data. In addition, there is growing evidence that intracranial neuromodulation is efficacious in the treatment of some primary generalized epilepsies. Expeditious referral to a comprehensive epilepsy surgery program is imperative to enable individuals with DRE to have access to the full spectrum of modern surgical treatments (**Fig. 1**). In light of this gap between what is possible and the surgical care actually received by the average patient with DRE, this article reviews 5 paradigm shifts in epilepsy surgery that are useful to consider for optimizing treatment.

PARADIGM SHIFT: BEYOND SEIZURE FREEDOM—QUALITY OF LIFE

Curing a patient's epilepsy through resection of the seizure onset zone traditionally has been considered the only goal of epilepsy surgery. Given that patients with poorly localized focal epilepsy, focal epilepsy arising from eloquent cortex, and patients with primary generalized epilepsy are not candidates for resection, there is growing awareness that intracranial neuromodulation can produce meaningful quality-of-life improvements. The first Food and Drug Administration (FDA) -approved intracranial neuromodulation device for epilepsy was the responsive neurostimulation system (RNS). The RNS System ® (NeuroPace, Inc., Mountain View, CA) is a completely cranial implant, consisting of a programmable onboard processor with 4 recording channels coupled to 2 bidirectional leads capable of both recording and stimulating, as well as storing electrographic data for offline analysis. Since approval in 2013, several publications have described the long-term outcomes of patients who participated in both the feasibility and the pivotal clinical trials of RNS therapy. Nair and colleagues[12] reported outcomes from 162 patients who participated in these trials and completed 9 years of follow-up. The median percent reduction at the end of 3 years was 58%, improving to 75% by the end of 9 years of treatment. Importantly, 35% experienced ≥90% seizure reduction and 21% were seizure free in the last 6 months of follow-up. A separate publication tackled the question of whether the timing of clinical

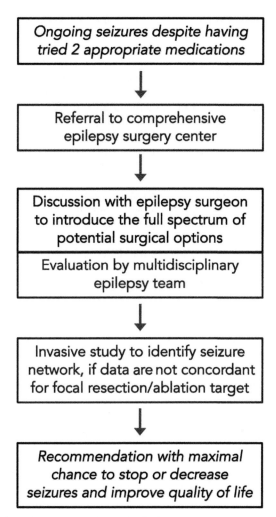

Fig. 1. Efficient presurgical evaluation. Individuals whose seizures are not controlled after having tried 2 appropriate medications should be referred for presurgical evaluation. Patients often benefit from an early introductory discussion with an epilepsy surgeon to explain how the presurgical evaluation is used to recommend a diagnostic and/or therapeutic surgery.

improvements in RNS therapy has accelerated in the field's posttrial experience. Based on a multicenter retrospective analysis, the answer appears to be yes: a median 75% seizure reduction was found at 2 years, and 82% reduction was achieved at ≥ 3 years.[13] The percentages of patients experiencing greater than 90% seizure reduction or no seizures in the last 6 months of follow-up also were similar to that previously reported at 9 years.

Deep brain stimulation (DBS) of the anterior nucleus of the thalamus (ANT), because of its involvement in common seizure propagating circuitry, was proposed by Upton and colleagues[14] for suppression of epileptiform discharges within the limbic system. In 1987, they reported significant seizure control in 4 of 6 patients with drug-resistant complex partial seizures who underwent bilateral ANT stimulation.[15] ANT-DBS was FDA approved in 2018, with outcomes having been followed out to 10 years. At 7 years, median seizure frequency percent reduction from baseline was 75%.[16] It is important to note that patients in the pivotal trials for DBS and RNS were highly refractory, averaging an approximately 20-year history of epilepsy, 20 to 50 disabling seizures a month at baseline, and having failed multiple other epilepsy treatments.[12,17]

The benefit-versus-risk profile of intracranial neuromodulation is impressive. No intraparenchymal hemorrhages were reported in either pivotal trial.[17,18] The infection rate with RNS was 3% and with DBS was 10%, the latter's higher rate likely being secondary to the additional incisions and surgical site needed for DBS pulse generator placement in the chest. Remarkably, the SUDEP rate decreased by two-thirds for each therapy ($\sim$3 per 1000 patient-years), compared with the expected rate in the DRE population ($\sim$9 per 1000 patient-years). In addition to reduced seizure burden, low morbidity, and the prevention of mortality, these therapies produce measurable improvements in quality of life. Mean quality-of-life scores were significantly improved at 1 year for patients with RNS, and these improvements were maintained through at least 9 years of treatment.[12] For patients with DBS, improvements in quality of life at 5 years remained stable at 7 years, whereby 43% of subjects experienced a clinically meaningful improvement.[16] A separate study of the RNS clinical trial patients found no significant cognitive declines for any neuropsychological measure, whereas improvements were found in the Boston Naming Test and Rey Auditory Verbal Learning tests, in patients with neocortical and mesial temporal seizure onset zones, respectively.[19] Importantly, patients treated with RNS earlier in the course of their epilepsy exhibited significant improvements in multiple mood and quality-of-life measures that were not seen in patients treated later in the course of their disease, despite similar efficacy in seizure reduction.[20] Thus, quality-of-life data also support the need to apply urgency in the presurgical evaluation process.

PARADIGM SHIFT: EPILEPSY SURGERY AS NETWORK SURGERY

For several decades, there has been accumulating evidence that specific cortical and subcortical networks enable the onset and propagation of both partial and generalized-onset seizures.[21] The need to emphasize a network approach for epilepsy surgery in most American epilepsy centers stems from the deep-rooted tradition of considering primarily an electrical-anatomic, focus-oriented approach to epilepsy surgery. In the 1950s, Penfield and Jasper[22] established surface electrocorticography as the mainstay for defining an "epileptogenic focus," and Bailey and Gibbs[23] wrote that "surgical eradication of focal seizure activity was comparable to eradicating a tumor." In contrast, the stereo-electroencephalography (SEEG) philosophy originated by Talairach and Bancaud focuses on determining the regions of cortex generating the clinical manifestation of the seizure[24] whereby the chronologic occurrence of ictal clinical signs (semiology) is crucial for elucidating the "anatomo-electro-clinical" organization of seizures.[25] This approach facilitates the conception of seizures as an emergent property of brain networks and requires that epilepsy surgery address a patient's network rather than solely 1 potential focus.

Resecting a critical seizure network node that may render a patient seizure free is always the first treatment of choice, but a network-oriented approach may best prepare the clinical team to make that assessment (**Fig. 2**). One downfall of approaching epilepsy surgery solely from the perspective of focus hunting is that if a resection is performed and the patient is not seizure free, the interpretation is that one "didn't get enough" or did not find "the right focus." When the overall goal of epilepsy surgery

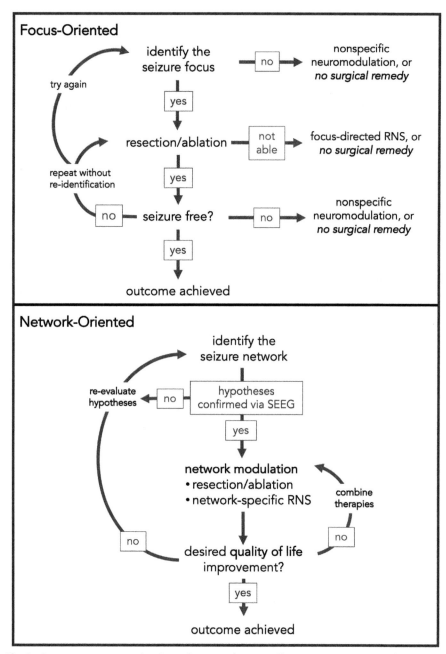

Fig. 2. Focus- versus network-oriented approaches to epilepsy surgery. A network-oriented surgical approach increases opportunities for therapeutic success.

is to take the seizure network offline, that is, to prevent emergence of seizures by disrupting the critical nodes of seizure organization, the emphasis is shifted from resection and seizure freedom to modulation and improved quality of life, with the ultimate goal of arresting seizures indefinitely. In addition, when the desired outcome of intracranial monitoring extends beyond whether a resection can be accomplished and considers how to take the network offline, the opportunity to use more than 1 therapeutic approach is presented.[26] This type of multimodal surgical approach has been enabled by the advent of recent advances in epilepsy surgery in the United States: increased use of SEEG, the development of MRI-guided laser interstitial thermal therapy (LITT), and FDA approval of both RNS and ANT DBS. For instance, LITT may be used in combination with RNS.[26] Others have reported the upfront combination of open craniotomy for partial resection of the epileptogenic zone with implantation of RNS, in cases whereby the epileptogenic zone encompasses eloquent cortex.[27]

Regarding complex seizure networks, therapeutic modulation of difficult-to-localize, multifocal, or generalized epilepsies can be accomplished by influencing cortical seizure onset zones via diffuse cortical projections from the thalamus. This is the general premise underlying open-loop stimulation with ANT-DBS. Several groups have developed closed-loop paradigms using the RNS system, involving a recording contact in the thalamus, and a stimulating contact in the ANT,[28,29] centromedian nucleus (CM),[30,31] or pulvinar.[32] In the largest case series to date, Burdette and colleagues[31] reported the outcomes of 7 patients with regional neocortical focal seizures, treated with responsive cortical-CM thalamic stimulation. All patients achieved ≥50% reduction in disabling seizures, with 3 patients achieving greater than 90% reduction, at a median follow-up duration of 17 months. These investigators achieved similar results using responsive cortical-pulvinar stimulation to treat regional neocortical seizures having onsets in the posterior quadrant,[32] given the strong functional-anatomic connectivity between the pulvinar and posterior brain regions.[33] The fact that responsive stimulation in 3 different thalamic nuclei each could achieve greater than 50% seizure reduction in these highly refractory patients highlights the potential of attaining even better outcomes as techniques evolve and the understanding of the role of specific thalamic nuclei in a given individual's seizure network improves.

In a focus-oriented approach to epilepsy surgery, these outcomes without seizure freedom often are referred to as "palliative." Palliative means alleviating symptoms but not treating the underlying disease. Given the evidence that intracranial neuromodulation has a neuroplastic effect on brain circuitry,[34,35] and that multimodal therapy in multifocal epilepsy can take individual nodes offline, characterization of these therapies as palliative is incorrect and unhelpful. With a network-oriented approach, the goal of surgery is to reduce seizures as maximally as possible, whereby a clinically significant reduction in seizures after surgical therapy represents successful modulation of the seizure circuit. Whether seizure reduction in the absence of seizure freedom would improve the patient's quality of life to an extent that justifies the full application of available surgical therapies is an important component of the presurgical discussion between the patient and the multidisciplinary team. The practical implications of combining this philosophy with recent technological advances in surgical care is described in the following sections.

PARADIGM SHIFT: SURGICAL TREATMENT OF PRIMARY GENERALIZED EPILEPSIES

Given this favorable risk-benefit profile, attention in the intracranial neuromodulation field has expanded to primary generalized epilepsies, for which there currently is no FDA-approved surgical intervention. Likewise, the role of thalamic nuclei in generalized epilepsies has been a longstanding area of focus in both animal and human models, since the work of Hunter and Jasper,[36] who showed that seizures could be induced by electrical stimulation of the thalamus. Subsequently, Monnier and colleagues[37] showed that medial thalamic stimulation could desynchronize cortical electroencephalography (EEG). In the 1980s, Velasco and colleagues[38–40] explored the CM as a DBS target for idiopathic generalized epilepsy (IGE), reporting excellent results. Subsequent feasibility studies and case series demonstrated equivocal findings, until a clinical trial by Valentín and colleagues[41,42] redemonstrated significant therapeutic benefit in patients with IGE. Recently, the University of Melbourne group reported results from a prospective, double-blind, randomized study of continuous, cycling stimulation of CM-DBS, in patients with Lennox-Gastaut syndrome.[43] The DBS device used in that study was not sensing-enabled, but subjects demonstrated significantly reduced electrographic activity on 24-hour ambulatory EEG at the end of the 3-month blinded stimulation phase.

Given that at least 20% of patients with IGE are refractory to pharmacologic treatment[44] (~35% of those with juvenile myoclonic epilepsy are refractory[45]) and evidence that the CM participates in the early propagation of generalized seizures, the author's group hypothesized that bilateral CM responsive neurostimulation with the RNS system would be effective in modulating the thalamocortical seizure network in individuals with IGE. Functional MRI studies have demonstrated increased signal in the thalamus both before[46] and at the onset of[47] generalized spike wave discharges (GSWD). Likewise, intracranial EEG (iEEG) recordings from externalized DBS leads implanted in patients with primary generalized epilepsy in previous studies have demonstrated that GSWD are present in the thalamus simultaneous with onset in the cortex.[48,49] The author reported the first use of bilateral CM RNS in a patient with IGE, a 19-year-old woman, diagnosed with eyelid myoclonia with absences.[50] iEEG recordings during the baseline prestimulation period revealed a multitude of transient (2- to 5-second duration) bilateral 3- to 5-Hz spike-wave discharges in the CM region, recapitulating the morphology and spectral signature of presurgical scalp EEG ictal discharges (**Fig. 3**). After 1 year of RNS therapy, the patient stopped taking all medications, and at 2 years, she continued to report a nearly 90% reduction in seizures, which manifest only as brief episodes of eyelid myoclonia, without loss of consciousness. The first 4 adult patients in the author's IGE CM-region RNS case series have all exhibited significant seizure reduction and improved quality of life (**Table 1**). Bilateral CM-RNS also has been reported in 2 pediatric patients with drug-resistant epilepsy secondary to Lennox-Gastaut syndrome and autism spectrum disorder,[51] and in a pediatric patient with primary generalized epilepsy,[52] all of whom experienced greater than 75% reduction in clinical seizures.

This intracranial neuromodulation experience in IGE demonstrates that it is important to think beyond the Engel score, which was created to assess outcomes relative to seizure freedom following surgical resection. The scale does not capture extensive quality-of-life changes that can occur in patients with intracranial neuromodulation without seizure freedom, such as a reduction in emergency room visits and hospitalizations, work/school days missed, and improvements in behavioral and developmental indices in younger patients. A multicenter, single-blind, randomized, sham stimulation-controlled pivotal study has been initiated with the goal of validating responsive thalamic stimulation as a surgical option for primary generalized seizures (NCT05147571).

PARADIGM SHIFT: VALUE OF CHRONIC INTRACRANIAL DATA

The advent of recording-enabled intracranial neuromodulation systems has opened an entirely new realm of clinical care in epilepsy, that of evaluating and responding

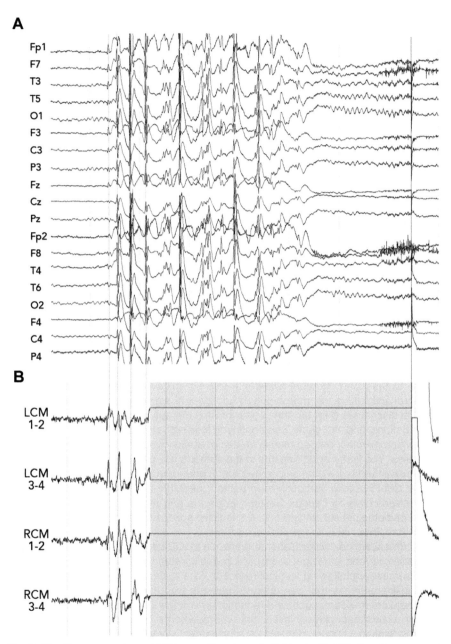

Fig. 3. Simultaneous scalp and iEEG recordings in an individual with IGE. Simultaneous scalp EEG (*A*) and intracranial thalamic EEG recordings on the 4 channels of the RNS device (*B*), during a generalized discharge, exhibit a similar pattern of GSWDs. Responsive stimulation (*green block*) is seen to suppress GSWDs in this example. LCM, left centromedian; RCM, right centromedian.

Table 1
First cohort of patients with idiopathic generalized epilepsy with 2-y follow-up after bilateral centromedian nucleus–region responsive neurostimulation

	Age					No. AEDs			Seizure Frequency			Seizure Severity	
Case	Seizure Onset	RNS Implant	Months Implanted	Sex	Seizure Type	Trialed	At RNS Implant	At MRFU	Pre-RNS	Post-RNS	Engel Score	Pre-RNS	Post-RNS
1	11	19	33	F	Absence with eyelid myoclonia	6	2	0	60/d	6/d	IB	4	2
2	11	22	27	M	Absence, GTC	9	4	2	3/wk, 1/mo	<1/mo, <1/y	IIA	5	2
3	16	21	25	F	Absence, GTC	3	1	1	3/wk, 2–4/m	<1/mo, <1/y	IIIA	5	2
4	17	31	24	F	Myoclonic, Absence, GTC	5	2	2	1/d, 1/wk, 1/y	<1/d, <1/wk, <1/y	IC	4	1

Abbreviations: F, female; GTC, generalized tonic clonic; M, male.

to data obtained from chronic iEEG recordings. The value of these data so far is evident in at least 6 domains: informing additional surgical procedures, seizure forecasting, medication management, lifestyle management, spell characterization, and biomarker detection.

Using iEEG recorded in 37 individuals with focal epilepsy implanted with RNS for up to 10 years, Baud and colleagues[53] first showed that interictal epileptiform activity oscillates with subject-specific multidien (multiday) periodicity, in addition to the well-known circadian rhythms. Seizures were found to occur preferentially during the rising phase of these multidien rhythms of interictal activity. In a follow-up study of 222 individuals with focal epilepsy implanted with RNS, it was reported that 60% of individuals exhibited multidien seizure cycles,[54] and 89% had a circadian cycle. This type of individualized data has the potential to greatly impact patients, given that self-reported and electrographic seizures occurred during the days-long rising phase of interictal activity, regardless of the length of the multidien period. Thus, it eventually should be possible to forecast the risk of seizure at any given timepoint to the patient, and additionally, to use this information to adjust medication timing to increase efficacy and reduce side effects.

Analysis of chronic iEEG data also can lead to evolution of the predominate seizure network hypothesis, enabling additional and highly effective surgery. Hirsch and colleagues[55] reported that among 157 patients with presumed bilateral epilepsy, 25 patients (16%) had a mesial temporal lobe resection informed by chronic ambulatory iEEG (mean duration of data storage = 24 months). Subsequently, the mean reduction in disabling seizures was 94% (range: 50%–100%) at last follow-up.

The ability to get an objective readout on medication efficacy and effects of medication adjustments in the patient's real-world environment also is unprecedented.[56] Quraishi and colleagues[57] recently demonstrated that in patients with RNS with stable detection settings, rates of interictal epileptiform and ictal detections predicted whether a new antiseizure drug would be efficacious, within the first 1 to 2 weeks. Given that most individuals with epilepsy are bothered constantly by physical or psychological effects of antiseizure medications,[58] the ability alone to track changes to medication, including medication withdrawal, can render RNS therapy worthwhile. The availability of this objective iEEG data creates the need for increased effort on the part of epilepsy practitioners. For example, gauging medication response by patient seizure report alone in an individual with RNS without looking at the data would be akin to flying an airplane without looking at the instruments. Fortunately, in the

United States, a procedure code (CPT 95836) has been developed that provides reimbursement for RNS iEEG review.

Patients with epilepsy also often experience episodic increases in seizure activity that sometimes are related to lifestyle choices. In 1 case, increased seizures were linked to increased caffeine consumption, by correlating trends in the iEEG data with the patient's behavior.[59] In that case, eliminating caffeine intake significantly reduced iEEG activity. Used in this manner, chronic iEEG monitoring can provide objective data with which to counsel patients regarding lifestyle choices in the areas of sleep hygiene, recreational drug use, and medication compliance. Similarly, the RNS system allows patients to trigger the storage of an iEEG record with use of a patient magnet that facilitates accurate characterization of patient-reported events, such as differentiating seizures from nonepileptic events, panic attacks, somatization disorders, and psychosis.[60]

Chronic iEEG recordings also are providing new opportunities to assess response to RNS therapy itself. Using RNS recordings from individuals with mesial temporal lobe implantations, Desai and colleagues[61] showed that the interictal spike rate was a strong differentiator of upper- versus lower-quartile clinical responders. Interictal spike rate was positively correlated with seizure rates at 7 years of therapy, suggesting that it could be used as a control signal to adapt stimulation delivered in a closed loop system. Kokkinos and colleagues[34] made the first discovery of putative ictal electrophysiological biomarkers that indicate and potentially predict therapeutic response in individual patients. By visually inspecting the spectral content of greater than 5000 RNS recordings that captured putative seizures, distinct categories of electrographic seizure pattern modulation (ESPM) were detected that were always present in responders and never present in nonresponders. In some cases, these ESPMs were observed in RNS recordings before patient-reported seizure reduction, suggesting their potential utilization in predicting therapeutic response. Subsequently, Khambhati and colleagues[35] identified another type of potential treatment response biomarker. By assessing interictal network reorganization during RNS therapy, they found that clinical seizure reduction was associated with changes in frequency-dependent functional connectivity within, between, and outside seizure foci. Since the extent of this reorganization scaled with seizure reduction and emerged within the first year of treatment, this network measure also may contribute to future strategies for prediction of therapeutic response.

In addition to the RNS system, a second sensing-enabled system with the ability for chronic recording of local field potentials is available clinically, the Medtronic Percept. The FDA-approved functionality of this system currently is limited to following the recording of peaks in the magnitude of the local field potential in the frequency domain (without ability for closed-loop stimulation), but other systems have been used in several preclinical studies of sensing-enabled DBS that explored the electrophysiology of seizure circuits in the time-frequency domain.[62–65] Use of the investigational Medtronic Summit RC+S research device, which can provide continuous iEEG (up to 1000 Hz) from any of 4 contacts on 4 leads, was recently reported for the optimization of automated seizure detection using ANT recordings, in individuals with bilateral ANT and hippocampus DBS leads.[66] This work presages opportunities that will emerge to characterize and modulate seizure networks, as device technologies evolve to include wireless data-streaming capabilities and increasing numbers of recording and stimulating channels.

PARADIGM SHIFT: GOALS AND STRATEGIES OF DIAGNOSTIC EPILEPSY SURGERY

The increased use of intracranial neuromodulation of both cortical and subcortical regions has expanded the scope of diagnostic epilepsy surgery. Given the safety profile of intracranial neuromodulation, the different avenues it offers for potential improvement in quality of life, and its potential use in multifocal and generalized epilepsies, intracranial monitoring surgery, specifically SEEG, has evolved to test a broader range of hypotheses about seizure onset zones and networks. SEEG typically is more versatile for hypothesis testing than subdural grid implantation (unless the phase 1 data are overwhelmingly concordant with a surface lesion).[67,68] The ability to offer a surgical treatment that does not require choosing which brain region to resect has created the need to expand hypothesis testing about the seizure network in ways that inform clinical decisions involving intracranial neuromodulation (**Table 2**). If there is the potential for RNS therapy, one must consider whether sensing should occur in the same location as stimulation. For instance, the author's practice now incorporates thalamic monitoring during SEEG, in cases whereby an eventual recommendation for RNS seems more likely than resection alone, and when it is not clear whether there may be early thalamic involvement in the seizure onset. Others have also evaluated thalamic activity with SEEG to inform RNS implantation.[32] As 1 example, a 31-year-old man presented with a 30-year history of seizures having semiologies that suggested posterior frontal (left hand dystonia and left arm tonic posturing, head drops) and anterior frontal (hypermotor, integrated motor activity) onsets. His MRI showed bilateral extended polymicrogyria, and his ictal EEG showed diffuse onset. With this information, it was not clear whether the patient would be best suited for cortical RNS or where cortical leads would best be placed, versus potentially undergoing bilateral thalamic RNS. The SEEG implantation included leads targeting the CM bilaterally, to test the hypothesis that the thalamus was involved very early in seizure onset and thus would be appropriate to serve as a location for both seizure detection and stimulation. Leads were implanted using the same trajectory and orientation in which they

Table 2
Clinical scenarios in which thalamic implantation during stereo-electroencephalography informs surgical decisions

Clinical Scenario	SEEG Implantation	Seizure Onset Zone Interpretation	Surgical Options Informed by SEEG
1	Standard	Bilateral localized	Bilateral region-specific RNS, bilateral ANT DBS
	+ Thalamic	**Above with ETI**	**Above + bilateral thalamic RNS**
		Above without ETI	Bilateral cortical RNS, bilateral ANT DBS
2	Standard	Unilateral broad onset	Unilateral cortical RNS
	+ Thalamic	**Above with ETI**	**Above + unilateral thalamocortical RNS**
		Above without ETI	Unilateral cortical RNS
3	Standard	Bilateral multifocal onset	Bilateral cortical RNS, bilateral ANT DBS
	+ Thalamic	**Above with ETI**	**Above**
		Above without ETI	**Bilateral thalamic RNS**, bilateral ANT DBS
4	Standard	Primary generalized	Bilateral thalamic RNS, bilateral ANT DBS
	+ Thalamic	**CM > ANT at onset**	**Bilateral CM RNS**
		ANT > CM at onset	**Bilateral ANT DBS**

Bold text denotes changes in management informed by recording from the thalamus during intracranial monitoring.
Abbreviation: ETI, early thalamic involvement.

would be used if implanted therapeutically, in order to simulate recordings that would be captured by an RNS system in which the leads were implanted in a transfrontal approach (**Fig. 4**). In each seizure recorded, the onsets recorded from thalamic contacts were temporally indistinguishable from those recorded on cortical contacts (**Fig. 5**A), resulting in a recommendation for thalamic RNS. After implantation, seizures were detected readily (**Fig. 5**B). Using the thalamic signal to trigger stimulation, in cases such as this one, allows stimulation to affect widespread cortical networks, without having to choose a subterritory of cortex for detection and stimulation, as would be required with the placement of cortical leads. At 14 months of therapy, this patient's seizure frequency had been stably reduced from daily to weekly, with concomitant reduction in seizure severity.

Other centers have explored the value of including the thalamus in diagnostic SEEG surgery. The Marseille group reported very early involvement of the thalamus in 4 patients and delayed involvement in 7 patients, among 13 patients with temporal lobe epilepsy in whom an electrode contact had entered the thalamus through an extended cortical trajectory.[69] Likewise, the University of Alabama group reported data from 11 patients undergoing SEEG for suspected temporal lobe epilepsy, who were implanted in the ANT. Seizure onset was reported to be preceded by a decrease in the mean

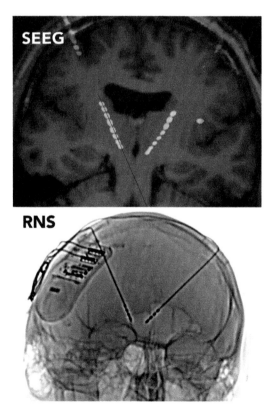

Fig. 4. Thalamic implantation during SEEG. Post-SEEG implantation CT fused to the preoperative brain MRI, demonstrating the position of the frontothalamic SEEG leads (*top*). The orientation and SEEG lead trajectories chosen for this patient were the same as that planned for use with transfrontal implantation of bilateral thalamic leads for RNS (*bottom*).

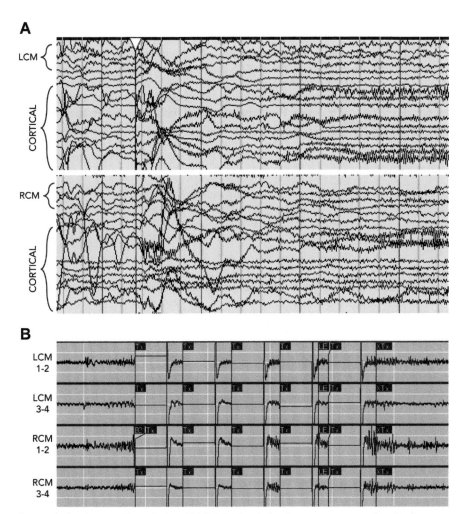

Fig. 5. Thalamic recordings during SEEG. (*A*) The thalamic contacts are active simultaneous with the cortical contacts at seizure onset. (*B*) Similar low-voltage fast activity subsequently was detected on the device and programmed to trigger stimulation.

power spectral density in both the thalamus and the seizure onset zone.[70] These investigators also observed early ictal recruitment of the midline thalamus in 3 cases of mesial temporal lobe epilepsy, where stimulation of either the thalamus or the hippocampus induced similar habitual seizures.[71] These results demonstrating the variable participation of thalamic nuclei in cases of temporal lobe epilepsy indicate the utility of mapping the involvement of potential thalamic nodes in an individual's seizure network, before including the thalamus in an intracranial neuromodulation strategy. Yu and colleagues[72] additionally demonstrated that high-frequency stimulation of the ANT during SEEG can desynchronize epileptic networks in a position-specific manner, implying that thalamic stimulation mapping may be useful for guiding clinically optimal lead placement.

Finally, it is important to note that although less frequent in epilepsy surgery before the approval of ANT-DBS, implantation of the thalamus and basal ganglia is an everyday occurrence in movement disorders DBS surgery. Thus, there is a known safety profile for inserting leads in these subcortical structures,[73] most importantly, an approximately 1% chance of symptomatic hemorrhage.[74] This risk is not different from the general risk of hemorrhage in SEEG procedures.[75] Indeed, the safety of modifying the trajectory of 1 electrode planned for clinical sampling to extend to the thalamus, which obviates implanting an additional electrode for thalamic sampling, was recently described.[70] The event most likely to affect the clinical assessment may be a temporary lesion effect that can occur with thalamic implantation that could prevent the patient from having a seizure during the intracranial monitoring admission.[42]

SUMMARY

Approaches to the evaluation and surgical treatment of individuals with epilepsy are evolving, especially with regard to epilepsy networks, quality of life, primary generalized epilepsies, the utility of chronic intracranial recordings, and goals of diagnostic surgery. These paradigm shifts may facilitate closure of the surgical treatment gap in DRE.

CLINICS CARE POINTS

- Intracranial neuromodulation can reduce seizure frequency by 75%.
- Thalamic implantation in stereo-electroencephalography may inform intracranial neuromodulation treatment strategy.
- Implantation of the thalamus is safe.
- Responsive neurostimulation of the thalamus may be effective in treating idiopathic generalized epilepsy.

DISCLOSURE

The author has current funding support from the NIH via U01NS117836, R01NS110424, U01NS121471, and R01NS119483.

REFERENCES

1. MM Z RK. National and state estimates of the numbers of adults and children with active epilepsy — United States, 2015. MMWR Morb Mortal Wkly Rep 2017;66: 821–5. https://doi.org/10.15585/mmwr.mm6631a1.
2. Yoon D, Frick KD, Carr DA, et al. Economic impact of epilepsy in the United States. Epilepsia 2009;50(10):2186–91. https://doi.org/10.1111/j.1528-1167.2009.02159.x.
3. Manjunath R, Paradis PE, Parisé H, et al. Burden of uncontrolled epilepsy in patients requiring an emergency room visit or hospitalization. Neurology 2012; 79(18):1908–16. https://doi.org/10.1212/wnl.0b013e318271f77e.
4. Kwan P, Brodie MJ. Early identification of refractory epilepsy. New Engl J Med 2000;342:314–9. https://doi.org/10.1056/nejm200002033420503.
5. Engel J, Wiebe S, French J, et al. Practice parameter: temporal lobe and localized neocortical resections for epilepsy. Epilepsia 2003;44(6):741–51. https://doi.org/10.1046/j.1528-1157.2003.48202.x.
6. Kwon C, Blank L, Mu L, et al. Trends in lobectomy/amygdalohippocampectomy over time and the impact of hospital surgical volume on hospitalization outcomes:

a population-based study. Epilepsia 2020;61(10):2173–82. https://doi.org/10.1111/epi.16664.

7. Englot DJ, Ouyang D, Wang DD, et al. Relationship between hospital surgical volume, lobectomy rates, and adverse perioperative events at US epilepsy centers: clinical article. J Neurosurg 2013;118(1):169–74. https://doi.org/10.3171/2012.9.jns12776.

8. Rolston JD, Englot DJ, Knowlton RC, et al. Rate and complications of adult epilepsy surgery in North America: analysis of multiple databases. Epilepsy Res 2016;124:55–62. https://doi.org/10.1016/j.eplepsyres.2016.05.001.

9. Haneef Z, Stern J, Dewar S, et al. Referral pattern for epilepsy surgery after evidence-based recommendations. Neurology 2010;75(8):699–704. https://doi.org/10.1212/wnl.0b013e3181eee457.

10. Epilepsies C on the PHD of the, Policy B on HS, Medicine I of. Epilepsy across the spectrum. 2012. doi:10.17226/13379

11. Samanta D, Ostendorf AP, Willis E, et al. Underutilization of epilepsy surgery: part I: a scoping review of barriers. Epilepsy Behav 2021;117:107837. https://doi.org/10.1016/j.yebeh.2021.107837.

12. Nair DR, Laxer KD, Weber PB, et al. Nine-year prospective efficacy and safety of brain-responsive neurostimulation for focal epilepsy. Neurology 2020;95(9). https://doi.org/10.1212/wnl.0000000000010154.

13. Razavi B, Rao VR, Lin C, et al. Real-world experience with direct brain-responsive neurostimulation for focal onset seizures. Epilepsia 2020;61(8):1749–57. https://doi.org/10.1111/epi.16593.

14. Upton AR, Cooper IS, Springman M, et al. Suppression of seizures and psychosis of limbic system origin by chronic stimulation of anterior nucleus of the thalamus. Int J Neurol 1985;19-20:223–30.

15. Upton ARM, Amin I, Garnett S, et al. Evoked metabolic responses in the LimbicStriate System produced by stimulation of anterior thalamic nucleus in man. Pacing Clin Electrophysiol 1987;10(1):217–25. https://doi.org/10.1111/j.1540-8159.1987.tb05952.x.

16. Salanova V, Sperling MR, Gross RE, et al. The SANTÉ study at 10 years of follow-up: effectiveness, safety, and sudden unexpected death in epilepsy. Epilepsia 2021;62(6):1306–17. https://doi.org/10.1111/epi.16895.

17. Salanova V, Witt T, Worth R, et al. Long-term efficacy and safety of thalamic stimulation for drug-resistant partial epilepsy. Neurology 2015;84(10):1017–25. https://doi.org/10.1212/wnl.0000000000001334.

18. Heck CN, King-Stephens D, Massey AD, et al. Two-year seizure reduction in adults with medically intractable partial onset epilepsy treated with responsive neurostimulation: final results of the RNS System Pivotal trial. Epilepsia 2014;55(3):432–41. https://doi.org/10.1111/epi.12534.

19. Loring DW, Kapur R, Meador KJ, et al. Differential neuropsychological outcomes following targeted responsive neurostimulation for partial-onset epilepsy. Epilepsia 2015;56(11):1836–44. https://doi.org/10.1111/epi.13191.

20. Loring DW, Jarosiewicz B, Meador KJ, et al. Mood and quality of life in patients treated with brain-responsive neurostimulation: the value of earlier intervention. Epilepsy Behav 2021;117:107868. https://doi.org/10.1016/j.yebeh.2021.107868.

21. Spencer SS. Neural networks in human epilepsy: evidence of and implications for treatment. Epilepsia 2002;43(3):219–27. https://doi.org/10.1046/j.1528-1157.2002.26901.x.

22. Penfield W, Jasper H. Epilepsy and the functional anatomy of the human brain. Little, Brown; 1954.

23. Bailey P, Gibbs FA. The surgical treatment of psychomotor epilepsy. J Amer Med Assoc 1951;145(6):365–70. https://doi.org/10.1001/jama.1951.02920240001001.

24. Kahane P, Landré E, Minotti L, et al. The Bancaud and Talairach view on the epileptogenic zone: a working hypothesis. Epileptic Disord Int Epilepsy J Video-tape 2006;8(Suppl 2):S16–26.

25. Bonini F, McGonigal A, Trébuchon A, et al. Frontal lobe seizures: from clinical semiology to localization. Epilepsia 2014;55(2):264–77. https://doi.org/10.1111/epi.12490.

26. Richardson RM. Decision making in epilepsy surgery. Neurosurg Clin N Am 2020;31(3):471–9. https://doi.org/10.1016/j.nec.2020.03.014.

27. Ma BB, Fields MC, Knowlton RC, et al. Responsive neurostimulation for regional neocortical epilepsy. Epilepsia 2020;61(1):96–106. https://doi.org/10.1111/epi.16409.

28. Herlopian A, Cash SS, Eskandar EM, et al. Responsive neurostimulation targeting anterior thalamic nucleus in generalized epilepsy. Ann Clin Transl Neur 2019;6(10):2104–9. https://doi.org/10.1002/acn3.50858.

29. Elder C, Friedman D, Devinsky O, et al. Responsive neurostimulation targeting the anterior nucleus of the thalamus in 3 patients with treatment-resistant multi-focal epilepsy. Epilepsia Open 2019;4(1):187–92. https://doi.org/10.1002/epi4.12300.

30. Gummadavelli A, Zaveri HP, Spencer DD, et al. Expanding brain–computer inter-faces for controlling epilepsy networks: novel thalamic responsive neurostimula-tion in refractory epilepsy. Front Neurosci 2018;12:474. https://doi.org/10.3389/fnins.2018.00474.

31. Burdette DE, Haykal MA, Jarosiewicz B, et al. Brain-responsive corticothalamic stimulation in the centromedian nucleus for the treatment of regional neocortical epilepsy. Epilepsy Behav 2020;112:107354. https://doi.org/10.1016/j.yebeh.2020.107354.

32. Burdette D, Mirro EA, Lawrence M, et al. Brain-responsive corticothalamic stimu-lation in the pulvinar nucleus for the treatment of regional neocortical epilepsy: a case series. Epilepsia Open 2021;6(3):611–7. https://doi.org/10.1002/epi4.12524.

33. Homman-Ludiye J, Bourne JA. The medial pulvinar: function, origin and associ-ation with neurodevelopmental disorders. J Anat 2019;235(3):507–20. https://doi.org/10.1111/joa.12932.

34. Kokkinos V, Sisterson ND, Wozny TA, et al. Association of closed-loop brain stim-ulation neurophysiological features with seizure control among patients with focal epilepsy. Jama Neurol 2019;76(7):800–8. https://doi.org/10.1001/jamaneurol.2019.0658.

35. Khambhati AN, Shafi A, Rao VR, et al. Long-term brain network reorganization predicts responsive neurostimulation outcomes for focal epilepsy. Sci Transl Med 2021;13(608):eabf6588. https://doi.org/10.1126/scitranslmed.abf6588.

36. Hunter J, Jasper HH. Effects of thalamic stimulation in unanaesthetised animals; the arrest reaction and petit mal-like seizures, activation patterns and generalized convulsions. Electroen Clin Neuro 1949;1(3):305–24. https://doi.org/10.1016/0013-4694(49)90043-7.

37. Monnier M, Kalberer M, Krupp P. Functional antagonism between diffuse reticular and intralaminary recruiting projections in the medial thalamus. Exp Neurol 1960;2(3):271–89. https://doi.org/10.1016/0014-4886(60)90014-5.

38. Velasco F, Velasco M, Ogarrio C, et al. Electrical stimulation of the centromedian thalamic nucleus in the treatment of convulsive seizures: a preliminary report. Epilepsia 1987;28(4):421–30. https://doi.org/10.1111/j.1528-1157.1987.tb03668.x.

39. Velasco F, Velasco AL, Velasco M, et al. Operative neuromodulation. Acta Neurochir Suppl 2007;97(Pt 2):337–42. https://doi.org/10.1007/978-3-211-33081-4_38.

40. Velasco F, Velasco M, Velasco AL, et al. Electrical stimulation of the centromedian thalamic nucleus in control of seizures: long-term studies. Epilepsia 1995;36(1): 63–71. https://doi.org/10.1111/j.1528-1157.1995.tb01667.x.

41. Fisher RS, Uematsu S, Krauss GL, et al. Placebo-controlled pilot study of centromedian thalamic stimulation in treatment of intractable seizures. Epilepsia 1992; 33(5):841–51. https://doi.org/10.1111/j.1528-1157.1992.tb02192.x.

42. Valentín A, Navarrete EG, Chelvarajah R, et al. Deep brain stimulation of the centromedian thalamic nucleus for the treatment of generalized and frontal epilepsies. Epilepsia 2013;54(10):1823–33. https://doi.org/10.1111/epi.12352.

43. Dalic LJ, Warren AEL, Bulluss KJ, et al. DBS of thalamic centromedian nucleus for Lennox–Gastaut syndrome (ESTEL trial). Ann Neurol 2021. https://doi.org/10.1002/ana.26280.

44. Panayiotopoulos CP. A clinical guide to epileptic syndromes and their treatment. Springer, London. 2010:377-421. doi:10.1007/978-1-84628-644-5_13

45. Stevelink R, Koeleman BPC, Sander JW, et al. Refractory juvenile myoclonic epilepsy: a meta-analysis of prevalence and risk factors. Eur J Neurol 2019;26(6): 856–64. https://doi.org/10.1111/ene.13811.

46. Moeller F, Siebner HR, Wolff S, et al. Changes in activity of striato–thalamo–cortical network precede generalized spike wave discharges. Neuroimage 2008;39(4):1839–49. https://doi.org/10.1016/j.neuroimage.2007.10.058.

47. Benuzzi F, Mirandola L, Pugnaghi M, et al. Increased cortical BOLD signal anticipates generalized spike and wave discharges in adolescents and adults with idiopathic generalized epilepsies. Epilepsia 2012;53(4):622–30. https://doi.org/10.1111/j.1528-1167.2011.03385.x.

48. Velasco M, Velasco F, Velasco AL, et al. Epileptiform EEG activities of the centromedian thalamic nuclei in patients with intractable partial motor, complex partial, and generalized seizures. Epilepsia 1989;30(3):295–306. https://doi.org/10.1111/j.1528-1157.1989.tb05301.x.

49. Martín-López D, Jiménez-Jiménez D, Cabañés-Martínez L, et al. The role of thalamus versus cortex in epilepsy: evidence from human ictal centromedian recordings in patients assessed for deep brain stimulation. Int J Neural Syst 2017; 27(07):1750010. https://doi.org/10.1142/s0129065717500101.

50. Kokkinos V, Urban A, Sisterson ND, et al. Responsive neurostimulation of the thalamus improves seizure control in idiopathic generalized epilepsy: a case report. Neurosurgery 2020;87(5):E578–83. https://doi.org/10.1093/neuros/nyaa001.

51. Kwon C, Schupper AJ, Fields MC, et al. Centromedian thalamic responsive neurostimulation for Lennox-Gastaut epilepsy and autism. Ann Clin Transl Neur 2020; 7(10):2035–40. https://doi.org/10.1002/acn3.51173.

52. Welch WP, Hect JL, Abel TJ. Case report: responsive neurostimulation of the centromedian thalamic nucleus for the detection and treatment of seizures in pediatric primary generalized epilepsy. Front Neurol 2021;12:656585. https://doi.org/10.3389/fneur.2021.656585.

53. Baud MO, Kleen JK, Mirro EA, et al. Multi-day rhythms modulate seizure risk in epilepsy. Nat Commun 2018;9(1):88. https://doi.org/10.1038/s41467-017-02577-y.

54. Leguia MG, Andrzejak RG, Rummel C, et al. Seizure cycles in focal epilepsy. JAMA Neurol 2021;78(4):454–63. https://doi.org/10.1001/jamaneurol.2020.5370.

55. Hirsch LJ, Mirro EA, Salanova V, et al. Mesial temporal resection following long-term ambulatory intracranial EEG monitoring with a direct brain-responsive neurostimulation system. Epilepsia 2020;61(3):408–20. https://doi.org/10.1111/epi.16442.

56. Skarpaas TL, Tcheng TK, Morrell MJ. Clinical and electrocorticographic response to antiepileptic drugs in patients treated with responsive stimulation. Epilepsy Behav 2018;83:192–200. https://doi.org/10.1016/j.yebeh.2018.04.003.

57. Quraishi IH, Mercier MR, Skarpaas TL, et al. Early detection rate changes from a brain-responsive neurostimulation system predict efficacy of newly added anti-seizure drugs. Epilepsia 2020;61(1):138–48. https://doi.org/10.1111/epi.16412.

58. Sajobi TT, Josephson CB, Sawatzky R, et al. Quality of life in epilepsy: same questions, but different meaning to different people. Epilepsia 2021;62(9):2094–102. https://doi.org/10.1111/epi.17012.

59. Mackow MJ, Krishnan B, Bingaman WE, et al. Increased caffeine intake leads to worsening of electrocorticographic epileptiform discharges as recorded with a responsive neurostimulation device. Clin Neurophysiol 2016;127(6):2341–2. https://doi.org/10.1016/j.clinph.2016.03.012.

60. Roach ATI, Chaitanya G, Riley KO, et al. Optimizing therapies for neurobehavioral comorbidities of epilepsy using chronic ambulatory electrocorticography. Epilepsy Behav 2020;102:106814. https://doi.org/10.1016/j.yebeh.2019.106814.

61. Desai SA, Tcheng TK, Morrell MJ. Quantitative electrocorticographic biomarkers of clinical outcomes in mesial temporal lobe epileptic patients treated with the RNS® system. Clin Neurophysiol 2019;130(8):1364–74.

62. Stypulkowski PH, Stanslaski SR, Jensen RM, et al. Brain stimulation for epilepsy – local and remote modulation of network excitability. Brain Stimul 2014;7(3):350–8. https://doi.org/10.1016/j.brs.2014.02.002.

63. Stanslaski S, Afshar P, Cong P, et al. Design and validation of a fully implantable, chronic, closed-loop neuromodulation device with concurrent sensing and stimulation. IEEE Trans Neural Syst Rehabil Eng 2012;20(4):410–21. https://doi.org/10.1109/tnsre.2012.2183617.

64. Lipski WJ, DeStefino VJ, Stanslaski SR, et al. Sensing-enabled hippocampal deep brain stimulation in idiopathic nonhuman primate epilepsy. J Neurophysiol 2015;113(4):1051–62. https://doi.org/10.1152/jn.00619.2014.

65. Wozny TA, Lipski WJ, Alhourani A, et al. Effects of hippocampal low-frequency stimulation in idiopathic non-human primate epilepsy assessed via a remote-sensing-enabled neurostimulator. Exp Neurol 2017;294:68–77. https://doi.org/10.1016/j.expneurol.2017.05.003.

66. Gregg NM, Marks VS, Sladky V, et al. Anterior nucleus of the thalamus seizure detection in ambulatory humans. Epilepsia 2021;62(10):e158–64. https://doi.org/10.1111/epi.17047.

67. Sokolov E, Sisterson ND, Hussein H, et al. Intracranial monitoring contributes to seizure freedom for temporal lobectomy patients with non-concordant pre-operative data. Epilepsia Open 2021. https://doi.org/10.1002/epi4.12483.

68. Tandon N, Tong BA, Friedman ER, et al. Analysis of morbidity and outcomes associated with use of subdural grids vs stereoelectroencephalography in patients with intractable epilepsy. JAMA Neurol 2019;76(6):672–81. https://doi.org/10.1001/jamaneurol.2019.0098.

69. Guye M, Régis J, Tamura M, et al. The role of corticothalamic coupling in human temporal lobe epilepsy. Brain 2006;129(7):1917–28. https://doi.org/10.1093/brain/awl151.

70. Pizarro D, Ilyas A, Chaitanya G, et al. Spectral organization of focal seizures within the thalamotemporal network. Ann Clin Transl Neur 2019;6(9):1836–48. https://doi.org/10.1002/acn3.50880.

71. Romeo A, Roach ATI, Toth E, et al. Early ictal recruitment of midline thalamus in mesial temporal lobe epilepsy. Ann Clin Transl Neur 2019;6(8):1552–8. https://doi.org/10.1002/acn3.50835.

72. Yu T, Wang X, Li Y, et al. High-frequency stimulation of anterior nucleus of thalamus desynchronizes epileptic network in humans. Brain 2018;141(9):2631–43. https://doi.org/10.1093/brain/awy187.

73. Zhang K, Bhatia S, Oh MY, et al. Long-term results of thalamic deep brain stimulation for essential tremor: clinical article. J Neurosurg 2010;112(6):1271–6. https://doi.org/10.3171/2009.10.jns09371.

74. Martin AJ, Starr PA, Ostrem JL, et al. Hemorrhage detection and incidence during magnetic resonance-guided deep brain stimulator implantations. Stereot Funct Neuros 2017;95(5):307–14. https://doi.org/10.1159/000479287.

75. McGovern RA, Ruggieri P, Bulacio J, et al. Risk analysis of hemorrhage in stereoelectroencephalography procedures. Epilepsia 2019;60(3):571–80. https://doi.org/10.1111/epi.14668.

Intraoperative Neuromonitoring

Andrew K. Wong, MD[a], Jay L. Shils, PhD[b], Sepehr B. Sani, MD[a],
Richard W. Byrne, MD[a,*]

KEYWORDS

- Somatosensory evoked potentials • Motor evoked potentials
- Electroencephalogram • Electromyography • Brainstem auditory evoked response
- Direct cortical stimulation

KEY POINTS

- Intraoperative neuromonitoring provides critical real-time information regarding surgical anatomic eloquence.
- The different intraoperative neuromonitoring modalities monitor specific neuropathways. Understanding the goal and anatomic relationships involved in the surgical procedure is critical in determining not only which modalities to use but also how they should be used and interpreted.
- Patient selection is key in the successful implementation of intraoperative neuromonitoring and considerations such as integrity of monitored neuropathway and patient tolerance, particularly for modalities that require the patient to be awake, must be taken into account.

INTRODUCTION

Intraoperative neurophysiological monitoring (IONM) is the evaluation of the nervous system during surgical procedures where injury to critical neurologic structures is possible. IONM can be divided into 2 classes: (1) detection of an iatrogenic injury allowing for reversal or minimization of the injury; and (2) localization (mapping) of critical neural structures during the procedure to avoid damaging those structures.[1] IONM is fast becoming a mainstay in a variety of surgical procedures, including scoliosis correction surgery, intramedullary spinal cord tumor resection, and acoustic neuroma resection. In other procedures, it is used to improve surgical decision making.[1–5] To properly interpret IONM data, the neurophysiologist needs to know the physiologic state of the patient, the competency of the technologist operating the equipment, the

[a] Department of Neurosurgery, Rush University, 1725 West Harrison Street #855, Chicago, IL 60612, USA; [b] Department of Anesthesiology, Rush University, 1653 West Congress Pkwy, Jelke 7, Chicago, IL 60612, USA
* Corresponding author:
E-mail address: Richard_Byrne@Rush.edu

Neurol Clin 40 (2022) 375–389
https://doi.org/10.1016/j.ncl.2021.11.010
0733-8619/22/© 2022 Elsevier Inc. All rights reserved.
neurologic.theclinics.com

state of the monitoring equipment, what the surgeon is doing, the preoperative examination of the patient (including the patient's history), and the anesthesia administered to the patient.[6]

IONM data are either obtained quasi continuously (somatosensory and motor evoked potentials [SSEP and MEP], electroencephalography [EEG], and free-run electromyography [fEMG]) or at specific time points such as for functional-anatomic localization (direct nerve and cortical stimulation). Evoked potentials require a stimulus applied at one point at the nervous system while recording the response at another point. To achieve optimal responses, all neural elements (axon, synapse, and neuromuscular junction) in the signal pathway need to be functioning at some minimal level.

All time-locked electrophysiological signals have 3 distinct properties: (1) the amplitude of the response; (2) the latency, or time of the response from the start of the stimulation; and (3) the morphology.

MODALITIES

Common IONM modalities include: (1) SSEPs which evaluate the sensory pathway from a point distal to surgical intervention to the sensory nuclei or cortex in the brain or brainstem; (2) MEPs which evaluate the largest 2% of fibers in the corticospinal tract from the brain to the muscle via the alpha motor neuron connecting the primary and secondary motor neurons; (3) fEMG records muscle activity resulting from potential irritation of a nerve innervating that muscle; (4) triggered EMG (tEMG) records muscle activity in response to stimulation of a nerve; (5) brainstem auditory evoked responses (BAERs) evaluate the sensory pathways of the auditory system from the cochlea through the auditory brainstem nuclei; (6) direct nerve recordings evaluate signal conduction through specific nerve segments; (7) EEG records the background activity of the superficial cortical layers of the brain; (8) single cell microelectrode recordings record the activity of individual neurons for localization purposes; and (9) direct cortical stimulation and mapping whereby cortical and subcortical structures are stimulated directly to localize eloquent regions.

Given that the main areas of anesthetic action are at the synapse, the overall effects of anesthetic agents on axonal membrane properties (ie, nerve conduction) are negligible, except at extremely high doses. The usual rule is that the more synapses a neural signal has to travel through, the greater the anesthetic effect. Yet, even a signal synapse, such as the one between the upper and lower motor neuron (αMN) can significantly be affected by anesthesia. Each monitoring modality is affected differently by anesthetic agents depending on the drug effects on specific neurotransmitters and the types of synapses involved in the monitored pathway. Responses are also affected differently depending on the location and mechanism of neural dysfunction or injury (eg, neural or vascular).

ELECTROENCEPHALOGRAM

The EEG records the averaged extracellular field potentials of the spontaneous activity of cortical neurons near the recording electrodes. The number of neurons recorded is a function of the location of the electrode (scalp, cortical, or intraparenchymal), the size of the electrode, the distance between the electrode and the neurons, and the tissue between the neurons and the electrode. For recordings, there is an "active" and "reference" electrode, such that the total activity recorded is the difference in activity between these electrodes. The activity in locations distant from the electrodes will have no impact on the recorded data. Thus, changes in cortical activity that are distant from the electrodes will be missed. Hence, the EEG is usually recorded using several pairs of electrodes over the areas of interest. EEG is recorded using a standard 21-channel electrode set, with placement based on the 10 to 20 electrode localization system,[7] (**Fig. 1**), the spatial resolution of each electrode placed on the scalp is approximately 6 cm.[8] A common intraoperative technique is to use 8 electrodes, which approximate a spatial resolution of approximately 10 to 12 cm (extrapolating from Gevins and colleagues[9]), thus focal effects may be missed.

The overall electrical activity of the brain is dependent on the availability of metabolites, including oxygen. When these are compromised, it is reflected quickly in loss of synaptic function. Intraoperative EEG can therefore be an indirect measure of cortical ischemia (**Fig. 2**). EEG is also helpful in detecting electrical seizure activity. Thus, the most common procedures where EEG is used are where the chance of vascular insult is high and during intracranial motor mapping procedures to identify seizure activity resulting from cortical stimulation.

As the spectral content of the EEG is critical to localizing insult to the brain, many systems include tempero/spectral plots to show the energy in the key EEG spectral

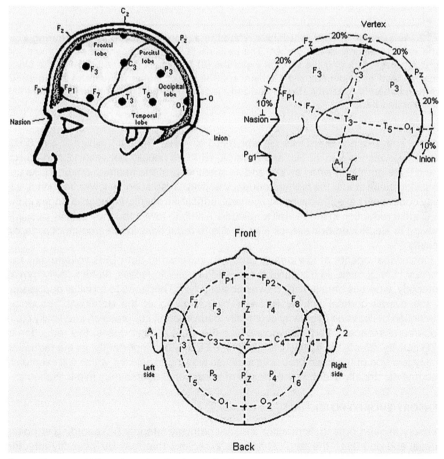

Fig. 1. The 10 to 20 location of scalp electrodes for EEG and SSEP recordings. Common placement of SSEP electrodes are at Fp, C3′ (about 2 cm behind C3), Cz′, and C4′, whereas for EEG, a full set will use all electrodes shown on the right image. MEP stimulation electrodes are usually placed just in front of C3-C4 or C1-C2.

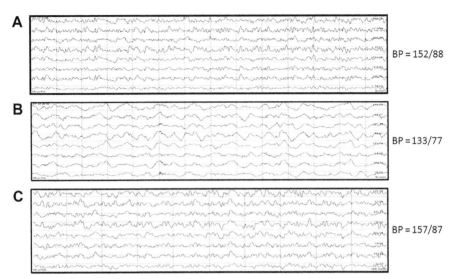

Fig. 2. An example of cortical ischemia related to a change in blood pressure during a carotid endarterectomy procedure. (*A*) The baseline EEG under general anesthesia with no burst suppression during the surgical exposure. (*B*) The effect of a reduction in the blood pressure. Notice the generalized δ activity and the loss of higher frequencies (θ and α). (*C*) A return to baseline activity. The generalized δ is gone and the higher frequency θ and small α are coming back.

bands. These bands are: Delta (δ), which is 1 to 4 Hz; Theta (θ), which is 4 to 8 Hz; Alpha (α), which is 8 to 12 Hz; and Beta (β), which is usually between 12 and 30 Hz. α and β are dominant when awake and as anesthesia starts to affect the brain. As unconsciousness starts, the higher frequency activity is replaced by lower frequency activity commonly called "slowing." In general, critical iatrogenic-induced changes in the EEG are a reduction in the overall amplitude, a shift to low-frequency activity possible moving to electrocerebral silence (**Fig. 3**) due to reductions in the amount of synaptic activity.[10]

Inhalational agents at low doses cause an increase in both EEG voltage and frequency.[11] In general, as the patient moves to unconsciousness, alpha activity moves anteriorly, whereas beta activity moves posteriorly.[12] This leads to an initial depression in the overall cortical activity followed by a slowing of the dominant frequency. Continued depression of activity eventually leads to burst suppression and finally electrocerebral silence at very high doses (see **Fig. 3**).[13] At high doses, this reduction in EEG activity affects the ability to interpret the EEG. Most importantly, as the reduction in oxygenation of the brain produces a diffuse slowing of activity, which will eventually become electrically silent, higher doses of inhalational agents may mimic ischemia.

SENSORY EVOKED POTENTIALS

Sensory evoked potentials monitor sensory pathway integrity by recording at points cranial and caudal to the surgical field, or in regions that may be indirectly affected by surgery (ie, aneurysm surgery potentially causing ischemic effects at the sensory cortex). A distal nerve is stimulated and responses are recorded at specific neural junctures along the ascending sensory pathway. Given the low amplitude of this response, it is very difficult to obtain a quality response using a single stimulus, thus

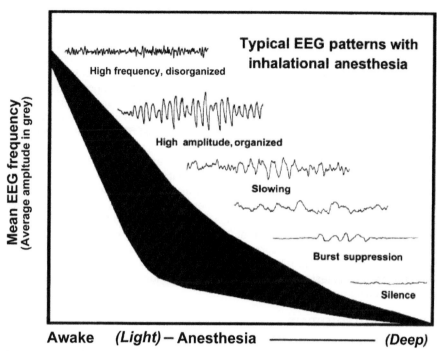

Awake   *(Light)* – Anesthesia ———————— *(Deep)*

Fig. 3. A generalized image of the EEG at different anesthetic states. In the awake state, the EEG shows low-amplitude higher frequency activity (in this case, the EEG is showing a predominant α activity). As the anesthetic starts to take effect, the α is reduced and the low-amplitude β activity starts shifting eventually to higher amplitude activity modulated by some lower frequency θ and δ activity. As the patient gets deeper, the higher frequencies are completely lost and the most predominant activity moves from θ and δ activity to burst suppression and finally electrocerebral silence. (*From* Shils JL, Sloan TB. Intraoperative neuromonitoring. Int Anesthesiol Clin. 2015;53(1):53 to 73. https://doi.org/10.1097/AIA. 0000000000000043; with permission).

multiple trials are performed and the results of those trials are averaged to remove the noise and enhance the signal.

The location of the surgery dictates the stimulus and recording locations. Common SSEP stimulation sites are as follows: (1) posterior tibial nerve at the medial ankle; (2) the common peroneal nerve behind the knee; (3) the median nerve at the wrist; (4) the ulnar nerve at the wrist; and (5) the ulnar nerve at the cubital tunnel in the elbow. Recording electrodes are placed at peripheral locations (popliteal fossa and Erb's point), along the spine (cervical spine [C7] and/or thoracolumbar spine [T12]), and over the sensory cortex [Fpz and C3′, C4′, Cz′] [see **]**).

Multiple factors affect the transmission of these signals, such as height, temperature, nerve compression, neural perfusion, anesthetic type, and dose, as well as some metabolic diseases. Given the primary effect of anesthetic agents is on synaptic transmission, the greater the number of synapses between the stimulus and recording sites the greater the effect of the anesthetic agent on that response.

ELECTROMYOGRAPHY

Electromyography monitors the spontaneous (background) (fEMG) or "triggered" (tEMG) activity in muscles by placing 2 electrodes into the body of the muscle approximately 1 cm apart. The *fEMG* method allows for continuous monitoring of any mechanical or metabolic iatrogenic irritation of nerves without the need for the surgeon to use an instrument to stimulate the nerve. In some surgical procedures, the surgeon needs to be able to accurately locate nervous tissue that may not easily be differentiated in the surgical field or to "map" the nervous structures in the surgical field. This is done using a probe that applies a focused stimulus ("trigger") to the tissue while monitoring for time-locked responses that indicate the nervous tissue was activated. Procedures where this technique is invaluable include skull base and/or ENT procedures where cranial, and most commonly, the facial nerves may not be easily identified or entry points may need to be localized. Using variations in stimulus intensity needed to activate the nerve, response amplitude, and response delay help determine the relative position of the nerve to the stimulator probe.

The EMG requires the neural signal to pass through the neuromuscular junction which is where the muscle relaxants block nerve transmission. The most common method to assess the degree of neuromuscular blockade is the train-of-four (TOF) response where 4 stimuli are applied at 2 Hz and the number of responses and their amplitudes are analyzed. To assure the best possible EMG response, a majority of groups recommend that the TOF response should be 4 of 4.[14] To get the most appropriate TOF result, the test should be performed in the muscles where the critical EMG response is being observed.[14]

MOTOR EVOKED POTENTIALS

MEPs monitor the efferent motor pathways from the motor cortex and fibers in the internal capsule to the muscle via the largest 1% to 2% of axons in corticospinal (or corticobulbar) tracts.[15] To evoke the MEP, transcranial electrical stimulation using a cathode (−electrode) placed on the ipsilateral scalp overlying the motor strip referenced to an anode (+electrode) placed on the contralateral scalp. Transcranial motor evoked potentials are produced when stimuli directly activate the axons of the large Betz cells located in the motor cortex, not the cell bodies. This fact is important because stronger stimulation activates the motor pathway deeper in the brain. Hence for monitoring when the motor cortex is at risk, "large" stimulation amplitude may activate corticospinal axons by *jumping* over the actual area of surgical interest to deeper structures, thus missing iatrogenic injury in the cortex[15,16] (**Fig. 4**). During open cranial procedures, MEPs may also be generated by directly stimulating the cortex and/or subcortical white matter.

Once an action potential is initiated, the activity travels down the corticospinal tract to activate the alpha-motor neurons (αMN) in laminae IX of the spinal cord to produce muscle compound action potentials (**Fig. 5**).

The effect of anesthetics on the motor pathway at the αMN is sufficient to prevent the recording of myogenic MEPs with a single transcranial stimulation pulse. To overcome this problem, a multipulse technique consisting of a train of 3 to 9 pulses with an interstimulus interval between 1 and 4 milliseconds[17,18] is used. This multipulse technique can cause significant patient movement. In most cases, this movement is acceptable yet, a key precaution is the addition of bite blocks to minimize tongue and lip lacerations.[19]

BRAINSTEM AUDITORY EVOKED RESPONSES

BAERs monitor the auditory pathway from the distal VIIIth to the auditory radiations although for cranial surgery applications monitoring is done to the inferior colliculus (see **Fig. 5**). This response is also known as the auditory brainstem response and

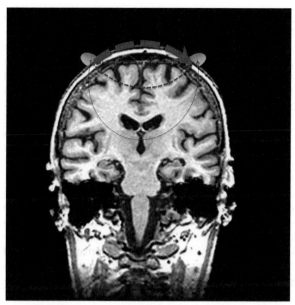

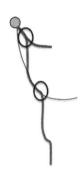

Fig. 4. The left image shows the penetration of the stimulation current into the brain (represented by the thickness of the red current *lines*). As can be seen, most of the energy is lost in the scalp and skull. This is about 80% of the stimulation current. As one looks deeper in the brain, the current becomes much less. There is a specific threshold that the axons will fire at. As the current increases, the location of the activation will be deeper in the brain. The image on the right demonstrates this. The most likely activation point is at bends in the axon. If the current reaching the deeper structure is strong enough that is the point of activation irrespective of what happens above that point.

- Wave I: distal cochlear nerve
- Wave II: proximal cochlear nerve   } Ipsilateral
- Wave III: cochlear nucleus

- Wave IV: superior olivary nucleus/lateral lemniscus
- Wave V: lateral lemniscus / inferior colliculus   }

Contralateral

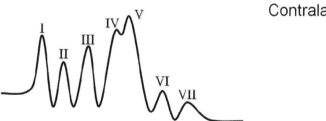

Fig. 5. A graphical representation of the brainstem auditory response with the location of the peak generators. Using this information, the IONM team can determine the potential location of the iatrogenic injury to the system.

the brainstem auditory evoked potentials. BAERs are performed by applying a full band click to the patient and recording responses from the distal VIIIth nerve (wave I), the proximal VIIIth nerve and the cochlear nucleus (wave II), the cochlear nucleus (wave III), the superior olivary nucleus and the nuclei of the lateral lemniscus (wave IV), and the lateral lemniscus and inferior colliculus (wave V). It should be noted that the actual location of each peak is still debated so you may find different generators in different texts. Waves I through III are recorded from the ipsilateral nerve and brainstem nuclei, whereas waves IV and V are recorded from the contralateral brainstem. It is also possible to record directly from the VIIIth nerve. BAER can be used to monitor the integrity of the VIIIth nerve, the integrity of the labyrinthian artery, and segments of the brainstem.

The applied clicks are usually of 100 to 200 microseconds in duration and 130 dB normal hearing level and a rate of 0.5 to 100 clicks per second (although a 11–13 Hz is what is commonly used in the operating room). In some cases, masking noise is used in the contralateral ear to minimize the effects from that ear on the recordings but many times in the OR masking noise is not used. The clicks can either be rarefaction (initial portion of the click "pulls" the eardrum), condensation (the initial click "pushes" the eardrum), or alternating which can be used to help minimize the stimulation artifact. Each of these polarities can affect the latency and shape of the responses, which need to be taken into account when switching between them in the operating room. Changing the polarity can help minimize noise that obscures the results.

Waves I, III, and V are the most prominent waves and are thus the primary waves used in evaluating potential iatrogenic injury. Both amplitude and latency changes are indicators of potential injury to some part of the system. Changes in the latency between waves I and III can indicate a problem in the VIIIth nerve, whereas changes in the latency between waves III and V can indicate issues in the brainstem. The temperature has a significant effect on the BAER latency with colder temperatures increasing the latency of each wave, thus this would not be related to iatrogenic injury. Latency and interpeak intervals increase by about 7% for each 1° C drop in temperature.[20] Traction or compression of the VIIIth nerve usually show as progressive changes over time with an increase in latency between waves I and III with little to no change in the latency between waves III and V.[20] These changes can be reversible. Damage to the labyrinthian artery or anterior inferior cerebellar artery on the other hand is usually not reversible and can show as a quick loss of all responses (waves I through V). In a systematic review of the literature, Thirumala and colleagues showed that specificity was high (98%), indicating that patients who woke with a deficit had a change in the BAER, whereas sensitivity was low (74%), indicating that even with a change in the OR some patient still woke with hearing intact.[21] Loss of wave V alone does not necessarily mean hearing will be lost at the end of surgery because temporary dispersion of responses do inflict minor mechanical injury.[20,21]

DIRECT CORTICAL STIMULATION

Intracranial surgery requires intimate knowledge of cortical and subcortical function to minimize postoperative neurologic deficits. Understanding the anatomic relationship of these areas with both surface and deep landmarks allows the surgeon to determine the safety of a planned resection. However, even with an extensive understanding of such relationships, individual variations in functional arrangement exist.[22–27] Furthermore, pathologic distortion of cortical eloquence either through mass effect or functional rearrangement often makes reliance on normal anatomic functional arrangement unacceptably inaccurate.[28–30] Though advanced imaging such as functional MRI, tractography, and magnetoencephalography provides patient-specific anatomic and functional detail, the lack of adequate granularity in such data often precludes them from being authoritative methods in determining surgical approaches and influencing intraoperative decision making. Direct cortical stimulation and mapping provide real-time information regarding the cortical or subcortical region of interest allowing for informed decision making by the surgeon. In this section, we will discuss the indications and benefits of this intraoperative neuromonitoring technique as well as its limitations.

Indication and Patient Selection

When eloquent regions of the brain are suspected to be intimately involved in the pathologic process, direct intraoperative cortical mapping should be considered. Cortical mapping is particularly informative when delineating areas involved in motor, sensory, and speech functions. Although advanced imaging modalities are often not detailed enough to direct operative decision making, they nevertheless are useful in approximating these eloquent areas and determining the need for cortical mapping. Therefore, cortical mapping is not a replacement for these preoperative investigations but rather a consequence of them. Although mapping of the motor cortex can be done with the patient fully anesthetized, mapping of the sensory and language cortex must be done with the patient awake. As such, the capacity of the patient's ability to tolerate an awake craniotomy should be assessed when considering sensory and language mapping. Extensive neuropsychiatric testing of language function must also be completed as language mapping requires adequate baseline function to provide a reliable and reproducible reference.

Surgical Considerations

Intraoperative cortical mapping requires considerable coordination among many different teams, including neurosurgeon, anesthesiologists, neurophysiologists, speech therapists, operating room nurses, and surgical technicians. The expectations and goals of surgery should be thoroughly reviewed with all teams involved to ensure optimal surgical outcomes. Premedication with an anxiolytic is typically given in the preoperative area before arrival in the operating room. A local anesthetic is then injected subcutaneously circumferentially in the scalp. If frameless intraoperative neuronavigation is used, the patient is placed in a skull clamp for rigid fixation with a further local anesthetic injected at the pin sites. After the surgical site is prepped and sterilized, the surgical drapes are placed in a fashion that allows ancillary staff to access the patient's face and contralateral extremities for assessment of function.

Stimulation Mapping

Identification of the central sulcus
An important landmark in many intracranial surgeries is the central sulcus as it defines the sensory and motor cortices. Although preoperative imaging and intraoperative observations of gyri and sulci can provide an approximation of the central sulcus, definitive identification is sometimes needed. SSEPs using a cortical electrode strip can be used in such situations to identify the central sulcus.[31,32] After identification of the Sylvian fissure, the electrode strip is placed over the cortical surface perpendicular to the presumed central sulcus approximately 3 cm above the Sylvian. An N20 wave is recorded using a stimulus to the contralateral median nerve. A phase reversal in the wave is seen in the recordings from the sensory cortex to the motor cortex, identifying the central sulcus (**Fig. 6**). This process is repeated 2 to 3 times moving rostrally to

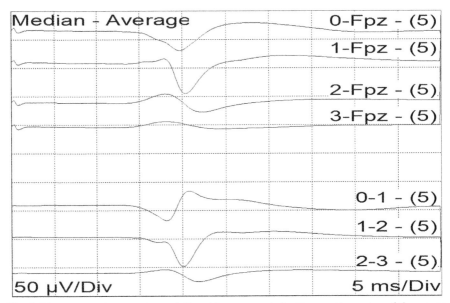

Fig. 6. Phase reversal across channels 2 and 3 seen as a deflection and inversion of the waves as you move sequentially across the electrode strip that is placed perpendicularly and traversing across the presumed central sulcus.

further delineate the central sulcus, which is then labeled for identification (**Fig. 7**). Phase reversal is particularly useful in identifying the central sulcus when there is distorting pathology and is a technique that can be done in a fully anesthetized or awake patient.

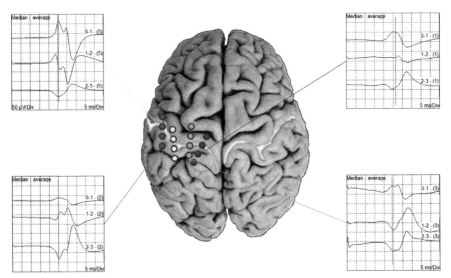

Fig. 7. Mapping of the central sulcus laterally using phase reversal by sequentially moving the electrode strip laterally (as represented by the colored dots).

Sensorimotor stimulation

After the central sulcus is determined through phase reversal on SSEP recordings, direct cortical stimulation can then be used for specific mapping of functional regions of the sensory and motor cortex. This is particularly of use when pathology has caused distortion in the normal anatomy. Stimulation of the sensory cortex begins in the suprasylvian area and must be done while the patient is awake. A unipolar or bipolar stimulator is used to provide a 1 to 2 mA stimulus at a 60 Hz frequency and 0.5 to 1 ms pulse duration. The cortex in question is sequentially stimulated in ∼1 cm^2 plots where the stimulator is placed for 3 seconds and the patient is asked to report changes in sensation such as paresthesias. This can be repeated to map out the tongue, lip, and hand somatotopic areas. To map lower extremity cortical representation, an electrode strip may be used to stimulate the difficult-to-reach interhemispheric fissure.

Mapping of the motor cortex can be done with the patient awake or fully anesthetized.[33] Stimulation is conducted in a similar fashion beginning at the suprasylvian area of the precentral gyrus. Higher amplitudes of stimulation may be required in a fully anesthetized patient to reach the threshold for response, though amplitudes above 6 mA are not recommended. The amplitude is increased gradually until movement in the contralateral limb is noted. Alternatively, changes in electromyography recordings of the contralateral limb can be noted for response.

After discharges immediately following stimulus should be carefully monitored and treated. Focal or generalized seizures as a result of intraoperative cortical mapping occur with an incidence of 8.8% to 35%.[34,35] These can typically be terminated by irrigating the cortex with chilled Ringer's solution for 5 to 10 seconds. If this does not terminate the seizures, a bolus of propofol can be given followed by methohexital for continued refractory seizures.[36] As with the treatment of any seizures, careful and continued assessment for the need to secure the patient's airway via intubation is paramount.

Language mapping

Language mapping is used in patients with pathology in the region of the dominant perisylvian frontotemporal lobes. Like sensory mapping, language mapping must be done in an awake patient. As it requires constant assessment of the patient's language function, extensive preoperative testing of the patient's baseline language function must be conducted. Patients with existing significant language deficits or those who cannot tolerate a physically demanding awake surgery would not benefit from language mapping.

Both unipolar and bipolar stimulation has been described though recent trends have shifted toward the former. Although bipolar stimulation is considered more sensitive in detecting clinically eloquent areas, unipolar stimulation has demonstrated a lower incidence of seizure induction. After discharges induced by stimulation, as measured by an electrocorticography grid, can lead to false-positive readings. Stimulation typically begins with an amplitude of 1 mA at 60 Hz with a pulse duration of 1 millisecond and is carried out in a similar fashion to sensory mapping wherein the stimulus is applied for approximately 3 seconds and speech arrest is monitored. Stimulus amplitude should be tailored such that it remains just below levels that would induce after discharges. Each cortical plot is stimulated 3 times. Counting, object naming, and word reading are tested with each sequential stimulus application. If the patient is unable to complete these tasks for 2 of 3 stimuli, the cortical plot is considered eloquent and positive for language function.[37] As opposed to sensory or motor mapping, the cortex is mapped out in comparatively smaller 3 mm^2 plots.

Once mapping is completed and all relevant cortical areas are labeled, resection can commence in a cortically "silent" area. All areas positive for language function should be avoided with a 1 cm margin or up to an adjacent sulcus. Anterior temporal lobe resections of the dominant hemisphere within 2 cm of identified language areas may result in mild aphasia that tends to improve over time.[38–40]

Should no surgically exposed area test positive for language function, a consensus should be reached among the neurosurgeon, anesthesiologist, and neurophysiologist that all aspects of mapping from sedation level to technique and equipment functionality were satisfactory and appropriate. It is also critical in such scenarios to have determined the after-discharge threshold as a positive control and to identify the maximal safe stimulus amplitude.

Subcortical stimulation mapping
Some intracranial procedures require exploration beyond the cortical surface, particularly in tumor resection surgery. Subcortical white matter tracts can be just as clinically relevant as the cortex and, when suspected, their preservation should be of equal importance. Mapping of the subcortical white matter can be completed in a similar fashion to determine eloquence before surgical manipulation or resection. Subcortical mapping is often carried out using unipolar stimulation and requires higher amplitude stimulation when compared with cortical mapping.

Subcortical mapping
As the surgical dissection and resection continues beyond the cortical surface and gray matter, it is critical to maintain an understanding of the eloquent deep white matter tracts. In fact, successful cortical mapping-directed dissection can be undermined if deeper subcortical tracts are disrupted. Subcortical stimulation mapping refers to the stimulation of subcortical white matter to identify descending or ascending white matter tracts that connect cortical gray matter with deep gray nuclei. Pathologic distortion in normal anatomy holds especially true within the more grossly homogenous subcortical white matter, making subcortical stimulation mapping and intraoperative neuronavigation especially important in identifying and maintaining the integrity of important subcortical pathways.[41] The technical aspects of subcortical stimulation mapping are much the same as cortical mapping though typically entails higher stimulation parameters and requires incremental resection and frequent confirmation with stimulation and neuronavigation before proceeding.

CLINICS CARE POINTS

- The use of intraoperative neuromonitoring must be tailored for each case.
- Prior to the utilization of any intraoperative neuromonitoring modality, careful consideration should be paid to its specific clinical utility, if any, and how it may affect operative decision making.
- A team-based approach among the neurosurgeon, anesthesiologist, neuromonitoring technician, and neurologist is key to the successful implementation and use of intraoperative neuromonitoring.

REFERENCES

1. Sala F, Manganotti P, Grossauer S, et al. Intraoperative neurophysiology of the motor system in children: a tailored approach. Childs Nerv Syst 2010;26(4): 473–90. https://doi.org/10.1007/s00381-009-1081-6.

2. Arle JE, Shils JL. Neurosurgical decision-making with IOM: DBS surgery. Neurophysiol Clin 2007;37(6):449–55. https://doi.org/10.1016/j.neucli.2007.09.010.

3. Deletis V, Sala F. Intraoperative neurophysiological monitoring of the spinal cord during spinal cord and spine surgery: a review focus on the corticospinal tracts. Clin Neurophysiol 2008;119(2):248–64. https://doi.org/10.1016/j.clinph.2007.09.135.

4. Sala F, Palandri G, Basso E, et al. Motor evoked potential monitoring improves outcome after surgery for intramedullary spinal cord tumors: a historical control study. Neurosurgery 2006;58(6):1129–43. https://doi.org/10.1227/01.Neu.0000215948.97195.58 [discussion 1129–43].

5. Nuwer MR. Handbook of clinical neurophysiology, vol. 8. New York: Elsevier; 2008.

6. Skinner SA, Cohen BA, Morledge DE, et al. Practice guidelines for the supervising professional: intraoperative neurophysiological monitoring. J Clin Monit Comput 2014;28(2):103–11. https://doi.org/10.1007/s10877-013-9496-8.

7. Fazel-Rezai R. Brain-computer interface systems - recent progress and future prospects. Norderstedt, Germany: BoD – Books on Demand; 2013.

8. Aguiar P, David A, Paulo S, et al. EEG solver- brain activity and genetic algorithms 2000. Available at: http://www.acm.org/conferences/sac/sac2000/Proceed/FinalPapers/BC-07/.

9. Gevins A, Le J, Martin NK, et al. High resolution EEG: 124-channel recording, spatial deblurring and MRI integration methods. Electroencephalogr Clin Neurophysiol 1994;90(5):337–58. https://doi.org/10.1016/0013-4694(94)90050-7.

10. Jameson LC, Janik DJ, Sloan TB. Electrophysiologic monitoring in neurosurgery. Anesthesiol Clin 2007;25(3):605–30. https://doi.org/10.1016/j.anclin.2007.05.004, x.

11. Nuwer MR, Emerson RG, Galloway G, et al. Evidence-based guideline update: intraoperative spinal monitoring with somatosensory and transcranial electrical motor evoked potentials. J Clin Neurophysiol 2012;29(1):101–8. https://doi.org/10.1097/WNP.0b013e31824a397e.

12. Jameson LC, Sloan TB. Using EEG to monitor anesthesia drug effects during surgery. J Clin Monit Comput 2006;20(6):445–72. https://doi.org/10.1007/s10877-006-9044-x.

13. Rampil IJ, Lockhart SH, Eger EI 2nd, et al. The electroencephalographic effects of desflurane in humans. Anesthesiology 1991;74(3):434–9. https://doi.org/10.1097/00000542-199103000-00008.

14. Leppanen RE. Intraoperative monitoring of segmental spinal nerve root function with free-run and electrically-triggered electromyography and spinal cord function with reflexes and F-responses. A position statement by the American Society of Neurophysiological Monitoring. J Clin Monit Comput 2005;19(6):437–61. https://doi.org/10.1007/s10877-005-0086-2.

15. Kaye AD. Principles of neurophysiological assessment. New York: Springer; 2013.

16. Macdonald DB, Skinner S, Shils J, et al. Intraoperative motor evoked potential monitoring - a position statement by the American Society of Neurophysiological Monitoring. Clin Neurophysiol 2013;124(12):2291–316. https://doi.org/10.1016/j.clinph.2013.07.025.

17. Szelényi A, Kothbauer KF, Deletis V. Transcranial electric stimulation for intraoperative motor evoked potential monitoring: stimulation parameters and electrode montages. Clin Neurophysiol 2007;118(7):1586–95. https://doi.org/10.1016/j.clinph.2007.04.008.

18. Taniguchi M, Cedzich C, Schramm J. Modification of cortical stimulation for motor evoked potentials under general anesthesia: technical description. Neurosurgery 1993;32(2):219–26. https://doi.org/10.1227/00006123-199302000-00011.

19. MacDonald DB. Safety of intraoperative transcranial electrical stimulation motor evoked potential monitoring. J Clin Neurophysiol 2002;19(5):416–29. https://doi.org/10.1097/00004691-200210000-00005.

20. Legatt AD. Mechanisms of intraoperative brainstem auditory evoked potential changes. J Clin Neurophysiol 2002;19(5):396–408. https://doi.org/10.1097/00004691-200210000-00003.

21. Thirumala PD, Carnovale G, Loke Y, et al. Brainstem auditory evoked potentials' diagnostic accuracy for hearing loss: systematic review and meta-analysis. J Neurol Surg B Skull Base 2017;78(1):43–51. https://doi.org/10.1055/s-0036-1584557.

22. Arora J, Pugh K, Westerveld M, et al. Language lateralization in epilepsy patients: fMRI validated with the Wada procedure. Epilepsia 2009;50(10):2225–41. https://doi.org/10.1111/j.1528-1167.2009.02136.x.

23. Bizzi A, Blasi V, Falini A, et al. Presurgical functional MR imaging of language and motor functions: validation with intraoperative electrocortical mapping. Radiology 2008;248(2):579–89. https://doi.org/10.1148/radiol.2482071214.

24. Bowyer SM, Moran JE, Weiland BJ, et al. Language laterality determined by MEG mapping with MR-FOCUSS. Epilepsy Behav 2005;6(2):235–41. https://doi.org/10.1016/j.yebeh.2004.12.002.

25. Chang EF, Raygor KP, Berger MS. Contemporary model of language organization: an overview for neurosurgeons. J Neurosurg 2015;122(2):250–61. https://doi.org/10.3171/2014.10.Jns132647.

26. Drane DL, Roraback-Carson J, Hebb AO, et al. Cortical stimulation mapping and Wada results demonstrate a normal variant of right hemisphere language organization. Epilepsia 2012;53(10):1790–8. https://doi.org/10.1111/j.1528-1167.2012.03573.x.

27. Roux FE, Boulanouar K, Lotterie JA, et al. Language functional magnetic resonance imaging in preoperative assessment of language areas: correlation with direct cortical stimulation. Neurosurgery 2003;52(6):1335–45. https://doi.org/10.1227/01.neu.0000064803.05077.40 [discussion 1337–45].

28. Duffau H, Capelle L. Preferential brain locations of low-grade gliomas. Cancer 2004;100(12):2622–6. https://doi.org/10.1002/cncr.20297.

29. Duffau H, Denvil D, Capelle L. Long term reshaping of language, sensory, and motor maps after glioma resection: a new parameter to integrate in the surgical strategy. J Neurol Neurosurg Psychiatry 2002;72(4):511–6. https://doi.org/10.1136/jnnp.72.4.511.

30. Wunderlich G, Knorr U, Herzog H, et al. Precentral glioma location determines the displacement of cortical hand representation. Neurosurgery 1998;42(1):18–26. https://doi.org/10.1097/00006123-199801000-00005 [discussion 17–26].

31. Lueders H, Lesser RP, Hahn J, et al. Cortical somatosensory evoked potentials in response to hand stimulation. J Neurosurg 1983;58(6):885–94. https://doi.org/10.3171/jns.1983.58.6.0885.

32. Wood CC, Spencer DD, Allison T, et al. Localization of human sensorimotor cortex during surgery by cortical surface recording of somatosensory evoked potentials. J Neurosurg 1988;68(1):99–111. https://doi.org/10.3171/jns.1988.68.1.0099.

33. Berger MS. Lesions in functional ("eloquent") cortex and subcortical white matter. Clin Neurosurg 1994;41:444–63.

34. Sartorius CJ, Wright G. Intraoperative brain mapping in a community setting-technical considerations. Surg Neurol 1997;47(4):380–8. https://doi.org/10.1016/s0090-3019(96)00340-0.
35. Yingling CD, Ojemann S, Dodson B, et al. Identification of motor pathways during tumor surgery facilitated by multichannel electromyographic recording. J Neurosurg 1999;91(6):922–7. https://doi.org/10.3171/jns.1999.91.6.0922.
36. Sartorius CJ, Berger MS. Rapid termination of intraoperative stimulation-evoked seizures with application of cold Ringer's lactate to the cortex. Technical note. J Neurosurg 1998;88(2):349–51. https://doi.org/10.3171/jns.1998.88.2.0349.
37. Ojemann G, Ojemann J, Lettich E, et al. Cortical language localization in left, dominant hemisphere. An electrical stimulation mapping investigation in 117 patients. 1989. J Neurosurg 2008;108(2):411–21. https://doi.org/10.3171/jns/2008/108/2/0411.
38. Gil-Robles S, Duffau H. Surgical management of World Health Organization Grade II gliomas in eloquent areas: the necessity of preserving a margin around functional structures. Neurosurg focus 2010;28(2):E8. https://doi.org/10.3171/2009.12.Focus09236.
39. Haglund MM, Berger MS, Shamseldin M, et al. Cortical localization of temporal lobe language sites in patients with gliomas. Neurosurgery 1994;34(4):567–76. https://doi.org/10.1227/00006123-199404000-00001 [discussion 576].
40. Krishnan R, Raabe A, Hattingen E, et al. Functional magnetic resonance imaging-integrated neuronavigation: correlation between lesion-to-motor cortex distance and outcome. Neurosurgery 2004;55(4):904–14. https://doi.org/10.1227/01.neu.0000137331.35014.5c [discussion 905–914].
41. Han SJ, Morshed RA, Troncon I, et al. Subcortical stimulation mapping of descending motor pathways for perirolandic gliomas: assessment of morbidity and functional outcome in 702 cases. J Neurosurg 2018;131(1):201–8. https://doi.org/10.3171/2018.3.Jns172494.

Current Indications for Management Options in Pseudotumor Cerebri

Asad Akhter, MD[a], Lauren Schulz, MD[a], Hilliary E. Inger, MD[b,c], John M. McGregor, MD[a],*

KEYWORDS

- Idiopathic intracranial hypertension • Pseudotumor cerebri • Venous sinus stenting
- Shunt • Optic nerve sheath fenestration • Complication

KEY POINTS

- There are surgical options available for those patients with IIH who have significant visual threat or visual deterioration despite best medical management or whose visual deterioration is rapid enough to warrant urgent intervention.
- ONSF, VSS, and CSF diversion via ventriculoperitoneal and lumboperitoneal shunting are useful adjuncts in the management of this condition. They are associated with successful visual preservation, moderately successful in headache amelioration, but require frequent monitoring because of known failures and revision rates.
- IIH is a condition with intense resource utilizatioin including radiation exposure.
- Further understanding of the pathophysiology of IIH will likely direct future treatment options to more targeted therapeutics including surgery for IIH in the future.

INTRODUCTION

The condition of idiopathic intracranial hypertension (IIH) has gone by several names over the years. Many of them are associated with the presenting symptoms that tend to occur when a patient develops elevated intracranial pressures (ICP), either acutely or over a very prolonged course. These names include pseudotumor cerebri, benign intracranial hypertension, primary intracranial hypertension, pseudotumor cerebri syndrome, hypertensive meningeal hydrops, otitic hydrocephalus, toxic hydrocephalus, serous meningitis, and the original term, meningitis serosa, coined by Quincke in 1897. There are several examples of intracranial hypertension (IH) that are found to

[a] Department of Neurological Surgery, The Ohio State University, N-1031 Doan Hall, 410 West 10th Avenue, Columbus, OH 43210, USA; [b] Department of Ophthalmology, The Ohio State University, 915 Olentangy River Rd, Ste 5000, Columbus, Ohio 43210, USA; [c] Department of Ophthalmology, Nationwide Children's Hospital Outpatient Care Center, 555 S. 18th S. 4th Floor, Columbus, Ohio 43205, USA
* Corresponding author.
E-mail address: john.mcgregor@osumc.edu

Neurol Clin 40 (2022) 391–404
https://doi.org/10.1016/j.ncl.2021.11.011
0733-8619/22/© 2021 Elsevier Inc. All rights reserved.
neurologic.theclinics.com

have underlying causes such as venous sinus thrombosis. When a cause for IH is identified, the condition is often termed secondary intracranial hypertension. The management scheme is often very similar between patients with either secondary IH or IIH. We can only hope that as more information as to pathophysiology of IIH unfolds, the term idiopathic will no longer apply. Still, the consistent condition found in all patients with IIH is elevated intracranial pressure without an anatomic or neurologic cause.

IIH is a relatively rare condition; however, the incidence has been increasing over the years. Treatment options continue to evolve and improve, and there continue to be slow advances in diagnostics, management strategies, and improved options for treatment. Symptomatic presentation varies. The possibilities of visual deterioration and blindness drive therapeutic interventions. When patients are unable to be effectively managed by medical means and lifestyle adjustments, procedural strategies and surgical interventions are available to assist in disease management.

PATHOPHYSIOLOGY

The pathophysiology of IIH remains unclear. Proposed hypotheses have been developed over the years with lines of evidence to support them. ICP has been shown to be elevated in known conditions of decreased absorption such as postinflammatory IH, or less likely, increased production of cerebrospinal fluid (CSF), as in choroid plexus papilloma.[1] Some investigators have suggested that cerebral blood volume fluctuations may be responsible for the increased pressure, the so-called hyperemic hydrocephalus hypothesis.[2,3] There has been some pathologic evidence that identifies the possibility that there is an increase in brain extracellular space fluid.[4] A common set of anatomic findings in IIH are that these patients tend to have small cerebral ventricles and small sulcal subarachnoid spaces (**Fig. 1**). With decompression procedures,

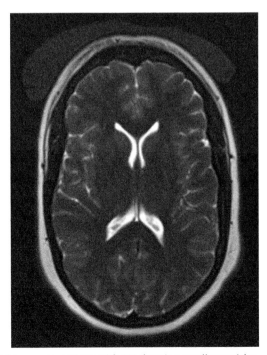

Fig. 1. MRI T2 axial image in patient with IIH showing small ventricles.

either through shunting of CSF in the lateral ventricles or by bony decompression through removal of the squamous temporal bone, the brain tends to expand into those spaces.[4] Although there has been mixed evidence on MRI equivalent studies regarding extracellular fluid, Alperin and colleagues, demonstrated significantly increased extraventricular CSF and interstitial fluid volumes in patients with IIH.[5,6] There has been a recent accumulation of evidence that an alteration in CSF glymphatic function is found in patients with IIH.[7–9] There is also evidence that elevated pressure differentials between CSF and central venous blood pressures are a mechanism for IIH. These may be a consequence of venous hypertension or venous outflow obstruction as in cases of venous sinus stenosis.[10] However, venous sinuses are noted to be narrow in many cases of IIH and may be either a contributor or an effect of IIH. Therefore, although there are many known causes of IH, so called secondary IH, there remain many patients whose pathophysiology is idiopathic.

DIAGNOSIS

The diagnosis of IIH is made using the 5 conditions set by the modified Dandy criteria.[11,12] For diagnosis, there needs to be signs and symptoms of elevated ICP, including headache, transient visual obscurations, tinnitus, papilledema, or possibly double vision secondary to a cranial nerve palsy. Second, there should be no localizing findings on neurologic examination. Third, all neurodiagnostic studies should be normal with several notable allowable exceptions. Allowable MRI findings that suggest elevated ICP include an empty sella turcica, type I Chiari malformation (**Fig. 2**), flattening of the globe, expansion of the optic nerve sheaths in the orbit (**Figs. 3**A and B), thinning or defects of the bone overlying the skull base, and smooth narrowing of the venous sinuses.[13] The finding of postcontrast FLAIR hyperintensity of the optic nerve and the optic nerve head have been shown to be correlated with IIH and are signs of papilledema.[14] Additional diagnostic imaging characteristics include optical coherence tomography findings of increased thickness of the retinal nerve fiber layer, which has been shown to correlate with grade of papilledema in these patients.[15] Finally, the ICP should be elevated greater than 25 cm H_2O, the patient should be

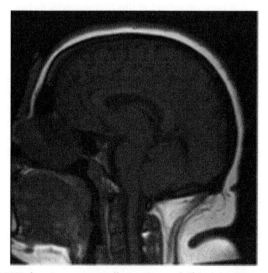

Fig. 2. Sagittal T1 MRI showing empty sella turcica and Chiari 1 anatomy.

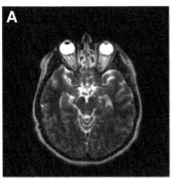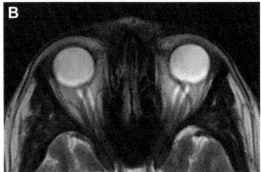

Fig. 3. (*A*) MRI T2 axial image in IIH patient showing dilated optic nerve sheaths and flattening of the posterior globes. (*B*) Axial orbital MRI T2 inpatient with IIH showing dilated optic nerve sheaths and swelling of the nerve heads consistent with papilledema.

awake and alert, and there should be no other identifiable causes of elevated intracranial pressure.

The IIH condition is noted to occur most frequently in patients who are obese women of childbearing age. The mean age is 30 years. Overall, the incidence is 0.9 per 100,000 persons, but 3.0/100,000 in women, and 19/100,000 in women whose weight is 20% greater than their ideal body weight. Of the primary patients with IIH, 90% are women and 90% are obese.[16] The World Health Organization Body Mass Index Comparisons have documented that the world population is growing heavier. We see patients with increased weight worldwide, particularly in the United States. The obesity prevalence (percent of adults > 30.0 kg/m^2) has gone from 18.7% in 1990 to 31.0% in 2008 and 36.2% in 2016 in the United States alone.[17]

The incidence in the pediatric population is beginning to be better understood. Gillson and colleagues were able to estimate the incidence of primary and secondary IH at 0.63 and 0.32 per 100,000 children, 69% were overweight or obese, and the female-to-male ratio for primary IIH was 1.3:1.[18,19] Of note, the classic association between IIH and obese women is best observed in the postpubertal population; in the prepubertal population the distribution was more equivalent.[20]

HEALTH CARE UTILIZATION

We have seen an increase in the diagnosis and health care utilization by patients with IIH. We identified an increasing frequency of emergency room (ER) visits due to the IIH condition. We analyzed our ER admissions and included only those whose primary diagnosis was IIH. We reviewed the numbers over a 3.5-year span, 2016 to 2019. One thousand two hundred twenty-three patient ER encounters were seen in our institution in patients with the diagnosis of IIH on their problem list and an additional ED diagnosis of

- Other headache syndromes
- New daily persistent headache
- Benign IH
- Papilledema associated with increased intracranial pressure
- Headache
- Other complicated headache syndromes
- Disorder of brain, unspecified

As expected, 90% were female patients. These patients required significant resources and time to conclude their ER visits. They spent an average of 9.7 hours from arrival to release, undergoing such evaluations as routine blood work; head computed tomography (CT) scans; MRI scans; radiographs of shunt implants; consultations with Neurology, Ophthalmology, and Neurosurgery; shunt adjustments; and lumbar punctures, many under fluoroscopy (**Tables 1** and **2**; **Figs. 4** and **5**).

We then looked at utilization in a retrospectively reviewed 100 randomly selected patient cohort with IIH and a prior CSF diversion procedure treated at our institution between July 2010 and August 2018. Radiological studies demonstrated no actionable findings in 82.5% CTs, 97.5% shunt radiographs, and 79.6% MRIs.[21] We have concluded that IIH is a resource intensive condition that is increasing in its incidence worldwide (**Table 3**).

After the initial diagnosis is suspected, patients undergo lumbar puncture, both for diagnostic and therapeutic purposes, followed by trials of medications, lifestyle changes, and close follow-up for examinations of vision. The Idiopathic Intracranial Hypertension Treatment Trial (IIHTT) has been able to show the effectiveness of acetazolamide in those adult patients with mild visual field loss.[22,23] Although most patients will be able to be treated successfully with medical therapy alone, there is a known incidence of disease progression or refractory symptoms despite medical management of IIH. The IIHTT trial of IIH in adults identified only one out of 86 patients treated in the acetazolamide arm who failed treatment with medical management.

SURGICAL INTERVENTIONS

Similar to adults, initial management in pediatrics is often successful with intracranial pressure–lowering medications. However, recurrence of disease and need for surgical intervention can occur. In the study by Alex and colleagues, there was a cumulative 20% risk of recurrence of disease within 6 months of weaning of intracranial pressure–lowering medications in the pediatric patient population.[24] Inger and colleagues noted a surgical rate of 9.8% in their pediatric population, with a presenting

---

Table 1
Emergency room visits for patients with primary diagnosis of idiopathic intracranial hypertension alone, 2013–2014

Measure	2013	2014	2013–2014
Volume of cases (encounters)	79	59	138
Male (%)	2.5%	10.2%	5.8%
Female (%)	97.5%	89.8%	94.2%
Mean Age (y)	33.3 y	34.6 y	33.9 y
Average ED arrival to disposition (h)	8.1 h	10.7 h	9.2 h
Average ED arrival to ED depart (h)	8.6 h	11.1 h	9.7 h
Average time from disposition to ED depart (min)	31.2 min	27.5 min	29.6 min
Percent that return within 30 d of ED depart	7.6%	2.5%	5.8%
Percent of ED patients admitted (%)	0%	1.7% (1 patient)	0.8%
Percent of ED patients placed in CDU (%)	5.1%	10.2%	7.2%
Percent of ED patients discharged from ED (%)	92.4%	81.4%	87.7%

Abbreviation: ED, emergency department.

Table 2
Average time to disposition in the emergency room of patients with primary diagnosis of idiopathic intracranial hypertension, 2016–17

Year/QTR	Average Hours from Arrival to ED Departure
2016 Q2	10 h 24 min
2016 Q3	11 h
2016 Q4	12 h
2017 Q1	12 h 6 min
2017 Q2	11 h
2017 Q3	13 h
2017 Q4	9 h 30 min

lumbar puncture opening pressure of greater than 52 cm H_2O being a significant indicator of progression to surgery.[25]

For those patients in whom medical management is no longer effective or becomes contraindicated due to side effects or allergies, surgical intervention is considered. The IIH patient who, despite medical management, continues with a significant threat of visual loss, has visual deterioration, and continues to suffer from intractable headaches that are moderated through temporary CSF diversion via lumbar puncture or drain may benefit from surgical strategies. These strategies include serial lumbar punctures, lumbar drain trials, subtemporal bony decompressions, optic nerve sheath fenestrations/decompressions (ONSF), CSF shunting, venous sinus stenting, and gastric bypass. In emergency situations in which patients have rapidly fulminant visual deterioration with significant elevated ICP admission and simultaneous medical

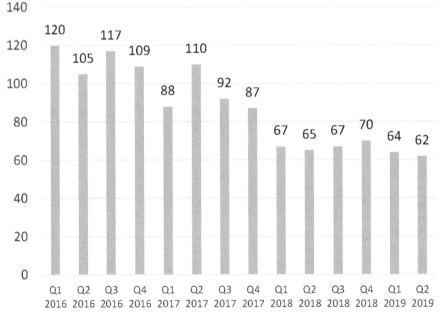

Fig. 4. Quarterly ER visits with the diagnosis of IIH, 2016–2019.

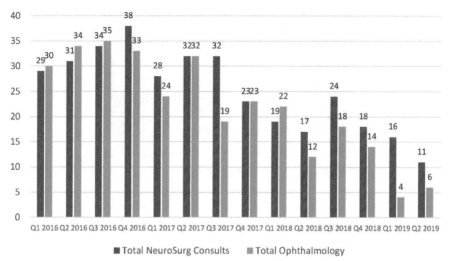

Fig. 5. Number of consults ordered per quarter in ED, 2016–2019.

management, the insertion of a lumbar drain may be used to stabilize a visual threatening emergency while surgical options are evaluated.[26]

The OSNF is a visually protecting surgery that diverts CSF from around the optic nerve via slits or windows created along the optic nerve sheath just posterior to the globe, allowing CSF to egress into the orbit and ultimately allowing the sheath to adhere to the nerve away from the nerve head, protecting the nerve head from damaging ICP pulsations (**Fig. 6**). The procedure has been shown to stabilize or improve vision in 89% of patients at 2 years.[27] Improvement in headache symptoms is less likely. There is an observed selection bias in ONSF studies toward surgical patients with primary visual difficulties and milder headache symptoms.

CSF diversion through shunts tends to be recommended more frequently in patients with intractable headache symptoms and visual threats. They have been shown to help preserve vision with 95% of patients noting visual stability or improvement at 4 years.[9] Visual deterioration can still occur, and shunted patients need to have ongoing follow-up visual evaluations. As a headache management tool, shunts are less effective. Ninety-five percent of shunted patients with IIH will note headache relief at 1 month, but only 52% continue to note headache relief at 2 years.[28]

The topic of shunting in pediatric patients with IIH requires some extra consideration. Children may be at a higher risk for developing complications such as shunt obstruction due to increased mechanical stress from growth, and correspondingly, many pediatric neurosurgeons are hesitant to commit a child to shunt.[29] Recently,

Table 3
Patient resource utilization and radiation exposure in 100 shunted patients with idiopathic intracranial hypertension, 2010–2018

Average Number of:						
Office Visits	ER Visits	Inpatient Admissions	Head CTs	Shunt radiographs	MRI Scans	Radiation Exposure
16.3	12.4	4.6	9.0	11.2	4.3	18.7 mSv

Average 4.8 y follow-up.

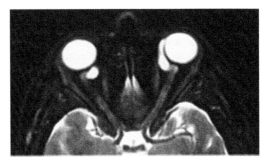

Fig. 6. T2 orbital MRI showing CSF signal in the orbits following bilateral ONSF surgery.

there has been some evidence to favor early placement of external lumbar drain (ELD) as a means of definitive treatment of IIH refractory to medication.[30] In select patient populations, external lumbar drains placed while visual acuity is relatively preserved have the potential to resolve IIH and avoid shunt placement altogether.[30]

The identification of venous hypertension due to sinus stenosis leading to the elevated ICP in IIH has opened another avenue of management for patients with refractory IIH. There are several studies that have indicated relief from IIH symptoms, both visual and headache improvement, with endovascular venous sinus stenting. Identifying these patients has been somewhat controversial. There is a known narrowing of the sinuses that can occur because of elevated ICP. There is also evidence that an effect of narrowed venous sinus outflow is to elevate ICP. Identifying which patients would be amenable to stent placement has been a challenge. Patients with suggestive stenosis on CT angiography or MR angiography (**Fig. 7**) must then undergo formal

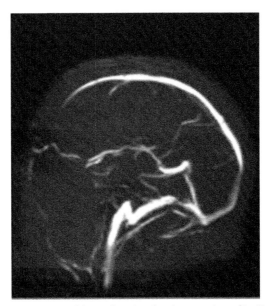

Fig. 7. MRV image in a patient with IIH showing focal narrowing of ipsilateral transverse sinus and congenital narrowing of the contralateral sinus, suggestive of possible venous sinus gradient. MRV, magnetic resonance venography.

cerebral venous angiography with venous pressure gradient measurements. Any sagittal sinus or bilateral transverse or sigmoid sinus segmental narrowing associated with a 10 mm Hg venous pressure difference across is considered a candidate for venous sinus stenting (VSS). Stented patients postoperatively are maintained on platelet inhibitors for 3 months, as well as long-term daily aspirin. Routine follow-up angiogram is performed to ensure patency of the stents (**Fig. 8**). Initial results are compelling with reduction of ICP elevations down to the normal ranges, 80% to 90% papilledema resolution and 80% to 100% headache improvement noted at 1.5 years.[31,32] Pulsatile tinnitus also showed improvement in up to 90% of patients.[33] Reported recurrence of IIH symptoms after stenting is roughly 10%, with the most common form of subsequent treatment being repeat endovascular procedure, followed by CSF diversion.[33] In addition, there is accumulating evidence as to the feasibility, the safety, and the effectiveness of VSS in the pediatric population.[34]

The indications for the placement of CSF-diverting shunts include intractable visual abnormalities despite nonoperative management, rapid visual deterioration amid the beginning of medical management, significant ICP elevation with papilledema and vision deficit, contraindications to diuretic therapy and/or antiplatelet therapy, absence of suitable venous pressure gradient, and intractable headaches. The decision on type of shunt and its locations can depend on several anatomic factors including ventricular size, abdominal size, previous surgeries, and the presence or absence of a Chiari malformation. CSF-diverting shunts use primarily either a lateral ventricle or the lumbar thecal sac as the proximal catheter insertion site. Distal catheter sites include the peritoneal cavity, the jugular vein, or more rarely the pleural cavity. The proximal catheter placement in the lateral ventricle for patients with IIH has become more successful and preferred over time with the advent of widely available stereotactic intraoperative image guidance catheter placements due to the small ventricular size that is typical in patients with IIH (**Fig. 9**). However, ventricle size in this patient population may be so small as to either obstruct a cerebral shunt too easily or drain too little volume to mitigate IIH symptoms successfully. In those situations, a lumbar shunt may be an alternative or additional option.

Lumboperitoneal shunts may be more difficult to place in the patient with larger abdominal girth. They may also be problematic in the patients with a known Chiari I

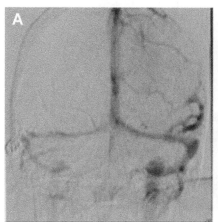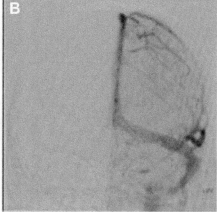

Fig. 8. Left transverse sinus at angiography. (*A*) Before stent placement. (*B*) After stenting procedure, for pressure gradient greater than 10 mm Hg.

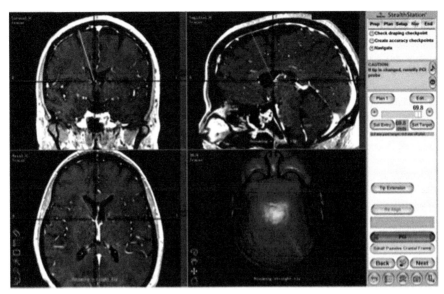

Fig. 9. Stereotactic guidance for ventricular catheter insertion in a patient with IIH and relatively small ventricles.

malformation. They may initiate or exacerbate symptoms referable to low-lying cerebellar tonsils, resulting in progressive Chiari signs and symptoms, including cervical syrinx formation, because of continuous CSF diversion from the thecal sac (**Fig. 10**). Previous abdominal surgeries or intraperitoneal infections may preclude peritoneal placement.

There are several choices for catheters and valves, but no evidence that any are particularly superior in this patient population. There are catheters of various

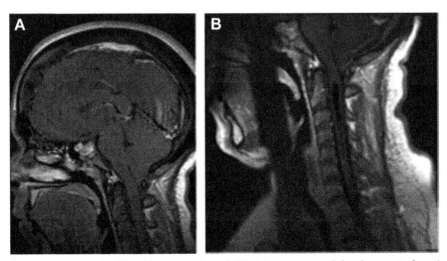

Fig. 10. A patient with IIH with progression of Chiari 1 anatomy and development of cervical syrinx 3 years following lumboperitoneal shunt placement. (*A*) Pre-LP shunt. (*B*) Post-LP shunt.

Table 4
Comparison of first-time shunt placements, lumboperitoneal and ventriculoperitoneal, for patients with idiopathic intracranial hypertension from 2003 to 2008

	VP (n = 15)	LP (n = 46)	P value
Age	33	31	.38
Female gender	13	42	—
Weight (lbs)	277	228	.02
Opening pressure	40.6	41.1	.89
Revision	7(47%)	24 (52%)	—
Median time to 1st revision	136 d (2–612)	111 d (1–354)	.69

Abbreviations: LP, lumboperitoneal; VP, ventriculoperitoneal.

diameters and some impregnated with antibiotics. There are valve systems that are either high-resistance or low-resistance systems, flow-controlled systems, fixed differential pressure valves, gravity compensation devices, incorporate anti-siphon devices, have adjustable differential pressures, and have locking mechanisms to prevent unexpected setting adjustments on exposures to magnetic fields. There are useful surgical adjuncts to the placement of shunts, including stereotactic image guidance and endoscopic assists for ventricular placement, laparoscopic techniques for peritoneal placements, and ultrasound guidance for percutaneous venous access for jugular vein placements.

As stated earlier, shunts are an effective treatment tool to assist with visual stabilization and improvement in patients with intractable IIH. They do require postoperative visits to assist with shunt pressure adjustments and evaluation for shunt dysfunction and the potential need for revision surgery.

We reviewed our series of 61 first-time shunt placements from 2003 to 2008 and identified a 51% revision rate irrespective of lumboperitoneal or ventriculoperitoneal configuration, on average at 4 months post-op, for such things as distal or proximal failure, persistent ICP elevation, intractable low-pressure symptoms, and infections (**Tables 4** and **5**).

In addition, we followed 35 consecutive lumboperitoneal shunt placement patients. We noted an acquired Chiari malformation rate from lumboperitoneal shunt placement of 29%, occurring between 3 months and 6.5 years post-op, the majority managed expectantly of by appropriate adjustments to the shunt setting where

Table 5
Complications following first-time ventriculoperitoneal (n = 15) and lumboperitoneal (n = 46) shunt placements, 2003–2008

Complications: Leading to 1st Revision	VP (7 Patients)	LP (24 Patients)
Distal catheter failure (migrations)	4(3)	13(9)
Proximal failure	1	3
CSF leak	1	1
Under drainage	2	5
Over drainage	0	2
Infection	0	1

Abbreviations: LP, lumboperitoneal; VP, ventriculoperitoneal.

Table 6
Percent of patients with idiopathic intracranial hypertension with listed results based on surgery performed

	VSS (%)	CSF Diversion (%)	ONSF (%)
Papilledema improved	87.1	78.9	90.5
Visual fields improved	72.7	66.8	65.2
Headaches improved	72.1	69.8	49.3
Severe complications	2.3	9.4	2.2
Failure rates	11.3	43.4	9.4

(*Data from* Kalyvas A, Neromyliotis E, Koutsarnakis C, et al. A systematic review of surgical treatments of idiopathic intracranial hypertension (IIH). Neurosurgical review 2021;44(2):773-92)

possible. There was a need for suboccipital decompression surgery in 14% of the patients.

Kalyvas and colleagues performed a metanalysis of the results of 109 controlled or observational studies of surgical intervention in the management of IIH from 1 January 1985 to 19 April 2019, and the results are tabulated in[35] **Table 6**. Cumulative analyses of the techniques of VSS, shunting, and ONSF all demonstrated success in the management of papilledema, visual fields, and headaches to varying degrees. Cumulative need for further interventions was highest in CSF diversion procedures during the observation periods.

SUMMARY

There are surgical options available for those patients with IIH who have significant visual threat or visual deterioration despite best medical management or whose visual deterioration is rapid enough to warrant urgent intervention. ONSF, VSS, and CSF diversion via ventriculoperitoneal and lumboperitoneal shunting are useful adjuncts in the management of this condition. They are associated with successful visual preservation, moderately successful in headache amelioration, but require frequent monitoring because of known failures and revision rates. Further understanding of the pathophysiology of IIH will likely direct future treatment options to more targeted therapeutics including surgery for IIH in the future.

CLINICS CARE POINTS

- Interventions including venous sinus stenting and cerebrospinal shunting are over 90% effective at preserving vision in IIH. Shunting is only 50% effective in controlling headache symptoms. Shunts have revision rates of 50%, irrespective of shunt type. Lumboperitoneal shunts have a 28% chance of developing an aquired Chiari 1 malformation.

DISCLOSURE

The authors have nothing to disclose.

REFERENCES

1. Boulton M, Amstrong D, Flessner M, et al. Raised intracranial pressure increases CSF drainage through arachnoid villi and extracranial lymphatics. Am J Physiol 1998;275:889–96.

2. Dandy WE. Intracranial pressure without brain tumor. Ann Surg 1937;106: 492–513.
3. Bateman GA. Association between arterial inflow and venous outflow in idiopathic and secondary intracranial hypertension. J Clin Neurosci 2006;13:550–7.
4. Sahs AL, Hyndman OR. Intracranial hypertension of unknown cause. Cerebral edema. Arch Surg 1939;38:428–42.
5. Bastin ME, Sinha S, Farrall AJ, et al. Diffuse brain oedema in idiopathic intracranial hypertension: a quantitative magnetic resonance imaging study. J Neurol Neurosurg Psychiatry 2003;74:1693–6.
6. Alperin N, Ranganathan S, Bagci AM, et al. MRI evidence of impaired CSF homeostasis in obesity-associated idiopathic intracranial hypertension. AJNR Am J Neuroradiol 2013;34:29–34.
7. Eide PK, Pripp AH, Ringstad G, et al. Impaired glymphatic function in idiopathic intracranial hypertension. Brain Commun 2021. https://doi.org/10.1093/braincomms/fcab043.
8. Mondejar V, Patsalides A. The role of arachnoid granulations and the glymphatic system in the pathophysiology of idiopathic intracranial hypertension. Curr Neurol Neurosci Rep 2020;20(7):20.
9. Nicholson P, Kedra A, Shotar E, et al. Idiopathic intracranial hypertension: glymphedema of the brain. J Neuroophthalmol 2021;41:93–7.
10. Karahalios DG, Rekate HL, Khayata MH, et al. Elevated intracranial venous pressure as a universal mechanism in pseudotumor cerebri of varying etiologies. Neurology 1996;46:198–202.
11. Wall M. Idiopathic intracranial hypertens. Neurol Clin 2010;28(3):593–617.
12. Wall M. Update on idiopathic intracranial hypertension. Neurol Clin 2017;35(1): 45–57.
13. Degnan AJ, Levy LM. Pseudotumor Cerebri: brief review of clinical syndrome and imaging findings. AJNR Am J Neuroradiol 2011;32(11):1986–93.
14. Golden E, Krivochenitser R, Mathews N, et al. Contrast-enhanced 3D-FLAIR imaging of the optic nerve and optic nerve head: novel neuroimaging findings of idiopathic intracranial hypertension. AJNR Am J Neuroradiol 2019;40:334–9.
15. Auinger P, Durbin M, Feldon S, et al. Baseline OCT measurements in the idiopathic intracranial hypertension treatment trial, part II: correlations and relationship to clinical features. Invest Ophthalmol Vis Sci 2014;55:8173–9.
16. Durcan FJ, Corbett JJ, Wall M. The incidence of pseudotumor cerebri. Population studies in Iowa and Louisiana. Arch Neurol 1988;45:875–7.
17. Available at: https://apps.who.int/gho/data/view.main.CTRY2450A?lang=en. August 23, 2021.
18. Gillson N, Jones C, Reem RE, et al. Incidence and demographics of pediatric intracranial hypertension. Pediatr Neurol 2017;73:42–7.
19. Jordan CO, Aylward SC. Intracranial hypertension: a current review. Curr Opin Pediatr 2018;30(6):764–74.
20. Malem A, Sheth T, Muthusamy B. Paediatric Idiopathic Intracranial Hypertension (IIH)-A review. Life (Basel) 2021;11(7):632.
21. Cho T, Kreatsoulas D, Fritz J, et al. An institutional review of hospital resource utilization and patient radiation exposure in shunted idiopathic intracranial hypertension. Neurosurg Rev. 10.1007/s10143-021-01502-8.
22. Friedman D, McDermott M, Kieburtz K, et al. The idiopathic intracranial hypertension treatment trial. J Neuroophthalmol 2014;34:107–17.

23. Wall M, McDermott MP, Kieburtz KD, et al. Effect of acetazolamide on visual function in patients with idiopathic intracranial hypertension and mild visual loss: the idiopathic intracranial hypertension treatment trial. JAMA 2014;311:1641–51.

24. Alex A, Jordan CO, Benedict MS, et al. Intracranial hypertension recurrence risk after wean of intracranial pressure-lowering medication. Pediatr Neurol 2021; 121:40–4.

25. Inger HE, McGregor ML, Jordan CO, et al. Surgical intervention in pediatric intracranial hypertension: incidence, risk factors, and visual outcomes. J AAPOS 2019;23:96.e1–7.

26. Ploof J, Aylward SC, Jordan CO, et al. Case series of rapid surgical interventions in fulminant intracranial hypertension. J Child Neurol 2021;14. 08830738211026798.

27. Feldon SE. Visual outcomes comparing surgical techniques for management of severe idiopathic intracranial hypertension. Neurosurg Focus 2007;23(5):E6.

28. McGirt MJ, Woodworth G, Thomas G, et al. Cerebrospinal fluid shunt placement for pseudotumor cerebri-associated intractable headache: predictors of treatment response and an analysis of long-term outcomes. J Neurosurg 2004;101: 627–32.

29. Ko MW, Liu GT. Pediatric idiopathic intracranial hypertension (Pseudotumor Cerebri). Horm Res Paediatr 2010;74:381–9.

30. Dotan G, Hadar Cohen N, Qureshi HM, et al. External lumbar drainage in progressive pediatric idiopathic intracranial hypertension. J Neurosurg Pediatr 2021;28(4):490–6.

31. Donnet A, Metellus P, Levrier O, et al. Endovascular treatment of idiopathic intracranial hypertension: clinical and radiologic outcome of 10 consecutive patients. Neurology 2008;70(8):641–7.

32. Bussière M, Falero R, Nicolleet D, et al. Unilateral transverse sinus stenting of patients with idiopathic intracranial hypertension. AJNR Am J Neuroradiol 2010; 31(4):645–50.

33. Nicholson P, Brinjikji W, Radovanovic I, et al. Venous sinus stenting for idiopathic intracranial hypertension: a systematic review and meta-analysis. J Neurointervent Surg 2019;11:380–5.

34. Lee KE, Zehri A, Soldozy S, et al. Dural venous sinus stenting for treatment of pediatric idiopathic intracranial hypertension. J Neurointerv Surg 2021;13(5): 465–70.

35. Kalyvas A, Neromyliotis E, Koutsarnakis C, et al. A systematic review of surgical treatments of idiopathic intracranial hypertension (IIH). Neurosurg Rev 2021; 44(2):773–92.

Familial Neoplastic Syndromes

Ryan G. Eaton, MD*, Russell R. Lonser, MD

KEYWORDS

- Neoplastic syndromes • Von Hippel–Lindau disease • Neurofibromatosis type 2
- Neurofibromatosis type 1 • Tuberous sclerosis • Phakomatoses

KEY POINTS

- Familial neoplastic syndromes frequently involve the central and peripheral nervous systems and are frequently caused by a germline mutation.
- Patients affected by neoplastic syndromes can develop associated tumors that require personalized management strategies.
- Because of the protean and widespread impact of familial neoplastic syndromes, a multidisciplinarily approach is critical for screening and management.

INTRODUCTION

The 3 most frequently encountered familial neoplastic syndromes that affect the central and/or peripheral nervous systems include neurofibromatosis type I (NF-1), neurofibromatosis type II (NF-2), and Von Hippel–Lindau disease (VHL). Less frequently seen familial tumor conditions that affect the nervous system include tuberous sclerosis, schwannomatosis, Li–Fraumeni syndrome, Cowden syndrome, and Lhermitte–Duclos disease. Each of these disorders can result in a diverse and unique array of characteristic neurologic and/or systemic manifestations. New insights into the genetic, biologic, natural history, and management of familial neoplastic conditions that affect the nervous system have been established. Here, we define the genetic, biologic, natural history, and management paradigms associated with familial neoplastic syndromes with associated nervous system tumors.

NEUROFIBROMATOSIS TYPE 1
Overview

NF-1, also known as *"von Recklinghausen disease,"* is a common neoplastic syndrome that affects approximately 1 in 3000 people worldwide.[1] NF-1 results from a germline mutation on the *NF1 tumor-suppressor* gene located on chromosome 17q11. This affects the function of a cytoplasmic protein called neurofibromin, which

Department of Neurological Surgery, The Ohio State University Wexner Medical Center, The Ohio State University, 410 West 10th Avenue, Doan Hall N1019, Columbus, Ohio 43210, USA
* Corresponding author.
E-mail address: ryan.eaton@osumc.edu

Neurol Clin 40 (2022) 405–420
https://doi.org/10.1016/j.ncl.2021.11.012
0733-8619/22/© 2021 Elsevier Inc. All rights reserved.
neurologic.theclinics.com

is a negative regulator of the *Ras pathway* for control of cell growth. The inherited form of NF-1 is passed down in an autosomal dominant pattern (100% penetrance). Approximately 50% of cases of NF-1 arise spontaneously.[2] Diagnosis is established through genetic testing and/or well-established clinical criteria (**Box 1**).[3]

Other common nonneoplastic manifestations of NF-1 include scoliosis (10%–26% of NF-1 patients), cardiovascular abnormalities (27%), and neurocognitive deficits (80%).[2] Patients with NF-1 are also suspectable to visceral malignancies including gastrointestinal stromal tumors (4%–25%), rhabdomyosarcoma (1%–6%), breast cancer (5-fold increase risk), leukemia (5-fold increase risk), and/or pheochromocytoma (up to 6%).[2] Central and peripheral nervous system neoplastic manifestations of NF-1 include optic pathway gliomas (15%–20%), other brain tumors (5-fold increase, including pilocytic astrocytoma, medulloblastoma, and high-grade glioma) and malignant peripheral nerve tumors (8%–13%).[2,4]

Optic Pathway Gliomas

NF-1-associated optic pathway gliomas typically present in patients less than 7 years of age. They represent approximately 80% of low-grade glial neoplasms in patients with NF-1. These are considered World Health Organization (WHO) grade 1 lesions histologically consistent with pilocytic astrocytoma and are often asymptomatic.[5] Clinical presentation for symptomatic lesions most frequently includes reduced vision and precocious puberty theorized to be due to the disruption of the hypothalamic–pituitary–gonadal axis.[6]

Beginning at 13 years of age, yearly ophthalmologic examinations are recommended in patients with NF-1. However, if an optic glioma is diagnosed magnetic resonance (MR)-imaging and ophthalmologic examinations should occur 4 times per year for the first year then lengthening the interval once stability is demonstrated.[2] First-line treatment of symptomatic tumors is chemotherapy with carboplatin and vincristine.[7] Surgery is generally reserved for atypical appearing lesions for tissue diagnosis or for debulking in refractory disease. Radiation therapy is generally avoided due to the potential risk of secondary malignancies.[8]

Brainstem Gliomas

Brainstem gliomas are the second most common intracranial tumor in patients with NF-1. They represent approximately 18% of NF-1 associated brain neoplasms.[9]

Box 1
National Institute of Health consensus criteria for the diagnosis of neurofibromatosis type I

The diagnostic criteria for NF-1 are met in an individual if 2 or more of the following are found:

- Six or more café-au-lait macules over 5 mm in greatest diameter in prepuberal individuals and over 15 mm in greatest diameter in postpubertal individuals.
- Two or more neurofibromas of any type or 1 plexiform neurofibroma.
- Freckling in the axillary or inguinal region.
- Optic glioma
- Two or more Lisch nodules (iris hamartomas).
- A distinctive osseous lesion such as sphenoid dysplasia or thinning of the long bone cortex with or without pseudoarthrosis.
- A first-degree relative (parent, sibling, or offspring) with NF-1 by the above criteria.

The majority (80%) of asymptomatic lesions are WHO grade I pilocytic astrocytoma and are managed conservatively.[10] Symptomatic tumors or tumors that demonstrate progression are managed more aggressively. Common presenting signs and symptoms include headaches, ataxia, nausea/vomiting, or cranial nerve deficits. MR-imaging is used to evaluate these lesions, which are often difficult to differentiate from "unidentified bright objects" that occur in up to half of patients with NF-1. A multicenter study of 133 NF-1 patients with brainstem gliomas found symptomatic patients were more likely to have high-grade lesions. Of the 12 out of 61 symptomatic patients who underwent biopsy, 8 (67%) were WHO grade II neoplasms, 3 (25%) were grade I, and 1 (8%) was a grade III glioma.[10] Only 5 of 72 asymptomatic patients underwent biopsy with 4 (80%) confirmed as grade I pilocytic astrocytoma, while the remaining (20%) tumor's biopsy was not available. Brainstem gliomas in NF-1 carry an overall favorable prognosis with an overall survival of 92% (123 of the 133 subjects) with a median progression-free survival of 67 months.

Other Gliomas

Patients with NF-1 are at a 5-fold increased risk for developing other brain tumors in addition to the optic pathway and brainstem gliomas.[2] These other tumors are often asymptomatic and typically occur in the temporal lobe, cerebellum, thalamus, basal ganglia, or spinal cord.[4] Cerebellar gliomas in children with NF-1 are most often pilocytic astrocytoma[11] and they are more likely to exist in the subependymal white matter of the fourth ventricle (compared with sporadic lesions that are usually found in the vermis or cerebellar hemispheres).[12] These are treated with surgical excision and adjunctive treatment is based on histologic grade. Lastly, WHO grade IV astrocytoma can occur in patients with NF-1. These tend to occur in early adulthood and patients with NF-1 are at a 50-fold increased risk relative to the general population.[4]

Peripheral Nerve Tumors

Neurofibromas are benign Schwann-cell tumors that are classified into 4 subtypes, including cutaneous, subcutaneous, spinal, and diffuse plexiform. Cutaneous lesions are fleshy tumors that arise on or near the surface of the skin. These can be numerous and disfiguring but do not undergo malignant transformation. Alternatively, subcutaneous lesions are firm and occur along the peripheral nerves below the skin surface. Subcutaneous lesions may contain atypical features and are at risk of undergoing malignant transformation.[5] Spinal neurofibromas are common and often exist in multiple nerve roots (**Fig. 1**). These present with sensory or motor deficits and are managed with surgical excision when symptomatic. Plexiform neurofibromas develop in 30% to 50% of patients with NF-1 and arise along the length of the nerve fascicle (**Fig. 2**).[13] They typically are present at birth and grow throughout the first decade causing pain and bony erosion. These lesions often become symptomatic and are removed/debulked to alleviate symptoms.[13,14]

Malignant peripheral nerve sheath tumors (MPNSTs) have a prevalence of 0.1% in NF-1 patients (compared with 0.001% in the general population). These tumors carry a poor prognosis.[15] They are a tumor of Schwann cell origin and patients with NF-1 have an overall lifetime risk of 10%.[16] Patients are at an increased risk if they have an existing internal plexiform neurofibroma, previous radiation therapy, or a large germline mutation of the NF1 gene.[2] The key presenting finding with MPNSTs is pain or the rapid enlargement of a neurofibroma. MR-imaging is useful in defining the location of the MPNST and ^{18}F-fuorodeoxyclucose-positron emission tomography can be useful for detection.[17] Complete surgical resection can be curative but the extent of invasion can preclude complete removal in some cases. Consequently, adjunct

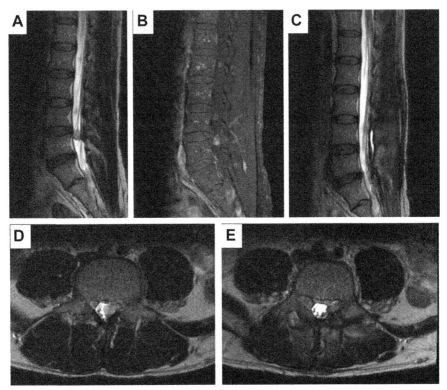

Fig. 1. 43-year-old NF-1 patient with several nerve sheath tumors of the lumbar nerve roots with the most prominent at L5 as seen on (*A*) T2-weighted MR-imaging sequence and (*B*) T1-weighted MR-imaging sequence with contrast. (*D*) T2-axial imaging shows the lesion beginning to extend into the left neural foramen. The top and bottom-right panels (*C*) and (*E*) show postoperative T2-weighted MR-imaging sequences 3 months after gross total resection. Pathology was consistent with neurofibroma.

radiotherapy and chemotherapy are often required. Mean length of survival with MPNSTs in patients with NF-1 is 2 to 3 years.[18]

NEUROFIBROMATOSIS TYPE 2
Overview

Neurofibromatosis type II is an autosomal dominant syndrome caused by a germline mutation of the *NF-2 tumor suppressor gene* on chromosome 22q12. The *NF-2 gene* encodes for the merlin or schwannomin protein product.[19] NF-2 affects 1 in 25,000 live births. Half of the cases are the result of a germline mutation and the other half arise from a *de novo* mutation.[19] There is almost 100% penetrance by age 60 with affected individuals developing a combination of nervous system tumors, neuropathy, ophthalmologic lesions, and/or cutaneous lesions. Clinical diagnostic criteria[20–22] have been defined previously (**Box 2**).[22] Management of lesions includes serial monitoring and timely directed treatment using a multi-disciplinary approach.[3]

Vestibular Schwannomas

Vestibular schwannomas are a major cause of morbidity in patients with NF-2. The most common presentation of these tumors is hearing loss in young adulthood.[23]

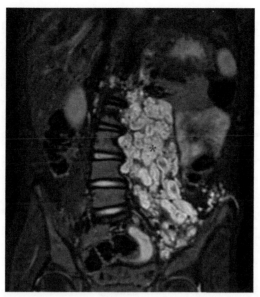

Fig. 2. 8-year-old male with an internal plexiform neurofibroma (*red star*). (*From* Hirbe AC, Gutmann DH. Neurofibromatosis type 1: a multidisciplinary approach to care. Lancet Neurol. 2014;13(8):834-843. doi:10.1016/S1474-4422(14)70063-8; Reprinted with permission of Elsevier.).

Nonvestibular cranial nerve schwannomas most commonly arise from oculomotor nerve, trigeminal nerve, and facial nerve and occur in up to 51% of patients with NF-2.[19] Bilateral vestibular schwannomas occur in 95% of patients with NF-2 and are nearly always benign lesions (**Fig. 3**).[23,24] Hearing generally remains stable for up to 2 years in a newly diagnosed tumor. However, individuals can develop rapid hearing loss that is not related to tumor size or progression.[25,26] Contrast-enhanced T1-weighted MR-imaging will demonstrate an enhancing lesion along the 8th cranial nerve in cases of vestibular schwannoma.

Complete resection of vestibular schwannomas is curative. However, the indications for surgery are varied and complex. Indications for resection can include brainstem compression and raised intracranial pressure from obstructive hydrocephalus.[27] Hearing preservation is another potential indication for resection. Lesions less than

---

Box 2
National Institute of Health consensus criteria for the diagnosis of neurofibromatosis type II

The criteria for NF-2 are met by an individual who has:

1. Bilateral eighth nerve masses seen with appropriate imaging techniques (eg, CT or MRI), *or*

2. A first-degree relative with NF-2 and either:
   a. Unilateral eighth nerve masses, *or*
   b. Two of the following:
      i. Neurofibroma.
      ii. Meningioma.
      iii. Glioma.
      iv. Schwannoma.
      v. Juvenile posterior subcapsular lenticular opacity.

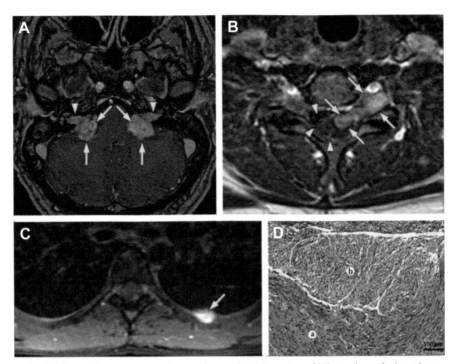

Fig. 3. (*A*) Axial T1-weighted contrast-enhanced MR-imaging of bilateral vestibular schwannomas (*arrows*) with intracanalicular extension (*arrowheads*). (*B*) Axial T1-weighted contrast-enhanced MR-imaging of spinal schwannoma of the cervical spine. (*C*) Intercostal nerve schwannoma seen on contrast-enhanced, fat-suppressed T1-weighted axial MR-image (*D*) classic appearance of vestibular schwannoma on hematoxylin and eosin-stained section with Antoni A (a) and Antoni B (b) arrangements. (*From* Asthagiri AR, Parry DM, Butman JA, et al. Neurofibromatosis type 2. Lancet. 2009;373(9679):1974-1986. doi:10.1016/S0140-6736(09)60259-2; Reprinted with permission of Elsevier.).

3 cm can be resected with 90% preservation of hearing.[28,29] If hearing is preserved in the first ear, resection of the contralateral lesion can be considered. Surgical resection is generally recommended for tumors 2 to 3 cm in size that have grown rapidly or if serviceable hearing loss has occurred.[19] Large lesions (greater than 3 cm) carry a higher operative risk of facial nerve paralysis. Stereotactic radiosurgery is an option for smaller lesions (less than 3 cm diameter).[30–33] Auditory brainstem implantation is an option for individuals who experience bilateral hearing loss.

Intracranial Meningiomas

Intracranial meningiomas are present in over 50% of patients with NF-2. These tumors are the second most common tumor in patients with NF-2.[19,23] Intracranial meningiomas present at a younger age in patients with NF-2 (mean age, 27 years) than sporadic meningiomas (median age, 66 years).[27,34,35] Approximately 20% of children with meningioma will have NF-2.[36] Intracranial meningiomas homogenously enhance on contrast-enhanced T1-weighted MR-imaging. Histologically, the fibroblastic variant is the most common histologic subtype.[34] Generally, these lesions demonstrated a saltatory growth pattern and unpredictable radiographic progression. Subsequently, resection is reserved for symptom-producing tumors.[27,37]

Spinal Tumors

Spinal cord ependymomas are the most common intramedullary spinal cord tumor in patients with NF-2. NF-2-associated ependymomas account for 75% of intramedullary lesions in this disorder.[38,39] These can affect up to half of the NF-2 patients and most commonly present with back pain (less commonly weakness or sensory disturbances).[40] MR-imaging demonstrates a homogenously contrast-enhancing lesion on T1-weighted sequences and hyperintensity on T2-weighted MRI.[24,38,39] Histopathology may show the characteristic perivascular pseudorosette and ependymal rosette with moderate cellularity. Surgical resection is reserved for symptomatic lesions.[41] These tumors are most often WHO grade II lesions and adjunctive therapy is usually unnecessary after complete resection.[42,43]

Intramedullary astrocytoma and schwannomas are less frequently found in patients with NF-2.[38,39] Intramedullary astrocytomas are most often pilocytic or diffuse astrocytoma.[44] Diffuse astrocytomas generally can be distinguished as an ill-defined T2-weighted hyperintensity that does not enhance on contrasted MR-imaging than intramedullary schwannomas which classically show significant enhancement with gadolinium.[39] While asymptomatic lesions should be observed, symptomatic lesions require microsurgical resection. Adjunct radiotherapy may improve survival for residual tumors but the survival benefit requires further investigation.[44]

Intradural extramedullary schwannomas (spinal nerve roots) and intradural extramedullary meningiomas are commonly related to NF-2. Neurofibromas may also occur in the intradural extramedullary region although are less frequent.[45] Symptomatic lesions are treated with surgical excision although lower-neuron findings must be differentiated from peripheral neuropathy that commonly found (67% of patients) patients with NF-2.[46]

Ocular and Cutaneous Manifestations

Cataracts and other lens opacities affect 75% of patients with NF-2.[19,47] Other ocular manifestation include epiretinal membranes (40%), disk gliomas (13%), and retinal hamartomas (3%).[47] Cataracts substantially interfere with vision in approximately 15% of patients with NF-2 and these cases can be treated with extraction.[48] Yearly ophthalmologic examinations starting in infancy are recommended for children of affected parents to enhance vision preservation.

Cutaneous tumors are present in approximately 60% of patients with NF-2. These lesions are often multiple and are categorized as skin plaques, subcutaneous tumors, or intradermal tumors. Most are histologically identified as schwannomas with subcutaneous tumors usually occurring along peripheral nerves generally presenting with pain and tenderness to palpation. Symptomatic lesions can be treated with surgical excision.[23,49]

VON HIPPEL–LINDAU DISEASE
Overview

VHL is an autosomal dominant multisystem tumor syndrome. It is associated with a germline mutation in the VHL tumor *suppressor gene* located on the short arm of chromosome 3.[50] It is a highly penetrant condition with more than 90% penetrance over the age of 65 years. The overall incidence is estimated to be 1 per 35,500 live births.[51] Affected individuals are at risk for the development of central nervous system lesions including retina, cerebellum, brainstem, spinal cord, and cauda equina hemangioblastomas, as well as endolymphatic sac tumors (ELST).

VHL-associated visceral manifestations include renal cysts and carcinoma, phaeochromocytomas, pancreatic cysts, and neuroendocrine tumors as well as epididymal and broad ligament cystadenomas. Interval screening for these conditions is required in high-risk individuals with a family history of VHL. Diagnosis is based on genetic evaluation or clinical criteria. Individuals with a family history and a central nervous system hemangioblastoma, or clear cell renal carcinoma are considered to have VHL. Individuals with no family history must have one central nervous system lesion with one visceral lesion or 2 or more central nervous system lesions to be diagnosed with VHL.[52]

Hemangioblastomas

Hemangioblastoma of the central nervous system is the most common tumor in VHL and affects more than 85% of patients. Related signs/symptoms have a mean age of onset of 33 years in VHL.[52] Hemangioblastomas can arise anywhere in the neuroaxis but 99% of hemangioblastomas are found below the level of the tentorium. They can be associated with peritumoral edema, cysts, or both. Hemangioblastomas most commonly arise in the cerebellum (38% of craniospinal hemangioblastomas), brainstem (10%), or spinal cord (50%). Spinal cord hemangioblastomas most commonly occur in the cervical (43%) and thoracic (47%) spine and less commonly the lumbar spine/cauda equina (11%).[52,53]

Hemangioblastomas are best assessed with contrast-enhanced T1-weighted MRI and characteristically show a vividly enhancing tumor with an associated homogenous dark region that represents the cyst (**Fig. 4**). When present, a peritumoral cyst often accounts for most of the mass effect and is frequently not related to tumor size. Peritumoral cysts are often present in symptomatic tumors (**Fig. 5**). Presentation varies based on tumor location. Brainstem tumors typically present with headache (83%) and singultus (67%). Cerebellar tumors are likely to present with headache (77%) and gait ataxia (57%). Spinal cord tumors present with paresthesia (74%) and pain (63%).[54]

Treatment of symptomatic hemangioblastomas is surgical excision.[55,56] Careful microsurgical technique obviates the need for angiographic embolization and its

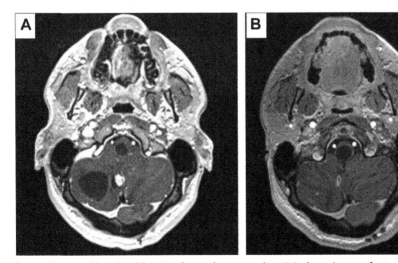

Fig. 4. 29-year-old male with VHL who underwent suboccipital craniotomy for resection of 2 VHL related hemangioblastomas. (*A*) The homogenous enhancing tumor can be well appreciated within the homogenous dark region of the cyst on the initial T1-weighted contrast-enhanced axial MR-imaging. (*B*) The same sequence 6-weeks postoperatively.

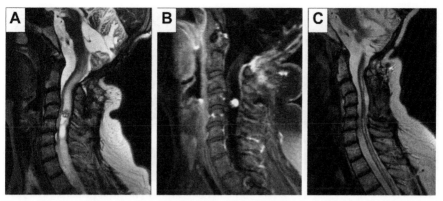

Fig. 5. 48-year-old female with VHL who underwent C3-C5 laminectomy for the resection of C4 hemangioblastoma. (*A*) T2-weighted MR-imaging sequence demonstrating a heterogenous mass with extensive peritumoral cyst formation. (*B*) The same homogenous contrast-enhancing lesion on T1-weighted MR-imaging.T2- (*C*) T2-weight MR-imaging obtained at 6-month post-operative follow-up with significant improvement in syrinx volume.

associated complications.[57] Patients with asymptomatic lesions of the central nervous system are monitored with interval MR-imaging conducted on a yearly basis starting at age 11. Radiosurgery and chemotherapy for hemangioblastomas have not shown long-term benefit/control.[58,59]

Other Central Nervous System Lesions

Retinal hemangioblastomas (retinal angiomas) are seen in as many as 60% of patients with VHL and have a mean age of presentation of 22.5 years.[60] Lesions can be found in the periphery or near the optic disc. They are often asymptomatic. Consequently, yearly ophthalmologic screening starting at age 1 is recommended. Early diagnosis and treatment are important for preventing visual loss. Generally, these lesions can be treated with laser photocoagulation.

Endolymphatic sac tumors (ELSTs) are present in 11% of patients and have a mean age of presentation of 22 years. Bilateral endolymphatic sac tumors are a unique characteristic finding of VHL.[61] Patients with VHL and ELSTs will most often experience hearing loss (100%), tinnitus (77%), and/or vertigo (62%). Less frequently patients have facial paresis (8%). Computed tomography scanning shows a destructive lesion in the endolymphatic duct that is usually isointense with brain parenchyma (**Fig. 6**). Surgery is curative when complete excision is achieved.

Visceral Tumors

Renal cell carcinomas are seen in 25% to 45% of patients and have a mean age of presentation of 39 years. These tumors are a major cause of morbidity in patients with VHL.[52] They often are asymptomatic. Consequently, patients are often screened with yearly abdominal MR-imaging or computed tomography scanning. Treatment is generally recommended for lesions greater than 3 cm in diameter. Pheochromocytoma arises in 10% to 20% of patients with VHL and has a mean age of presentation at 30 years.[62] These can be multiple and bilateral and are screened for yearly with plasma or 24-hour urine catecholamines and metanephrines. Pancreatic neuroendocrine tumors occur in 8% to 17% of patients and have a mean age of presentation at 37 years.[63] Pheochromocytoma and pancreatic neuroendocrine tumors can be

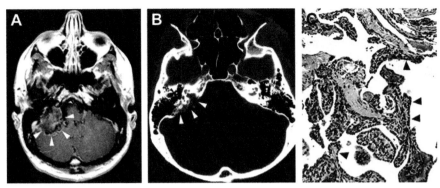

Fig. 6. Characteristic imaging and histologic findings of endolymphatic sac tumor in a 33-year-old man. (*A*) Axial T1-weighted postcontrast MRI with a large heterogeneously enhancing tumor of the cerebellopontine angle (*arrowheads*). (*B*) Axial CT scan with destructive lesion eroding posterior petrous region (*arrowheads*). (*C*) Hematoxylin and eosin-stained section showing cuboidal epithelium in a papillary pattern as typically seen (*arrowheads*). (*From* Lonser RR, Glenn GM, Walther M, et al. von Hippel-Lindau disease. Lancet. 2003;361(9374):2059-2067. doi:10.1016/S0140-6736(03)13643-4; Reprinted with permission of Elsevier.).

treated with surgical resection. Broad ligament cystadenomas and epididymal cystadenomas are commonly seen in VHL patients and are both benign and managed expectantly.

OTHER NEOPLASTIC SYNDROMES
Tuberous Sclerosis

Tuberous sclerosis is an autosomal dominant multisystem disorder caused by germline mutations in *TSC1* and *TSC2 genes* (chromosome 9 and 16, respectively) resulting in the dysregulation of cell proliferation and differentiation. Most cases are diagnosed in early childhood with the identification of characteristic skin findings such as hypomelanotic macules (present in 95%), facial angiofibromas, shagreen patches, and/or ungual fibromas.[64] Nervous system complications occur in 85% of children, including epilepsy, cognitive impairment, and behavior problems. Characteristic imaging findings include cortical tubers, subependymal giant-cell astrocytoma, and subependymal nodules. Intracranial aneurysms also occur at an increased rate compared with the general population.[65] Serial MR-imaging of brain is recommended to screen for giant-cell astrocytoma beginning at the age of 2 years.[66] These lesions are responsive to mTOR inhibitors, including rapamycin, which is considered first-line therapy in cases that are not complicated by obstructive hydrocephalus.[67] Other disease features include retinal hamartomas, cardiac rhabdomyomas, renal angiomyolipoma, and renal-cell carcinomas.

Schwannomatosis

Schwannomatosis is an autosomal dominant transmitted neoplastic syndrome that is defined by the predisposition to developing multiple schwannomas. The diagnosis of schwannomatosis is established with the identification of a germline variant of *SMARCB1* or *LZTR1* (both located on chromosome 22q11) in an individual with a schwannoma or meningioma. The peripheral and spinal nerves are most commonly affected. Presentation typically involves an asymptomatic mass discovered incidentally on imaging or a mass with associated pain. After diagnosis, annual MR-imaging is recommended to screen for intracranial or spinal schwannomas. Symptomatic lesions or lesions that demonstrate significant interval enlargement are treated with surgical excision.[68]

Li–Fraumeni Syndrome

Li–Fraumeni syndrome is a heritable genetic syndrome resulting from germline mutation in the *TP53 gene* resulting in deficient DNA repair (chromosome 17). Associated cancers typically occur before the age of 30 years and include sarcomas, adrenocortical carcinomas, central nervous system tumors (astrocytoma, glioblastoma, choroid plexus carcinoma, medulloblastoma), and early-onset breast cancer.[69] There are several causal *TP53 germline* variants and penetrance is variable making predicting individual cancer-risk challenging.[69] In the 0 to 15 year age group, choroid plexus carcinoma and medulloblastoma are the most common central nervous system tumors. In the 16 to 50 year age group, astrocytomas and glioblastoma are the most commonly found tumors.[70] To identify tumors early, it is recommended these individuals undergo annual MR-imaging of the brain starting at 1 year of age.[71]

Lhermitte–Duclos Disease and Cowden Syndrome

Lhermitte–Duclos disease (LD), also referred to as dysplastic cerebellar gangliocytoma, is a rare hamartomatous growth affecting the cerebellum.[72] It is associated with Cowden syndrome in 40% of cases, which is an autosomal dominant neoplastic syndrome affecting the breast, thyroid, gastrointestinal tract, and genito-urinary system.[73] Both syndromes are the result of mutations in the *phosphatase and tensin homolog gene (PTEN) gene* (chromosome 10q23). The LD lesion is best seen on MR-imaging which shows a T1 hypointense and T2 hyperintense expansile lesion with proton spectroscopy showing a lactate peak and a reduction in choline peak.[74] These are slowly progressive lesions that are generally observed unless they become symptomatic. Surgical resection is curative.

SUMMARY

Familial neoplastic syndromes commonly impact the central and peripheral nervous systems. Managing these neoplastic syndromes requires a multi-disciplinary approach to ensure appropriate interval screening and to address the myriad of systemic complicating features. An understanding of the genetics, pathophysiology, manifestations, and management of each condition is necessary for neurologist and neurosurgeons treating these conditions.

CLINICS CARE POINTS

- NF-1 is an autosomal dominant disorder due to germline mutations on chromosome 17 with 100% penetrance defined by café au lait spots, neurofibromas, axillary, or intertriginous hyperpigmentation, optic gliomas, iris hamartomas, and/or sphenoid dysplasia.
- NF-2 is associated with bilateral vestibular schwannomas. It is caused by a mutation on chromosome 22 and, like NF-1, is autosomal dominant. Other associated tumors include meningiomas, gliomas, and neurofibromas.
- VHL is a multisystem neoplastic disorder autosomal dominant condition caused by mutation at the chromosome 3p25 locus associated with hemangioblastomas formation within the cerebellum, retina, brainstem, and spinal cord.

- Tuberous sclerosis is inherited in an autosomal dominant fusion with a classic triad of seizures, intellectual disability, and sebaceous adenomas. CNS findings include subependymal nodules and subependymal giant cell astrocytoma.
- Other nervous system neoplastic syndromes include schwannomatosis, Li–Fraumeni syndrome, Lhermitte–Duclos disease, and Cowden syndrome.

DISCLOSURE

The authors have nothing to disclose.

REFERENCES

1. Lammert M, Friedman JM, Kluwe L, et al. Prevalence of neurofibromatosis 1 in German children at elementary school enrollment. Arch Dermatol 2005;141(1): 71–4. https://doi.org/10.1001/archderm.141.1.71.
2. Hirbe AC, Gutmann DH. Neurofibromatosis type 1: a multidisciplinary approach to care. Lancet Neurol 2014;13(8):834–43. https://doi.org/10.1016/s1474-4422(14)70063-8.
3. National Institutes of Health Consensus Development Conference Statement: neurofibromatosis. Bethesda, MD, USA, July 13-15, 1987. Neurofibromatosis 1988;1(3):172–8.
4. Costa AA, Gutmann DH. Brain tumors in Neurofibromatosis type 1. Neurooncol Adv 2019;1(1):vdz040. https://doi.org/10.1093/noajnl/vdz040.
5. Ferner RE, Huson SM, Thomas N, et al. Guidelines for the diagnosis and management of individuals with neurofibromatosis 1. J Med Genet 2007;44(2):81–8. https://doi.org/10.1136/jmg.2006.045906.
6. King A, Listernick R, Charrow J, et al. Optic pathway gliomas in neurofibromatosis type 1: the effect of presenting symptoms on outcome. Am J Med Genet A 2003; 122a(2):95–9. https://doi.org/10.1002/ajmg.a.20211.
7. Packer RJ, Ater J, Allen J, et al. Carboplatin and vincristine chemotherapy for children with newly diagnosed progressive low-grade gliomas. J Neurosurg 1997;86(5):747–54. https://doi.org/10.3171/jns.1997.86.5.0747.
8. Sharif S, Ferner R, Birch JM, et al. Second primary tumors in neurofibromatosis 1 patients treated for optic glioma: substantial risks after radiotherapy. J Clin Oncol 2006;24(16):2570–5. https://doi.org/10.1200/jco.2005.03.8349.
9. Ullrich NJ, Raja AI, Irons MB, et al. Brainstem lesions in neurofibromatosis type 1. Neurosurgery 2007;61(4):762–6. https://doi.org/10.1227/01.neu.0000298904.63635.2d [discussion 766–7].
10. Mahdi J, Shah AC, Sato A, et al. A multi-institutional study of brainstem gliomas in children with neurofibromatosis type 1. Neurology 2017;88(16):1584–9. https://doi.org/10.1212/wnl.0000000000003881.
11. Vinchon M, Soto-Ares G, Ruchoux MM, et al. Cerebellar gliomas in children with NF1: pathology and surgery. Childs Nerv Syst 2000;16(7):417–20. https://doi.org/10.1007/pl00007285.
12. Sevick RJ, Barkovich AJ, Edwards MS, et al. Evolution of white matter lesions in neurofibromatosis type 1: MR findings. AJR Am J Roentgenol 1992;159(1):171–5. https://doi.org/10.2214/ajr.159.1.1609692.
13. Nguyen R, Kluwe L, Fuensterer C, et al. Plexiform neurofibromas in children with neurofibromatosis type 1: frequency and associated clinical deficits. J Pediatr 2011;159(4):652–5.e2. https://doi.org/10.1016/j.jpeds.2011.04.008.

14. Pollack IF, Colak A, Fitz C, et al. Surgical management of spinal cord compression from plexiform neurofibromas in patients with neurofibromatosis 1. Neurosurgery 1998;43(2):248–55. https://doi.org/10.1097/00006123-199808000-00038 [discussion 255–6].

15. Ferner RE, Gutmann DH. International consensus statement on malignant peripheral nerve sheath tumors in neurofibromatosis. Cancer Res 2002;62(5):1573–7.

16. Evans DG, Baser ME, McGaughran J, et al. Malignant peripheral nerve sheath tumours in neurofibromatosis 1. J Med Genet 2002;39(5):311–4. https://doi.org/10.1136/jmg.39.5.311.

17. Ferner RE, Golding JF, Smith M, et al. [18F]2-fluoro-2-deoxy-D-glucose positron emission tomography (FDG PET) as a diagnostic tool for neurofibromatosis 1 (NF1) associated malignant peripheral nerve sheath tumours (MPNSTs): a long-term clinical study. Ann Oncol 2008;19(2):390–4. https://doi.org/10.1093/annonc/mdm450.

18. Watson KL, Al Sannaa GA, Kivlin CM, et al. Patterns of recurrence and survival in sporadic, neurofibromatosis Type 1-associated, and radiation-associated malignant peripheral nerve sheath tumors. J Neurosurg 2017;126(1):319–29. https://doi.org/10.3171/2015.12.jns152443.

19. Asthagiri AR, Parry DM, Butman JA, et al. Neurofibromatosis type 2. Lancet 2009;373(9679):1974–86. https://doi.org/10.1016/s0140-6736(09)60259-2.

20. Evans DG, Baser ME, O'Reilly B, et al. Management of the patient and family with neurofibromatosis 2: a consensus conference statement. Br J Neurosurg 2005;19(1):5–12. https://doi.org/10.1080/02688690500081206.

21. Baser ME, Friedman JM, Wallace AJ, et al. Evaluation of clinical diagnostic criteria for neurofibromatosis 2. Neurology 2002;59(11):1759–65. https://doi.org/10.1212/01.wnl.0000035638.74084.f4.

22. Acoustic neuroma. Consens Statement 1991;9(4):1–24.

23. Evans DG, Huson SM, Donnai D, et al. A clinical study of type 2 neurofibromatosis. Q J Med 1992;84(304):603–18.

24. Mautner VF, Lindenau M, Baser ME, et al. The neuroimaging and clinical spectrum of neurofibromatosis 2. Neurosurgery 1996;38(5):880–5. https://doi.org/10.1097/00006123-199605000-00004 [discussion 885–6].

25. Masuda A, Fisher LM, Oppenheimer ML, et al. Hearing changes after diagnosis in neurofibromatosis type 2. Otol Neurotol 2004;25(2):150–4. https://doi.org/10.1097/00129492-200403000-00012.

26. Asthagiri AR, Vasquez RA, Butman JA, et al. Mechanisms of hearing loss in neurofibromatosis type 2. PLoS One 2012;7(9):e46132. https://doi.org/10.1371/journal.pone.0046132.

27. Dirks MS, Butman JA, Kim HJ, et al. Long-term natural history of neurofibromatosis Type 2-associated intracranial tumors. J Neurosurg 2012;117(1):109–17. https://doi.org/10.3171/2012.3.jns111649.

28. Samii M, Matthies C, Tatagiba M. Management of vestibular schwannomas (acoustic neuromas): auditory and facial nerve function after resection of 120 vestibular schwannomas in patients with neurofibromatosis 2. Neurosurgery 1997;40(4):696–705. https://doi.org/10.1097/00006123-199704000-00007 [discussion 705–6].

29. Brackmann DE, Fayad JN, Slattery WH 3rd, et al. Early proactive management of vestibular schwannomas in neurofibromatosis type 2. Neurosurgery 2001;49(2):274–80. https://doi.org/10.1097/00006123-200108000-00007 [discussion 280–3].

30. Kida Y, Kobayashi T, Tanaka T, et al. Radiosurgery for bilateral neurinomas associated with neurofibromatosis type 2. Surg Neurol 2000;53(4):383–9. https://doi.org/10.1016/s0090-3019(00)00174-9 [discussion 389–90].

31. Mathieu D, Kondziolka D, Flickinger JC, et al. Stereotactic radiosurgery for vestibular schwannomas in patients with neurofibromatosis type 2: an analysis of tumor control, complications, and hearing preservation rates. Neurosurgery 2007;60(3):460–8. https://doi.org/10.1227/01.neu.0000255340.26027.53 [discussion 468–70].

32. Roche PH, Régis J, Pellet W, et al. [Neurofibromatosis type 2. Preliminary results of gamma knife radiosurgery of vestibular schwannomas]. [Neurofibromatose de type 2. Résultats préliminaires de la radiochirurgie gamma knife des schwannomes vestibulaires]. Neurochirurgie 2000;46(4):339–53 [discussion 354].

33. Rowe JG, Radatz MW, Walton L, et al. Clinical experience with gamma knife stereotactic radiosurgery in the management of vestibular schwannomas secondary to type 2 neurofibromatosis. J Neurol Neurosurg Psychiatry 2003;74(9):1288–93. https://doi.org/10.1136/jnnp.74.9.1288.

34. Perry A, Giannini C, Raghavan R, et al. Aggressive phenotypic and genotypic features in pediatric and NF2-associated meningiomas: a clinicopathologic study of 53 cases. J Neuropathol Exp Neurol 2001;60(10):994–1003. https://doi.org/10.1093/jnen/60.10.994.

35. Ostrom QT, Gittleman H, Truitt G, et al. CBTRUS statistical report: primary brain and other central nervous system tumors diagnosed in the United States in 2011-2015. Neuro Oncol 2018;20(suppl_4):iv1–86. https://doi.org/10.1093/neuonc/noy131.

36. Evans DG, Birch JM, Ramsden RT. Paediatric presentation of type 2 neurofibromatosis. Arch Dis Child 1999;81(6):496–9. https://doi.org/10.1136/adc.81.6.496.

37. Look A, Lonser RR. Inherited genetic syndromes and meningiomas. Handb Clin Neurol 2020;169:121–9. https://doi.org/10.1016/b978-0-12-804280-9.00007-x.

38. Dow G, Biggs N, Evans G, et al. Spinal tumors in neurofibromatosis type 2. Is emerging knowledge of genotype predictive of natural history? J Neurosurg Spine 2005;2(5):574–9. https://doi.org/10.3171/spi.2005.2.5.0574.

39. Patronas NJ, Courcoutsakis N, Bromley CM, et al. Intramedullary and spinal canal tumors in patients with neurofibromatosis 2: MR imaging findings and correlation with genotype. Radiology 2001;218(2):434–42. https://doi.org/10.1148/radiology.218.2.r01fe40434.

40. McCormick PC, Torres R, Post KD, et al. Intramedullary ependymoma of the spinal cord. J Neurosurg 1990;72(4):523–32. https://doi.org/10.3171/jns.1990.72.4.0523.

41. Plotkin SR, O'Donnell CC, Curry WT, et al. Spinal ependymomas in neurofibromatosis Type 2: a retrospective analysis of 55 patients. J Neurosurg Spine 2011;14(4):543–7. https://doi.org/10.3171/2010.11.spine10350.

42. Epstein FJ, Farmer JP, Freed D. Adult intramedullary spinal cord ependymomas: the result of surgery in 38 patients. J Neurosurg 1993;79(2):204–9. https://doi.org/10.3171/jns.1993.79.2.0204.

43. Hoshimaru M, Koyama T, Hashimoto N, et al. Results of microsurgical treatment for intramedullary spinal cord ependymomas: analysis of 36 cases. Neurosurgery 1999;44(2):264–9. https://doi.org/10.1097/00006123-199902000-00012.

44. Minehan KJ, Shaw EG, Scheithauer BW, et al. Spinal cord astrocytoma: pathological and treatment considerations. J Neurosurg 1995;83(4):590–5. https://doi.org/10.3171/jns.1995.83.4.0590.

45. Mautner VF, Tatagiba M, Lindenau M, et al. Spinal tumors in patients with neurofibromatosis type 2: MR imaging study of frequency, multiplicity, and variety. AJR Am J Roentgenol 1995;165(4):951–5. https://doi.org/10.2214/ajr.165.4.7676998.

46. Sperfeld AD, Hein C, Schröder JM, et al. Occurrence and characterization of peripheral nerve involvement in neurofibromatosis type 2. Brain 2002;125(Pt 5): 996–1004. https://doi.org/10.1093/brain/awf115.

47. Bosch MM, Boltshauser E, Harpes P, et al. Ophthalmologic findings and long-term course in patients with neurofibromatosis type 2. Am J Ophthalmol 2006; 141(6):1068–77. https://doi.org/10.1016/j.ajo.2005.12.042.

48. Bouzas EA, Parry DM, Eldridge R, et al. Visual impairment in patients with neurofibromatosis 2. Neurology 1993;43(3 Pt 1):622–3. https://doi.org/10.1212/wnl.43. 3_part_1.622.

49. Mautner VF, Lindenau M, Baser ME, et al. Skin abnormalities in neurofibromatosis 2. Arch Dermatol 1997;133(12):1539–43.

50. Latif F, Tory K, Gnarra J, et al. Identification of the von Hippel-Lindau disease tumor suppressor gene. Science 1993;260(5112):1317–20. https://doi.org/10.1126/ science.8493574.

51. Maddock IR, Moran A, Maher ER, et al. A genetic register for von Hippel-Lindau disease. J Med Genet 1996;33(2):120–7. https://doi.org/10.1136/jmg.33.2.120.

52. Lonser RR, Glenn GM, Walther M, et al. von Hippel-Lindau disease. Lancet 2003; 361(9374):2059–67. https://doi.org/10.1016/s0140-6736(03)13643-4.

53. Wanebo JE, Lonser RR, Glenn GM, et al. The natural history of hemangioblastomas of the central nervous system in patients with von Hippel-Lindau disease. J Neurosurg 2003;98(1):82–94. https://doi.org/10.3171/jns.2003.98.1.0082.

54. Lonser RR, Butman JA, Huntoon K, et al. Prospective natural history study of central nervous system hemangioblastomas in von Hippel-Lindau disease. J Neurosurg 2014;120(5):1055–62. https://doi.org/10.3171/2014.1.jns131431.

55. Lonser RR, Oldfield EH. Microsurgical resection of spinal cord hemangioblastomas. Neurosurgery 2005;57(4 Suppl):372–6. https://doi.org/10.1227/01.neu. 0000176849.76663.e4 [discussion 372–6].

56. Lonser RR, Weil RJ, Wanebo JE, et al. Surgical management of spinal cord hemangioblastomas in patients with von Hippel-Lindau disease. J Neurosurg 2003;98(1):106–16. https://doi.org/10.3171/jns.2003.98.1.0106.

57. Cornelius JF, Saint-Maurice JP, Bresson D, et al. Hemorrhage after particle embolization of hemangioblastomas: comparison of outcomes in spinal and cerebellar lesions. J Neurosurg 2007;106(6):994–8. https://doi.org/10.3171/jns.2007.106. 6.994.

58. Migliorini D, Haller S, Merkler D, et al. Recurrent multiple CNS hemangioblastomas with VHL disease treated with pazopanib: a case report and literature review. CNS Oncol 2015;4(6):387–92. https://doi.org/10.2217/cns.15.22.

59. Pan J, Ho AL, D'Astous M, et al. Image-guided stereotactic radiosurgery for treatment of spinal hemangioblastoma. Neurosurg Focus 2017;42(1):E12. https://doi. org/10.3171/2016.10.focus16361.

60. Dollfus H, Massin P, Taupin P, et al. Retinal hemangioblastoma in von Hippel-Lindau disease: a clinical and molecular study. Invest Ophthalmol Vis Sci 2002; 43(9):3067–74.

61. Manski TJ, Heffner DK, Glenn GM. Endolymphatic sac tumors. A source of morbid hearing loss in von Hippel-Lindau disease. JAMA 1997;277(18):1461–6.

62. Walther MM, Reiter R, Keiser HR, et al. Clinical and genetic characterization of pheochromocytoma in von Hippel-Lindau families: comparison with sporadic pheochromocytoma gives insight into natural history of pheochromocytoma.

J Urol 1999;162(3 Pt 1):659–64. https://doi.org/10.1097/00005392-199909010-00004.

63. Hammel PR, Vilgrain V, Terris B, et al. Pancreatic involvement in von Hippel-Lindau disease. The Groupe Francophone d'Etude de la Maladie de von Hippel-Lindau. Gastroenterology 2000;119(4):1087–95. https://doi.org/10.1053/gast.2000.18143.

64. Józwiak S, Schwartz RA, Janniger CK, et al. Usefulness of diagnostic criteria of tuberous sclerosis complex in pediatric patients. J Child Neurol 2000;15(10):652–9. https://doi.org/10.1177/088307380001501003.

65. Chihi M, Gembruch O, Darkwah Oppong M, et al. Intracranial aneurysms in patients with tuberous sclerosis complex: a systematic review. J Neurosurg Pediatr 2019;24(2):174–83. https://doi.org/10.3171/2019.2.peds18661.

66. Nabbout R, Santos M, Rolland Y, et al. Early diagnosis of subependymal giant cell astrocytoma in children with tuberous sclerosis. J Neurol Neurosurg Psychiatry 1999;66(3):370–5. https://doi.org/10.1136/jnnp.66.3.370.

67. Franz DN, Leonard J, Tudor C, et al. Rapamycin causes regression of astrocytomas in tuberous sclerosis complex. Ann Neurol 2006;59(3):490–8. https://doi.org/10.1002/ana.20784.

68. Dhamija R, Plotkin S, Asthagiri A, et al. Schwannomatosis. In: Adam MP, Ardinger HH, Pagon RA, et al, editors. GeneReviews(®). Seattle: University of Washington; 1993.

69. Frebourg T, Bajalica Lagercrantz S, Oliveira C, et al. Guidelines for the Li-Fraumeni and heritable TP53-related cancer syndromes. Eur J Hum Genet 2020;28(10):1379–86. https://doi.org/10.1038/s41431-020-0638-4.

70. Amadou A, Achatz MIW, Hainaut P. Revisiting tumor patterns and penetrance in germline TP53 mutation carriers: temporal phases of Li-Fraumeni syndrome. Curr Opin Oncol 2018;30(1):23–9. https://doi.org/10.1097/cco.0000000000000423.

71. Kratz CP, Achatz MI, Brugières L, et al. Cancer screening recommendations for individuals with Li-Fraumeni syndrome. Clin Cancer Res 2017;23(11):e38–45. https://doi.org/10.1158/1078-0432.ccr-17-0408.

72. Giorgianni A, Pellegrino C, De Benedictis A, et al. Lhermitte-Duclos disease. A case report. Neuroradiol J 2013;26(6):655–60. https://doi.org/10.1177/197140091302600608.

73. Murray C, Shipman P, Khangure M, et al. Lhermitte-Duclos disease associated with Cowden's syndrome: case report and literature review. Australas Radiol 2001;45(3):343–6. https://doi.org/10.1046/j.1440-1673.2001.00933.x.

74. Joo G, Doumanian J. Radiographic findings of dysplastic cerebellar Gangliocytoma (Lhermitte-Duclos Disease) in a woman with cowden syndrome: a case study and literature review. J Radiol Case Rep 2020;14(3):1–6. https://doi.org/10.3941/jrcr.v14i3.3814.

Surgery, Stereotactic Radiosurgery, and Systemic Therapy in the Management of Operable Brain Metastasis

Rupesh Kotecha, MD[a,b], Manmeet S. Ahluwalia, MD[b,c],
Vitaly Siomin, MD[b,d], Michael W. McDermott, MD[b,d],*

KEYWORDS

- Stereotactic radiosurgery • Surgery • Targeted therapy • Immunotherapy
- Brain metastases

KEY POINTS

- Brain metastases represent the most common brain tumors in adults.
- Recent advances in our understanding of the molecular biology of metastases versus primary tumors have allowed for tailoring systemic therapies in those with actionable alterations and the introduction of immunotherapies has provided additional treatment options for a broad range of malignancies.
- Technical advances in surgical techniques with intraoperative image guidance and electrophysiologic mapping have improved surgical outcomes and innovative radiotherapy approaches, such as preoperative or postoperative stereotactic radiosurgery, continue to improve local control rates.
- Given the complexity of managing operable patients with brain metastases in the modern era, multi-disciplinary care is critical to improving patient outcomes.

INTRODUCTION

With an increasing proportion of the population being of advanced age, the prevalence of brain metastasis is likely to become a more important part of the practice of future neurosurgeons and radiation oncologists. Many of the advances in surgical techniques and radiotherapy over the last 25 years are now part of the routine practice

[a] Department of Radiation Oncology, Miami Cancer Institute, Baptist Health South Florida, Miami, FL, USA; [b] Herbert Wertheim College of Medicine, Florida International University, Miami, FL, USA; [c] Department of Medical Oncology, Miami Cancer Institute, Baptist Health South Florida, Miami, FL, USA; [d] Division of Neurosurgery, Miami Neuroscience Institute, Baptist Health South Florida, 8950 North Kendall Drive Suite 407 West, Miami, FL, USA
* Corresponding author. Miami Neuroscience Institute, Baptist Health South Florida, 8950 North Kendall Drive Suite 407 West, Miami, FL 33176.
E-mail address: MWMCD@baptisthealth.net

Neurol Clin 40 (2022) 421–436
https://doi.org/10.1016/j.ncl.2021.11.002
0733-8619/22/© 2021 Elsevier Inc. All rights reserved.

in most Western medical systems. The new age of advanced molecular-based pharmaceuticals will provide further improved control of both primary tumors and extracranial metastatic disease as well as intracranial disease. This review will focus primarily on surgical and radiosurgical therapies for brain metastases with a special focus on the recent literature.

PATHOLOGIC DIAGNOSIS OF BRAIN METASTASIS: A REVIVAL

A recent comprehensive review of the Surveillance, Epidemiology, and End Results (SEER) Medicare program demonstrated that only 10% to 13% of patients with brain metastasis undergo surgery.[1] Although resection is traditionally performed in the setting of an unknown primary,[2] solitary brain metastasis,[3] large intracranial lesion (>3 cm),[4] or significant neurologic symptomatology due to associated vasogenic edema and mass effect, there is a resurgence in interest in performing a biopsy or resection outside of these common criteria given the increasing data resulting from molecular profiling analyses of intracranial metastases. Whole-exome sequencing studies have demonstrated key genomic alterations associated with brain metastases not present in primary tumors that have been successfully recapitulated in xenograft mouse models.[5] This understanding, coupled with the increasing availability of molecular-based therapies with central nervous system (CNS) penetration, has promoted an increased interest in sampling intracranial disease in selected patients with discordant responses to systemic therapy. For example, a study of whole-exome sequencing of 86 matched brain metastases to primary tumors and normal tissues revealed potentially clinically actionable alterations in 53% of brain metastases not detected in primary tumors.[6] Importantly, comparisons of multiple intracranial lesions in the same patient demonstrate similar actionable changes, yet these seem distinct from extracranial metastases. To date, this genomic variability has been most robustly demonstrated in patients with breast cancer brain metastasis. In a recent systematic review of the literature of 1373 patients who underwent biopsy or resection of at least one intracranial lesion compared with the primary tumor, approximately 43% exhibited discordance in any receptor.[7] Of particular note, the weighted pooled estimate of HER2 gain was 9.0%, potentially increasing therapeutic targets for this otherwise overlooked patient population. This becomes even more relevant in patients with lung cancer, who not only represent the largest proportion of patients with brain metastasis but also the patient population for whom actionable alterations are observed in approximately 33% to 45%.[8] A deeper understanding of the genomic drivers of brain metastasis development coupled with innovative drug development will result in consideration for surgical intervention in patients until more minimally invasive profiling procedures become available.

SURGICAL ADVANCES IN BRAIN METASTASIS

Of the close to 1.5 million patients who will be expectedly diagnosed with cancer this year, up to 15% will present with brain metastases.[9,10] Almost 80% are found in the cerebral hemispheres, 15% in the cerebellum, and 5% in the brainstem. Only 10% to 15% are located in deep or eloquent parts of the brain.[11] Therefore, the vast majority of brain metastases could be considered "operable." While most of the patients with well-controlled intracranial disease typically die from the systemic disease progression, the mortality in patients with poorly controlled brain metastases is commonly related to the progressive deterioration of CNS functions.[12] This factor could be potentially modified with further refinement of the strategies to achieve optimal local control of the brain metastases. Even though considerable changes in treatment paradigms have been observed over the past years, neurosurgeons continue to play a crucial role in the modern management of this group of patients and will likely remain an integral part of the multidisciplinary team in the foreseeable future.

Surgical Options for Newly Diagnosed Brain Metastasis

Surgical options in patients with newly diagnosed brain metastasis (BM) include biopsy and/or surgical resection of the mass via craniotomy. In select cases (especially when the brain metastasis is deep-seated or in an eloquent area), needle biopsy can be combined with an upfront laser interstitial thermal therapy (LITT).

Surgery can offer several advantages over nonsurgical approaches:

- In up to 15% of patients, intracranial disease may be the only manifestation of cancer.[13] In such cases, obtaining tissue for pathologic diagnosis may be the only way to determine further treatment steps.
- Patients presenting with neurologic deterioration (eg, mental status and cognitive changes, seizures, weakness, sensory, and visual changes) are typically discovered to have a significant focal mass effect related to the location of the brain metastasis, presence of perifocal brain edema, hydrocephalus, or their combination. Craniotomy for resection of as much of the metastasis as safely possible may lead to rapid decompression of the brain, resolution of symptoms, and potential discontinuation of corticosteroids.

Considering the invasive nature of any neurosurgical procedure, the surgical risks are inevitable and should be carefully considered when evaluating indications for various treatments. Mut and colleagues in their review of the results of the surgical treatment of brain metastasis mention an iatrogenic mortality of 0.7% to 1.9% and morbidity of 3.9% to 6%.[14] Additionally, a typical postoperative recovery process (taking up to several weeks) may not seem to be critical in many patients with nonmetastatic brain lesions or could significantly delay treatment in patients whose expected survival will be relatively short. Therefore, it is commonly agreed that brain metastasis resection should probably be avoided in patients with a life expectancy of fewer than 3 to 6 months.[15] The probability of a favorable outcome may increase if several critical prognostic factors, such as baseline performance status (typically measured using the Karnofsky Performance Scale [KPS]), age, histology, and the number of metastatic lesions are factored in. The first such set of recommendations was introduced by the Radiation Therapy Oncology Group (RTOG).[16] The recursive partitioning analysis (RPA) evaluated the impact of the above patient-specific pretreatment variables on the outcomes after radiotherapy with or without surgery. Of note, only 15% of the patients with RTOG ended up having surgery. Nonetheless, the study determined that patients with RPA class 1 (KPS $\geq$70 and < 65 years of age with controlled primary disease) may be "more likely to benefit from aggressive treatment strategies," including resection.[17] Although the utilization of the RTOG/RPA classes was found to be easy and reproducible, the advances in the treatment of brain metastasis over the past 2 decades and failure to address the importance of tumor histology, became the basis for the search for more relevant and versatile prognostic systems. More recently, the graded prognostic assessment (GPA) and disease-specific graded prognostic assessment (DS-GPA) scores were introduced and successfully validated as potentially more precise prognostication tools.[9] In the referenced studies, the median overall survival was stratified based on the histology of the most common cancers metastatic to the brain: small cell/nonsmall cell lung carcinoma, renal cell carcinoma, melanoma, and breast cancer. Other factors, such as KPS, age, number of brain metastasis, and the extent of extracranial disease are included as well. Even though

GPA scores seem to hold prognostic value in patients with brain metastasis, they do not seem to be predictive of short-term mortality, thereby limiting their usefulness in neurosurgical populations.[18] Therefore, the idea that prognostic indices could be used alone to decide whether surgery is warranted or not, seems to be premature.

Surgery for Recurrent Lesions After Radiation Therapy

Repeat craniotomy for previously resected and irradiated brain metastasis has been demonstrated to improve long-term local control and even survival in patients with RPA class 1.[19] Kenion and colleagues retrospectively summarized their experience with redo craniotomy in 29 patients. 90% of patients survived more than 3 months, and 65.5% survived at least half a year. Five patients had more than 2 craniotomies, but only 2 had serious complications.[20] Repeat craniotomy for brain metastasis may be associated with several significant risks and technical difficulties, including wound healing problems and dehiscence, prolonged surgical time, higher risk of infection, presence of scar tissue, and adhesions that make dissection and mapping difficult, among others.[21] Kamp and colleagues described the challenges associated with repeat craniotomy for brain metastasis. In their series of 36 patients, only 37.8% had a gross total resection but definitive local control was achieved in 92% of patients with utilization of adjuvant therapy. The authors concluded that the presence of residual tumor on an early postoperative MRI correlated with further local progression.[22] Considering the high rates of local tumor control after reoperation, especially when combined with adjuvant modalities as part of a multi-modal approach, redo surgery seems to be a viable option in properly selected cases.

Laser Interstitial Thermal Therapy

LITT is a relatively novel strategy that may be used in patients with recurrent/progressive disease after surgical resection, radiation therapy, or both. This is a minimally invasive procedure involving the placement of a burr hole and stereotactic insertion of a laser probe. Focally delivered thermal energy induces protein denaturation, membrane disruption, leak of enzymes, vascular sclerosis and eventually, conversion of highly reactogenic radiation necrosis to a much less reactogenic coagulative necrosis.[23] In our institution, the procedure is performed inside the intraoperative MRI unit. The duration and extent of thermal ablation are guided by MR thermography. LITT may be advantageous in debilitated patients, in whom craniotomy would be otherwise considered with caution. A small (often "stab") incision eliminates the issue of wound healing, while the utilization of a stereotactic path minimizes the chances of morbidity related to intradural manipulation. Additionally, LITT can be a reasonable alternative for patients with inaccessible lesions, or in whom other standard options have failed.[24] The disadvantages of laser ablation include challenges associated with the treatment of very superficial lesions, or tumors adjacent to large blood vessels or in periventricular location, as flowing blood and CSF can function as heat sinks. LITT may also be limited to lesions less than 3 cm in diameter, unless several probes are inserted, which can make the procedure longer and potentially more complicated.[21] The acquisition of high-quality prospective data has been lagging behind the enthusiasm about the utilization of this promising technology in patients with brain metastasis.

Technological Advances

Several modern technological advances recently made it to the mainstream of oncological neurosurgery, including utilization of diffusion tensor images (DTI) and functional MRI (fMRI), that can be merged with standard navigational sequences and provide the surgical team with invaluable information about the functional significance of the tissues adjacent to the tumor. Surgeons can also now develop plans superimposing motor, sensory, visual, and functional networks on intraoperative image-guided systems (**Fig. 1**). The use of neuromonitoring and awake craniotomy techniques, as well as fluorescence and intraoperative MRI have aided surgeons in achieving more aggressive resection of brain metastasis via smaller openings and with reduced complication rates, even in lesions involving the eloquent regions of the brain.[21,25]

Significance of the Extent of Resection

Several studies demonstrated that the extent of resection (EOR) is one of the important factors that can have an impact on the local disease control and the risk of recurrence. Despite utilization of the most advanced microsurgical techniques and essentially universal use of postoperative adjuvant radiotherapy, local recurrence remains a significant challenge and may occur in 10% to 34% of patients a year after surgery.[14] Baumert and colleagues reported that infiltrative growth beyond the radiographically and macroscopically visible border of the brain metastasis was demonstrated in 63% of the evaluated cases[26]; small cell lung cancer and melanoma were associated with a maximum extent of infiltration up to 3 mm. Consequently, a concept of "supramarginal" resection of brain metastasis was introduced around the same time when the concept of "supratotal" resection was introduced in glioblastoma surgery. Supramarginal resection implies the removal of approximately 3 mm of normal-appearing perifocal tissue commonly with the use of an ultrasonic aspirator. Limited and mostly retrospective data confirms the safety and feasibility of this technique, as well as suggest improved local control compared with historic series.[27] Yoo and colleagues demonstrated better local tumor control after supratotal resection than standard gross total resection with 1 and 2-year respective local control rates of 29.1% and 29.1% in the supratotal and 58.6% and 63.2% in the gross total resection groups.[28] Unfortunately, the supratotal resection technique is limited to noneloquent areas of the cerebral hemispheres and cerebellum. Whether seemingly improved local control after maximally aggressive surgical resection will translate into improved overall disease control and/or survival is yet to be determined with the acquisition of higher quality data.

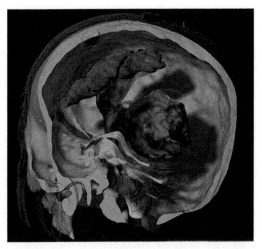

Fig. 1. Intraoperative image-guided system 3D representation of primary motor cortex (purple), descending motor fiber pathways (blue), visual fiber pathways (yellow).

RADIATION STRATEGIES IN THE MANAGEMENT OF RESECTABLE BRAIN METASTASIS

In patients with resectable brain metastasis, there are several treatment options and approaches from a radiotherapy standpoint, including postoperative whole-brain radiotherapy (WBRT), postoperative stereotactic radiosurgery (SRS), preoperative SRS, intraoperative radiotherapy (IORT), and CNS brachytherapy.

Historically, the addition of surgery to WBRT in patients with single brain metastasis was associated with an improvement in local control, neurologic survival, and functional independence.[3] On the other hand, for patients planning to undergo resection of brain metastasis, the addition of WBRT to surgery was associated with improvements in local control, distant intracranial control, and neurologic death, establishing the importance of adjuvant radiotherapy.[29] Even in the modern era, a reevaluation of the role of adjuvant radiotherapy has continued to demonstrate the benefit in disease control over resection alone.[30] Given the risks of neurocognitive decline in patients treated with WBRT and the increasing use of SRS for intact metastasis, there has been increasing interest in the use of postoperative SRS in patients undergoing resection. This led to the N107c trial in which patients who underwent resection of at least one brain metastasis were randomized to postoperative WBRT or SRS.[31] As compared with WBRT, postoperative SRS resulted in similar rates of local control, allowed for a shorter course of treatment, was associated with reduced toxicity and better quality-of-life, resulted in similar survival rates, and most importantly, improved neurocognitive preservation.[31] This has resulted in a key paradigm shift, illustrated best by patterns-of-care analyses which demonstrate that most of the postoperative patients in current practice now receive postoperative SRS rather than postoperative WBRT.[32]

Unlike postoperative WBRT, for which the entire cranial contents are treated to a relatively uniform prescription dose, postoperative SRS requires careful delineation of the target volume as well as consideration toward using additional microscopic disease extension margins. For example, as opposed to intact brain metastasis SRS cases, lower conformality indices were initially associated with improvements in local disease control, leading to a hypothesis that unintended margins beyond the surgical cavity itself were needed to reduce local failure rates.[33] Subsequent studies have demonstrated that a 2 mm clinical target volume (CTV) margin was associated with improved control compared with a 0 mm CTV margin[34] with others demonstrating no difference in local control with a margin of greater than 1 mm[35] and yet other studies demonstrating that a 3 mm margin is needed to cover at least 90% of tumor recurrences.[36] Additional work has demonstrated low rates of corridor recurrences with exclusion of the surgical tract.[37] Consensus contouring guidelines have been recently developed for target volume delineation and recommend inclusion of the entire surgical cavity, surgical tract, preoperative dural border, and sinus abutment with a 2 to 3 mm expansion (**Fig. 2**).[38] However, these are based on expert opinion and patterns-of-failure data are needed to validate these principles and guide clinical practice.

In addition to target volume delineation, selection of a dose/fractionation schedule based on the volume of the resection cavity is needed to balance the rate of tumor control with the risk of radiation necrosis (**Table 1**). Although single-fraction SRS has been used in the early postoperative SRS clinical trials, given the modest rates of disease recurrence (15%–39%),[30,31,39] several subsequent studies have evaluated the role of postoperative fractionated stereotactic radiosurgery (FSRS) to improve the local control rates while minimizing the risk of radiation necrosis.[40] To this end, the International Society of Stereotactic Radiosurgery (ISRS) consensus guidelines

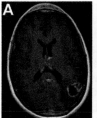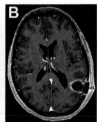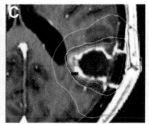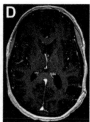

Fig. 2. Axial T1 postcontrast MRIs of the brain of a patient with adenosquamous carcinoma of the cervix found in a postictal state with a solitary left parietal lesion (*A*). She underwent gross total resection of the brain metastasis (*B*) and was subsequently treated with postoperative hypofractionated stereotactic radiosurgery to a dose of 27 Gy in 3 fractions (blue = cavity, red = 2 mm microscopic margin, yellow = 27 Gy prescription isodose *line*, green = 12 Gy isodose *line*) (*C*). Posttreatment imaging (*D*) demonstrates reduced enhancement of the surgical cavity without radiographic evidence of disease recurrence.

recommend postoperative dose and fractionation schedules of approximately 30 to 50 Gy $EQD2_{10}$, 50 to 70 $EQD2_5$, and 70 to 90 $EQD2_2$.[41] The ongoing A071801 trial (NCT04114981) randomizes patients with resected brain metastasis $\geq$2 cm to single-fraction SRS or FSRS with a primary endpoint of time to local recurrence and will provide additional prospective comparative data to guide clinical practice.

In addition to the challenges of target volume delineation and selection of an optimal dose and fractionation schedule, postoperative SRS has also been associated with a unique form of leptomeningeal disease failure—nodular leptomeningeal disease.[42] This occurs in approximately 7% to 23% of patients, with higher incidences in those with breast and lung cancer as well as those with metastases in infratentorial locations.[43] Nodular leptomeningeal disease development after surgery and postoperative SRS is not only challenging to salvage, it is also associated with an increased risk of neurologic death.[44] Focal therapy for these nodular failures is associated with further dural-based failures, albeit with similar overall survival to WBRT.[45]

Although postoperative SRS demonstrates significant advances over postoperative WBRT, preoperative SRS was developed as a focal therapy designed to overcome the limitations of postoperative SRS. First, preoperative SRS allows for accurate tumor volume delineation, similar to intact SRS treatments, with no additional microscopic margin additions required (**Fig. 3**). Although postoperative tumor cavities may often be smaller than preoperative tumor volumes, the inclusion of the surgical tract as

Table 1			
Recommended postoperative stereotactic radiosurgery guidelines for resected brain metastasis and associated risk of radiation necrosis[31,34,49,74–76]			
Cavity Volume[a]	Single Session SRS	Hypofractionated SRS[b]	Radiation Necrosis Risk
< 10 cc	18–20 Gy	27 Gy in 3 fx	15% (single fx); 10% (fractionated)
10–20 cc	15–17 Gy	27 Gy in 3 fx	10%
20–30 cc	14 Gy	27–30 Gy in 3–5 fx	10%–15%
> 30 cc	12 Gy	30 Gy in 3–5 fx	15%–20%

[a] 2 mm margin, adjacent/attached dura included in treatment volume, treatment week 3 to 4 from resection.
[b] dose-reduction performed for specific locations (brainstem, proximity to optic pathway, etc.).

well as microscopic margin addition may result in larger radiotherapy treatment volumes.[46] Second, preoperative SRS ensures that patients receive both the radiotherapy and surgery treatments for their intracranial disease without the need for coordinating logistics after resection. In a prospective phase II trial of postoperative SRS, 20% of patients did not receive treatment due to early disease recurrence, general medical decline, large-sized surgical cavities, and loss to follow-up.[39] Preliminary series of preoperative SRS with 20% dose-reduction from RTOG 90 to 05 dosing schema, no additional microscopic margins, and surgery planned within 48 hours of resection were associated with favorable local control rates (85% at 1 year) with no perioperative adverse events or leptomeningeal failures.[47] Retrospective comparative series has demonstrated similar rates of local recurrence and overall survival to postoperative WBRT[48] and reduced rates of radiation necrosis and leptomeningeal failure to postoperative SRS.[49] Given these promising results, preoperative dose-escalation studies have been recently performed to further improve local control rates (**Table 2**).[50] Ultimately, 2 ongoing trials (NCT03750227 and NCT03741673) will provide prospective comparative data of preoperative SRS to postoperative SRS for operable brain metastasis.

Although traditional radiotherapy options in the postoperative setting included WBRT and SRS/FSRS, there has been a resurgence in interest in IORT.[51] This allows for focal therapy to be delivered directly to the tumor cavity with no additional need for arranging logistics of postoperative radiotherapy, reduced ability for cancer regrowth before postoperative external beam radiotherapy, and faster initiation of systemic therapy. Retrospective series of intraoperative photon interstitial radiosurgery systems, which deliver approximately 1 to 2 Gy/min at a depth of 1 cm, have demonstrated favorable local control rates (>80% with a short median follow-up of 6 months), to metastases treated to a median dose of 16 Gy in 1 fraction.[52] However, prospective series using the same technology and a higher median dose of 18 Gy in 1 fraction have demonstrated surprisingly modest control rates (<50%), prompting questions regarding the true therapeutic benefit of this treatment approach.[53] Alternative IORT techniques have also been evaluated[54] and ongoing studies are evaluating the feasibility and local control rates with IORT in brain metastases (NCT03226483).

In addition to intraoperative external beam delivery technologies, brachytherapy is also gaining prominence in select patients who cannot undergo preoperative SRS or in those with recurrent disease. Early experience used iodine-125 (I-125) borrowing from extracranial indications and techniques, but although some series initially

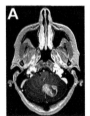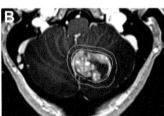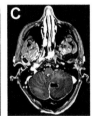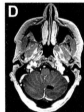

Fig. 3. Axial T1 postcontrast MRIs of the brain of a patient with a history of lung cancer who presented with occipital headaches and found to have a posterior fossa mass with effacement of the 4th ventricle (A). She underwent dose-escalated preoperative stereotactic radiosurgery to a dose of 18 Gy in 1 fraction (red = tumor, yellow = 18 Gy prescription isodose line, green = 12 Gy isodose line) (B). Immediate postoperative MRI of the brain (C) and subsequent follow-up image demonstrate retraction of the surgical bed and no radiographic evidence of disease recurrence (D).

Table 2
Recommended preoperative stereotactic radiosurgery guidelines for brain metastasis[47,50]

Lesion Diameter	Single Session SRS[a]	Hypofractionated SRS[a]
0–2 cm	18–20 Gy	27 Gy in 3 fx
2.1–3 cm	15–18 Gy	27 Gy in 3 fx
3.1–4 cm	15–18 Gy	27–30 Gy in 3–5 fx
> 4 cm	12–15 Gy	27–30 Gy in 3–5 fx

[a] dose-reduction performed for specific locations (brainstem, proximity to optic pathway, etc.).

demonstrated impressive local control rates,[55] the risk of radiation necrosis exceeded 20% in other series.[56] Alternatively, the utilization of Cesium-131 (C-131) over I-125 has proven advantageous for CNS brachytherapy applications given the faster dose rate (0.342 Gy/h vs 0.069 Gy/h) and limited half-life (9.69 days vs 59.4 days).[51] Wernicke evaluated the cost-effectiveness of surgical resection and brachytherapy versus surgical resection and SRS in a comparative series of 24 and 25 patients, respectively.[57] Direct hospital cost was significantly lower for the surgery/Cs-131 brachytherapy group, and quality-adjusted life years and incremental cost-effectiveness ratios favored surgery and brachytherapy over surgery and SRS. A prospective phase I/II trial in 24 newly-diagnosed brain metastasis (median size 2.7 cm) treated with resection and intraoperative C-131 implantation to a dose of 80 Gy prescribed to 5 mm depth demonstrated a 100% local control rate at a median follow-up of 19.3 months and no radiation necrosis events.[58] A subsequent trial in 42 patients treated to 46 large (all >2.0 cm, median size 3.0 cm) brain metastases demonstrated a 100% local control rate with no radiation necrosis events, albeit with a shorter median follow-up of 11.9 months.[59] Pham and colleagues demonstrated that patients with brain metastases who received cesium I-131 brachytherapy implants showed improvement in their neurocognitive status and self-assessment of quality of life at 4 and 6 months follow-up, compared with their baseline assessment.[60] Based on these promising results, a prospective phase III randomized trial is currently ongoing, evaluating postoperative CNS brachytherapy (C-131 carrier) to postoperative SRS/FSRS in patients with large (≥2.5 cm) resectable brain metastases (NCT04365374). However, given the limited options for patients with operable recurrent brain metastasis, especially after prior SRS, CNS brachytherapy is an additional tool in the armamentarium that should be considered in selected patients (**Fig. 4**).[61]

INTEGRATION OF SYSTEMIC THERAPY AND SURGERY: LESSONS LEARNED

Lung cancer is a leading cause of cancer death worldwide with more than 50% of patients diagnosed with advanced-stage disease at first diagnosis and is the leading cause of brain metastases.[62] Molecular diagnostic testing is routinely recommended for all patients with lung cancer to determine the possible use of targeted therapies for those with actionable alterations.[63] Given that there has been a transformational change in the genomically driven therapeutic management of lung cancer, there is an urgent need for more focused efforts to study the molecular drivers of brain metastases, and to identify new therapeutic targets with CNS penetration. In a recent effort to identify genomic alterations that promote lung cancer brain metastases, whole-exome sequencing of 73 lung cancer adenocarcinoma brain metastases cases was performed and compared with 503 primary lung adenocarcinomas.[5] The study identified significantly more frequent amplification of frequencies in MYC (12% vs 6%),

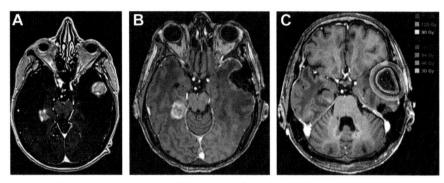

Fig. 4. Axial T1 postcontrast MRIs of the brain of a patient with nonsmall cell lung cancer metastatic to the brain with disease progression of a left anterior temporal lesion after whole-brain radiation therapy and salvage stereotactic radiosurgery (*A*). He underwent gross total resection of the brain metastasis (*B*) and implantation of Cesium-131 brachytherapy with isodose distribution displayed (*C*).

YAP1 (7% vs 0.8%), and MMP13 (10% vs 0.6%), and significantly higher deletions in CDKN2A/B (27% vs 13%) in brain metastases than primary lung tumors. The increased amplification frequencies of MYC and YAP1/MMP13 were confirmed in an independent cohort of 105 patients.[5] These findings confirm that somatic alterations can contribute to brain metastases and surgery plays a critical role in tissue acquisition to aid in such studies. In addition, there are known potential discordances between primary tumors and brain metastasis,[7,64] known recognition of the discordances in receptor status is a critical aspect of genomically driven therapeutic management of patients and surgery is needed for tissue acquisition in this scenario as well. Receptor expression profiles in cancer can alter during a disease course due to biological changes in the tumor, often as a result of selective pressure of systemic therapy, or because the metastatic lesions may be a result of clones with a molecular pattern for homing and growth conducive to a particular organ (in this case, the brain).[65,66] Epidermal growth factor receptor (EGFR) mutation occurs in 15% of the Caucasian population and higher incidence of up to 50% is seen in the Asian population.[67,68] Patients with exon 19 and 21 EGFR mutations have longer median progression-free survival (PFS) than wild-type EGFR disease (15.2 months vs 4.4 months) and hence it is important to know the receptor status on any craniotomy that is performed.[69]

Novel immunotherapeutic strategies targeting the PD-1/PD-L1 axis are promising in patients with metastatic lung cancer and have become the standard of care.[70] In patients without targetable oncogenic driver mutations, immune checkpoint inhibitors (ICIs) are commonly-used systemic therapeutic options for managing intracranial metastases. Corticosteroids are frequently used for symptomatic management of patients with brain metastases to manage edema; however, their immune-suppressive mechanism of action is can also antagonize immunotherapeutic strategies. The first evidence of the impact of corticosteroids was reported in a phase 2 clinical trial in melanoma brain metastases, which demonstrated a better response to immunotherapy in patients who did not receive upfront corticosteroids and were neurologically asymptomatic when compared with patients who received corticosteroid.[71] More recently, Checkmate 204 evaluated the response rates in previously untreated brain metastasis with dual immune checkpoint inhibitor therapy, and confirmed much lower response rates in patients who were on corticosteroid and were neurologically symptomatic compared with those not on corticosteroid or asymptomatic.[72] Two of 12 patients on corticosteroids had a complete response; 2 of 6 not on corticosteroids had a response. Hence, surgery can be helpful in symptomatic patients who would benefit from debulking mitigating the need for corticosteroids during systemic therapy. In addition, PD-L1 receptor discordance between the primary tumor and lung cancer brain metastasis has been well described. In an analysis of 146 paired primary lung cancers and brain metastases from 73 cases were identified and assessed for PD-L1, lesions with 5% or greater PD-L1 expression were considered positive.[73] There was discordance of tumor cell PD-L1 expression in 10 cases (14%), and disagreement of tumor-infiltrating lymphocytes PD-L1 expression in 19 cases (26%). Lesions with more discordant tumor cell expression of PD-L1 were obtained 6 or more months apart. This underscores the need for surgery to help in the recognition of the receptor status in such patients.

SUMMARY

Advances in the multi-disciplinary management of patients with brain metastasis have allowed for personalized treatment options for each patient in the modern era. Although surgery has remained a key role, advances in surgical techniques and the introduction of minimally invasive procedures have promoted its part in the multi-modal management. Further clinical trials will help determine the optimal radiotherapy approaches around resection as well as the introduction of novel agents with systemic penetration as we better learn the biological underpinnings of metastatic disease to the CNS.

AUTHORSHIP STATEMENT

Conception and Design: RK and McD. Critical Review of Manuscript: All authors.

DECLARATION OF INTERESTS

Conflicts of interest. R. Kotecha: Honoraria from Accuray Inc., Elekta AB, Viewray Inc., Novocure Inc., Elsevier Inc. Institutional research funding from Medtronic Inc., Blue Earth Diagnostics Ltd., Novocure, GT Medical Technologies, AstraZeneca, Exelixis, Viewray Inc. M. S. Ahluwalia: Receipt of grants/research supports: Astrazeneca, BMS, Bayer, Incyte, Pharmacyclics, Novocure, Mimivax, Merck. Receipt of honoraria or consultation fees: Bayer, Novocure, Kiyatec, Insightec, GSK, Xoft, Nuvation, Cellularity, SDP Oncology, Apollomics, Prelude, Janssen. Stock shareholder: Doctible, Mimivax, Cytodyn, MedInnovate Advisors LLC. V. Siomin: None. M. McDermott: Deinde Medical – consultant; Stryker - consultant. Cite Sources of Support (if applicable): None.

CLINICS CARE POINTS

- Resection of brain metastasis is performed in the setting of an unknown primary, solitary lesion, large lesion, or in those with significant neurologic symptomatology.
- Resection of brain metastasis may provide important molecular information on patients with discordant responses to systemic therapy or new actionable targets.
- Post-operative stereotactic radiosurgery preserves neurocognition and is associated with similar survival to post-operative whole-brain radiotherapy.

- Post-operative brachytherapy or pre-operative radiosurgery represents additional treatment options to improve local disease control rates.
- Surgery may be used in patients planned for systemic immunotherapy to relieve mass effect and reduce corticosteroid requirements.

ACKNOWLEDGMENTS

None

REFERENCES

1. Lamba N, Kearney RB, Catalano PJ, et al. Population-based estimates of survival among elderly patients with brain metastases. Neuro Oncol 2021;23(4): 661–76.
2. Giordana MT, Cordera S, Boghi A. Cerebral metastases as first symptom of cancer: a clinico-pathologic study. J Neurooncol 2000;50(3):265–73.
3. Patchell RA, Tibbs PA, Walsh JW, et al. A randomized trial of surgery in the treatment of single metastases to the brain. N Engl J Med 1990;322(8):494–500.
4. Prabhu RS, Press RH, Patel KR, et al. Single-fraction stereotactic radiosurgery (SRS) alone versus surgical resection and SRS for large brain metastases: a multi-institutional analysis. Int J Radiat Oncol Biol Phys 2017;99(2):459–67.
5. Shih DJH, Nayyar N, Bihun I, et al. Genomic characterization of human brain metastases identifies drivers of metastatic lung adenocarcinoma. Nat Genet 2020; 52(4):371–7.
6. Brastianos PK, Carter SL, Santagata S, et al. Genomic Characterization of Brain Metastases Reveals Branched Evolution and Potential Therapeutic Targets. Cancer Discov 2015;5(11):1164–77.
7. Kotecha R, Tonse R, Rubens M, et al. Systematic review and meta-analysis of breast cancer brain metastasis and primary tumor receptor expression discordance. Neurooncol Adv 2021;3(1):vdab010.
8. Lamba N, Wen PY, Aizer AA. Epidemiology of brain metastases and leptomeningeal disease. Neuro Oncol 2021;23(9):1447–56.
9. Sperduto PW, Chao ST, Sneed PK, et al. Diagnosis-specific prognostic factors, indexes, and treatment outcomes for patients with newly diagnosed brain metastases: a multi-institutional analysis of 4,259 patients. Int J Radiat Oncol Biol Phys 2010;77(3):655–61.
10. Zimm S, Wampler GL, Stablein D, et al. Intracerebral metastases in solid-tumor patients: natural history and results of treatment. Cancer 1981;48(2):384–94.
11. Colaco R, Martin P, Chiang V. Evolution of multidisciplinary brain metastasis management: case study and literature review. Yale J Biol Med 2015;88(2):157–65.
12. Arbit E, Wronski M, Burt M, et al. The treatment of patients with recurrent brain metastases. A retrospective analysis of 109 patients with nonsmall cell lung cancer. Cancer 1995;76(5):765–73.
13. Han HJ, Chang WS, Jung HH, et al. Optimal Treatment Decision for Brain Metastases of Unknown Primary Origin: The Role and Timing of Radiosurgery. Brain Tumor Res Treat 2016;4(2):107–10.
14. Mut M. Surgical treatment of brain metastasis: a review. Clin Neurol Neurosurg 2012;114(1):1–8.
15. Ranasinghe MG, Sheehan JM. Surgical management of brain metastases. Neurosurg Focus 2007;22(3):E2.

16. Gaspar LE, Scott C, Murray K, et al. Validation of the RTOG recursive partitioning analysis (RPA) classification for brain metastases. Int J Radiat Oncol Biol Phys 2000;47(4):1001–6.
17. Nieder C, Nestle U, Motaref B, et al. Prognostic factors in brain metastases: should patients be selected for aggressive treatment according to recursive partitioning analysis (RPA) classes? Int J Radiat Oncol Biol Phys 2000;46(2):297–302.
18. Jakola AS, Gulati S, Nerland US, et al. Surgical resection of brain metastases: the prognostic value of the graded prognostic assessment score. J Neurooncol 2011;105(3):573–81.
19. Vecil GG, Suki D, Maldaun MV, et al. Resection of brain metastases previously treated with stereotactic radiosurgery. J Neurosurg 2005;102(2):209–15.
20. Kennion O, Holliman D. Outcome after craniotomy for recurrent cranial metastases. Br J Neurosurg 2017;31(3):369–73.
21. Sankey EW, Tsvankin V, Grabowski MM, et al. Operative and peri-operative considerations in the management of brain metastasis. Cancer Med 2019;8(16):6809–31.
22. Kamp MA, Fischer I, Dibue-Adjei M, et al. Predictors for a further local in-brain progression after re-craniotomy of locally recurrent cerebral metastases. Neurosurg Rev 2018;41(3):813–23.
23. Lagman C, Chung LK, Pelargos PE, et al. Laser neurosurgery: A systematic analysis of magnetic resonance-guided laser interstitial thermal therapies. J Clin Neurosci 2017;36:20–6.
24. Salem U, Kumar VA, Madewell JE, et al. Neurosurgical applications of MRI guided laser interstitial thermal therapy (LITT). Cancer Imaging 2019;19(1):65.
25. Kamp MA, Slotty PJ, Cornelius JF, et al. The impact of cerebral metastases growth pattern on neurosurgical treatment. Neurosurg Rev 2018;41(1):77–86.
26. Baumert BG, Rutten I, Dehing-Oberije C, et al. A pathology-based substrate for target definition in radiosurgery of brain metastases. Int J Radiat Oncol Biol Phys 2006;66(1):187–94.
27. Kamp MA, Rapp M, Slotty PJ, et al. Incidence of local in-brain progression after supramarginal resection of cerebral metastases. Acta Neurochir (Wien) 2015;157(6):905–10.
28. Yoo H, Kim YZ, Nam BH, et al. Reduced local recurrence of a single brain metastasis through microscopic total resection. J Neurosurg 2009;110(4):730–6.
29. Patchell RA, Tibbs PA, Regine WF, et al. Postoperative radiotherapy in the treatment of single metastases to the brain: a randomized trial. JAMA 1998;280(17):1485–9.
30. Mahajan A, Ahmed S, McAleer MF, et al. Post-operative stereotactic radiosurgery versus observation for completely resected brain metastases: a single-centre, randomised, controlled, phase 3 trial. Lancet Oncol 2017;18(8):1040–8.
31. Brown PD, Ballman KV, Cerhan JH, et al. Postoperative stereotactic radiosurgery compared with whole brain radiotherapy for resected metastatic brain disease (NCCTG N107C/CEC.3): a multicentre, randomised, controlled, phase 3 trial. Lancet Oncol 2017;18(8):1049–60.
32. Chin AL, Li G, Gephart MH, et al. Stereotactic Radiosurgery After Resection of Brain Metastases: Changing Patterns of Care in the United States. World Neurosurg 2020;144:e797–806.
33. Soltys SG, Adler JR, Lipani JD, et al. Stereotactic radiosurgery of the postoperative resection cavity for brain metastases. Int J Radiat Oncol Biol Phys 2008;70(1):187–93.

34. Choi CY, Chang SD, Gibbs IC, et al. Stereotactic radiosurgery of the postoperative resection cavity for brain metastases: prospective evaluation of target margin on tumor control. Int J Radiat Oncol Biol Phys 2012;84(2):336–42.

35. Jhaveri J, Chowdhary M, Zhang X, et al. Does size matter? Investigating the optimal planning target volume margin for postoperative stereotactic radiosurgery to resected brain metastases. J Neurosurg 2018;130(3):797–803.

36. Gui C, Moore J, Grimm J, et al. Local recurrence patterns after postoperative stereotactic radiation surgery to resected brain metastases: A quantitative analysis to guide target delineation. Pract Radiat Oncol 2018;8(6):388–96.

37. Shi S, Sandhu N, Jin M, et al. Stereotactic Radiosurgery for Resected Brain Metastases: Does the Surgical Corridor Need to be Targeted? Pract Radiat Oncol 2020;10(5):e363–71.

38. Soliman H, Ruschin M, Angelov L, et al. Consensus Contouring Guidelines for Postoperative Completely Resected Cavity Stereotactic Radiosurgery for Brain Metastases. Int J Radiat Oncol Biol Phys 2018;100(2):436–42.

39. Brennan C, Yang TJ, Hilden P, et al. A phase 2 trial of stereotactic radiosurgery boost after surgical resection for brain metastases. Int J Radiat Oncol Biol Phys 2014;88(1):130–6.

40. Minniti G, Niyazi M, Andratschke N, et al. Current status and recent advances in resection cavity irradiation of brain metastases. Radiat Oncol 2021;16(1):73.

41. Redmond KJ, De Salles AAF, Fariselli L, et al. Stereotactic Radiosurgery for Postoperative Metastatic Surgical Cavities: A Critical Review and International Stereotactic Radiosurgery Society (ISRS) Practice Guidelines. Int J Radiat Oncol Biol Phys 2021;111(1):68–80.

42. Cagney DN, Lamba N, Sinha S, et al. Association of Neurosurgical Resection With Development of Pachymeningeal Seeding in Patients With Brain Metastases. JAMA Oncol 2019;5(5):703–9.

43. Shi S, Sandhu N, Jin MC, et al. Stereotactic Radiosurgery for Resected Brain Metastases: Single-Institutional Experience of Over 500 Cavities. Int J Radiat Oncol Biol Phys 2020;106(4):764–71.

44. Prabhu RS, Turner BE, Asher AL, et al. Leptomeningeal disease and neurologic death after surgical resection and radiosurgery for brain metastases: A multi-institutional analysis. Adv Radiat Oncol 2021;6(2):100644.

45. Prabhu RS, Turner BE, Asher AL, et al. A multi-institutional analysis of presentation and outcomes for leptomeningeal disease recurrence after surgical resection and radiosurgery for brain metastases. Neuro Oncol 2019;21(8):1049–59.

46. Routman DM, Yan E, Vora S, et al. Preoperative Stereotactic Radiosurgery for Brain Metastases. Front Neurol 2018;9:959.

47. Asher AL, Burri SH, Wiggins WF, et al. A new treatment paradigm: neoadjuvant radiosurgery before surgical resection of brain metastases with analysis of local tumor recurrence. Int J Radiat Oncol Biol Phys 2014;88(4):899–906.

48. Patel KR, Burri SH, Boselli D, et al. Comparing pre-operative stereotactic radiosurgery (SRS) to post-operative whole brain radiation therapy (WBRT) for resectable brain metastases: a multi-institutional analysis. J Neurooncol 2017;131(3):611–8.

49. Patel KR, Burri SH, Asher AL, et al. Comparing Preoperative With Postoperative Stereotactic Radiosurgery for Resectable Brain Metastases: A Multi-institutional Analysis. Neurosurgery 2016;79(2):279–85.

50. Murphy ES, Yang K, Suh JH, et al. Prospective Phase I Dose Escalation Study for Neoadjuvant Radiosurgery for Large Brain Metastases. Int J Radiat Oncol Biol Phys 2019;105(1):S10–1.

51. Tom MC, Joshi N, Vicini F, et al. The American Brachytherapy Society consensus statement on intraoperative radiation therapy. Brachytherapy 2019;18(3):242–57.
52. Curry WT Jr, Cosgrove GR, Hochberg FH, et al. Stereotactic interstitial radiosurgery for cerebral metastases. J Neurosurg 2005;103(4):630–5.
53. Pantazis G, Trippel M, Birg W, et al. Stereotactic interstitial radiosurgery with the Photon Radiosurgery System (PRS) for metastatic brain tumors: a prospective single-center clinical trial. Int J Radiat Oncol Biol Phys 2009;75(5):1392–400.
54. Weil RJ, Mavinkurve GG, Chao ST, et al. Intraoperative radiotherapy to treat newly diagnosed solitary brain metastasis: initial experience and long-term outcomes. J Neurosurg 2015;122(4):825–32.
55. Petr MJ, McPherson CM, Breneman JC, et al. Management of newly diagnosed single brain metastasis with surgical resection and permanent I-125 seeds without upfront whole brain radiotherapy. J Neurooncol 2009;92(3):393–400.
56. Huang K, Sneed PK, Kunwar S, et al. Surgical resection and permanent iodine-125 brachytherapy for brain metastases. J Neurooncol 2009;91(1):83–93.
57. Wernicke AG, Yondorf MZ, Parashar B, et al. The cost-effectiveness of surgical resection and cesium-131 intraoperative brachytherapy versus surgical resection and stereotactic radiosurgery in the treatment of metastatic brain tumors. J Neurooncol 2016;127(1):145–53.
58. Wernicke AG, Yondorf MZ, Peng L, et al. Phase I/II study of resection and intraoperative cesium-131 radioisotope brachytherapy in patients with newly diagnosed brain metastases. J Neurosurg 2014;121(2):338–48.
59. Wernicke AG, Hirschfeld CB, Smith AW, et al. Clinical Outcomes of Large Brain Metastases Treated With Neurosurgical Resection and Intraoperative Cesium-131 Brachytherapy: Results of a Prospective Trial. Int J Radiat Oncol Biol Phys 2017;98(5):1059–68.
60. Pham A, Yondorf MZ, Parashar B, et al. Neurocognitive function and quality of life in patients with newly diagnosed brain metastasis after treatment with intraoperative cesium-131 brachytherapy: a prospective trial. J Neurooncol 2016;127(1):63–71.
61. Raleigh DR, Seymour ZA, Tomlin B, et al. Resection and brain brachytherapy with permanent iodine-125 sources for brain metastasis. J Neurosurg 2017;126(6):1749–55.
62. Siegel RL, Miller KD, Fuchs HE, et al. Cancer Statistics, 2021. CA Cancer J Clin 2021;71(1):7–33.
63. Mayekar MK, Bivona TG. Current Landscape of Targeted Therapy in Lung Cancer. Clin Pharmacol Ther 2017;102(5):757–64.
64. Hulsbergen AFC, Claes A, Kavouridis VK, et al. Subtype switching in breast cancer brain metastases: a multicenter analysis. Neuro Oncol 2020;22(8):1173–81.
65. Thompson AM, Jordan LB, Quinlan P, et al. Prospective comparison of switches in biomarker status between primary and recurrent breast cancer: the Breast Recurrence In Tissues Study (BRITS). Breast Cancer Res 2010;12(6):R92.
66. Gong Y, Han EY, Guo M, et al. Stability of estrogen receptor status in breast carcinoma: a comparison between primary and metastatic tumors with regard to disease course and intervening systemic therapy. Cancer 2011;117(4):705–13.
67. Langer CJ, Mehta MP. Current management of brain metastases, with a focus on systemic options. J Clin Oncol 2005;23(25):6207–19.
68. Palmer JD, Trifiletti DM, Gondi V, et al. Multidisciplinary patient-centered management of brain metastases and future directions. Neurooncol Adv 2020;2(1):vdaa034.

69. Han G, Bi J, Tan W, et al. A retrospective analysis in patients with EGFR-mutant lung adenocarcinoma: is EGFR mutation associated with a higher incidence of brain metastasis? Oncotarget 2016;7(35):56998–7010.

70. Yu H, Boyle TA, Zhou C, et al. PD-L1 Expression in Lung Cancer. J Thorac Oncol 2016;11(7):964–75.

71. Margolin K, Ernstoff MS, Hamid O, et al. Ipilimumab in patients with melanoma and brain metastases: an open-label, phase 2 trial. Lancet Oncol 2012;13(5):459–65.

72. Tawbi HA, Forsyth PA, Hodi FS, et al. Safety and Efficacy of the Combination of Nivolumab Plus Ipilimumab in Patients With Melanoma and Asymptomatic or Symptomatic Brain Metastases (CheckMate 204). Neuro Oncol 2021;23(11):1961–73.

73. Mansfield AS, Aubry MC, Moser JC, et al. Temporal and spatial discordance of programmed cell death-ligand 1 expression and lymphocyte tumor infiltration between paired primary lesions and brain metastases in lung cancer. Ann Oncol 2016;27(10):1953–8.

74. Navarria P, Pessina F, Clerici E, et al. Surgery followed by hypofractionated radiosurgery on the tumor bed in oligometastatic patients with large brain metastases. Results of a Phase II study. Int J Radiat Oncol Biol Phys 2019;105(5):1095–105.

75. Minniti G, Esposito V, Clarke E, et al. Multidose stereotactic radiosurgery (9 Gy x 3) of the postoperative resection cavity for treatment of large brain metastases. Int J Radiat Oncol Biol Phys 2013;86(4):623–9.

76. Nguyen TK, Sahgal A, Detsky J, et al. Predictors of Leptomeningeal Disease Following Hypofractionated Stereotactic Radiotherapy for Intact and Resected Brain Metastases. Neuro Oncol 2019;22(1):84–93.

Surgical Neuro-Oncology
Management of Glioma

Dana Mitchell, MS[a,1], Jack M. Shireman, BS[b,1], Mahua Dey, MD[b,*]

KEYWORDS

- Glioma • Glioblastoma • Astrocytoma • Low-grade glioma • Oligodendroglioma
- Surgery • Management • Biopsy

KEY POINTS

- Gliomas are the most common primary CNS malignancy in adults and there are currently no effective treatment options.
- Surgical management of gliomas aids in tissue diagnosis, relieves mass effect, cytoreduction, and improves overall survival.
- Integrated histologic and molecular tissue diagnosis is of utmost importance for the management of gliomas and clinical trial eligibility.
- Modern surgical adjuncts such as functional mapping and improved intraoperative tumor visualization are critical to optimizing gross total resection without neurologic deficits.
- Surgical intervention plays a crucial role in innovative clinical trials involving intracavitary delivery of therapeutics, thus bypassing the limitations of BBB.

INTRODUCTION

According to the NCI's Surveillance, Epidemiology, and End Results program, brain and other nervous system tumors will account for an estimated 24,530 cancer diagnoses and 18,600 fatalities in 2021 (www.seer.cancer.gov). The average age of diagnosis for a CNS tumor is 60 years; however, this can vary widely with tumor type. Gliomas account for 25% of nonmalignant and 81% of malignant CNS lesions.[1] Tumors of astrocytic origin account for the majority of all gliomas (76%), with glioblastoma (GBM), accounting for 57% of all malignant gliomas diagnosed.[1] According to the Central Brain Tumor Registry of the United States (CBTRUS) data compiled from 2012 to 2016, GBM carried the highest age-adjusted annual incidence rate of any malignant tumor at 3.22 per 100,000 individuals. Based on this incidence rate, there will be roughly 11,000 new cases of GBM diagnosed yearly in the United States. CBTRUS

[a] Department of Pediatrics, Indiana University, Herman B. Wells Center for Pediatric Research 1044 W Walnut St, Indianapolis, IN 46202, USA; [b] Department of Neurosurgery, University of Wisconsin School of Medicine and Public Health, 600 Highland Avenue CSC K3/803, Madison, WI 53792, USA
[1] Coauthors: Both authors contributed equally to this work.
* Corresponding author.
E-mail address: dey@neurosurgery.wisc.edu

Neurol Clin 40 (2022) 437–453
https://doi.org/10.1016/j.ncl.2021.11.003
0733-8619/22/© 2021 Elsevier Inc. All rights reserved.

estimates the 5-year survival post-GBM diagnosis at 6.8%, meaning roughly only 750 of those 11,000 individuals diagnosed this year will survive until 2026.

Before 2016, the World Health Organization (WHO) classified gliomas based on histology alone (**Table 1**) to aid in therapeutic decision-making and predict prognosis. Highly proliferative high-grade gliomas (HGGs) were associated with rapid disease progression as well as poor overall survival (OS), whereas slow-growing low-grade gliomas (LGGs) were associated with better prognosis, but eventual recurrence. However, clinical data demonstrate that despite exhibiting similar histologic characteristics, there is significant variation within each tumor grade in terms of disease course, time to recurrence, response to therapy, and OS.[2]

Recent data suggest that the molecular classification of gliomas based on genetic and epigenetic changes is more predictive of clinical course than histologic classification.[2,3] For example, a high-grade tumor as defined by histology, such as GBM, that carries a molecular mutation in isocitrate dehydrogenase (IDH) has almost double the median OS of an IDH-wildtype (*wt*) tumor (15 months vs 31 months).[4] Other molecular markers have been recognized for their ability to predict prognosis and distinguish tumors that deviate significantly from typical survival patterns. 1p/19q codeletion typically co-occurs with IDH mutations and is indicative of a less aggressive tumor, regardless of histology.[5] O^6-Methylguanine-DNA methyltransferase (MGMT) gene methylation status has also emerged as a prognostic biomarker for the efficacy of alkylating therapies in the treatment of gliomas. In GBM specifically, MGMT promoter methylation increases survival from 15.3 months to 21.7 months.[6] Other therapeutic and prognostic markers important for glioma diagnosis are summarized in **Table 2**. Consequently, in 2016, the WHO revised the classification of gliomas to incorporate these molecular biomarkers together with histologic features, thereby introducing the concept of "integrated diagnosis" as a means to better guide therapeutic strategy and predict patient outcomes.[2]

CLINICAL PRESENTATION

Patients with gliomas most commonly present with focal neurologic deficits that have progressed over days to weeks in patients with HGGs, or over longer periods in those with LGGs.[7] Patients may also experience headaches (50%–60%) or seizures (20%–50%), with seizures occurring as a presenting symptom more commonly in patients

Table 1		
WHO grading of glioma		
Grade	Characteristics	Tumor Types
I	Low proliferative potential	Pilocytic astrocytoma
II	Low proliferative potential, but infiltrative. Often recur and can progress to higher grade tumors	Astrocytoma Oligodendroglioma Oligoastrocytoma
III	Demonstrate histologic evidence of malignancy: 1. Hypercellularity 2. Nuclear atypia 3. Increased mitotic activity	Anaplastic astrocytoma Anaplastic oligodendroglioma Anaplastic oligoastrocytoma
IV	Demonstrate histologic evidence of malignancy: 1. Hypercellularity 2. Nuclear atypia 3. Increased mitotic activity Plus vascular proliferation and presence of necrosis	Glioblastoma

Table 2
Molecular markers of glioma

Molecular Markers	Identification	Primary Outcome Difference	Comments
IDH1/IDH2 mutation	Histologic Stain DNA sequencing IDH1 (Codon 132) IDH2 (Codon 172)	Tumors harboring IDH mutations carry a much higher overall survival rate and may offer additional targeting or therapeutic strategies	The most common IDH mutation in glioma is IDH1 R132H
1p/19q codeletion	FISH NGS (with copy number information)	1p/19q codeletion is a defining feature of oligodendroglial tumors and a predictor of favorable response among other gliomas	Almost always co-occurs with IDH mutations so disagreement between the two should raise concerns for false positives in deletion detection
ATRX mutation	Histologic stain (loss of nuclear ATRX expression indicates the presence of ATRX mutation) DNA sequencing	Typically used as a broad classifier for well-differentiated astrocytic glioma No prognostic indication	ATRX mutation closely correlates with IDH and TP53 mutations but is mutually exclusive with 1p/19q codeletion
TP53 mutation	Histologic staining (nuclear localization) DNA sequencing	Supportive in diagnosis for IDH mutant astrocytoma No prognostic indication	Nuclear localization of TP53 can reflect mutation of the gene but sequencing should still confirm
H3K27m mutation	Histologic staining for specific mutation protein DNA sequencing	Prognostically can indicate poor survival in pediatric glioblastomas	Typically present in diffuse gliomas in midline locations such as DIPG
H3G34 mutation	Histologic staining for specific mutation proteins NGS	Associated with poor prognosis in mainly diffuse hemispheric gliomas in children and young adults	The mutations associated with H3G4 are missense and result in G34R or G34V alterations
BRAF alteration	Histologic stain for mutation-specific proteins (V600E Mutation) DNA sequencing FISH (KIAA1549-BRAF fusion)	BRAF V600E mutation typically correlates with an increased risk of recurrence in pediatric gliomas	BRAF V600E mutational IHC histologic stains can be difficult to interpret
RELA Fusion	FISH	RELA fusion clinically defines 70% of childhood supratentorial ependymomas No prognostic indication	Fusion is between RELA and C19orf95 L1CAM expression on histology can correlate with the presence of RELA fusion

(continued on next page)

Table 2 (continued)			
Molecular Markers	Identification	Primary Outcome Difference	Comments
YAP1 fusion	FISH NGS	Diagnostically characteristic of a subset of childhood supratentorial ependymomas No prognostic indication	Fusion typically occurs with MAMLD1 but is not exclusive

with LGGs harboring isocitrate dehydrogenase type 1 (IDH1) mutations.[7–9] Tumor location is the primary determinant of presenting signs and symptoms. Frontal tumors may present with weakness, those in the parietal lobe with numbness or hemineglect, and occipital tumors or masses along the optic radiations with visual field deficits. Gliomas within the temporal lobe, prefrontal cortex, or corpus callosum may present with less overt findings such as short-term memory deficits, personality changes, or mood disorders. Tumors within eloquent regions of the brain are likely to present at smaller size, whereas those in less eloquent areas, such as the frontal lobe, tend to be larger at presentation[10] (Box 1).

Box 1
Clinical evaluation for glioma

Clinical Evaluation for a Patient Presenting with Neurologic Deficits or Seizures:

- Thorough history of presentation, symptoms, and physical examination
- Computed tomography (CT) scan:
  Lesion that may be homogenous or heterogenous with vasogenic edema.
- MRI with and without gadolinium if suspected glioma on CT scan:
  Contrast enhancement, edema, and gyral enlargement strongly suggest high-grade tumor. Lack of contrast enhancement in the setting of edema and gyral enlargement suggest low-grade tumor.
- Diffusion tensor imaging allows for the visualization of tracts to assess tumor involvement in the displacement of critical structures.
- Functional MRI is helpful primarily for dominant hemisphere gliomas involving eloquent regions.
- MR spectroscopy can help delineate between glioma and other pathologies if the initial imaging and clinical presentation are not highly conclusive of glioma.

Initial Management

Symptom Management
- Antiepileptics if there is any suspicion for prior epileptic activity.
- In patients with new or worsening neurologic deficits, dexamethasone can improve clinical functioning by reducing vasogenic edema.
- Any signs or symptoms of increased intracranial pressure or impending hydrocephalus should prompt urgent neurosurgical evaluation and consideration for inpatient admission.
- Given the need for tissue diagnosis in most glioma patients, a thorough preoperative evaluation should be performed as well.

Imaging

Diagnosis and preoperative planning

Gadolinium-enhanced MRI remains the gold standard for the diagnosis of glioma. In adults, LGGs are typically nonenhancing on T1 and appear as hyperintense lesions on T2/FLAIR with an absence of vasogenic edema.[11,12] Alternatively, HGGs are hypointense masses and demonstrate heterogeneous contrast enhancement on T1-weighted sequences.[11,13] In contrast to LGGs, HGGs are associated with significant vasogenic edema, which appears hyperintense on T2/FLAIR.[11,13] Specifically, GBMs are characterized by a peripheral rim of enhancement surrounding a nonenhancing region of central necrosis[11,13] (**Fig. 1**). Gliomas with distinct molecular characteristics may demonstrate specific findings on imaging. For instance, compared with IDH-*wt* tumors, IDH-mutant gliomas demonstrate less contrast enhancement, larger tumor size, and the presence of cystic components.[6] 1p/19q Codeleted tumors may be distinguished by the presence of calcifications and indistinct tumor margins.[6] In addition, the T2/FLAIR mismatch sign, which describes homogeneous hyperintensity on T2-weighted imaging with a relatively hypointense signal on T2/FLAIR, is highly specific for IDH-*mutant*, 1p/19q noncodeleted astrocytoma.[6]

MR spectroscopy (MRS), which measures metabolite concentrations within the tissues, can also be used to predict glioma grade and differentiate residual tumor infiltration from surrounding normal tissues.[14] In the setting of LGG, a study using both intraoperative MRS (iMRS) and intraoperative MRI (iMRI) found that the sensitivity of iMRS for identifying residual tumor was 85.7%, and the specificity was 100%. Thus, this imaging modality may be used to limit unnecessary resections at the tumor border when gliomas are located in eloquent regions.

Functional MRI (fMRI) and MR tractography are used for determining the localization of important functional regions and white matter tracts.[11] However, the accuracy of fMRI in localizing language and motor functions is highly variable across studies.

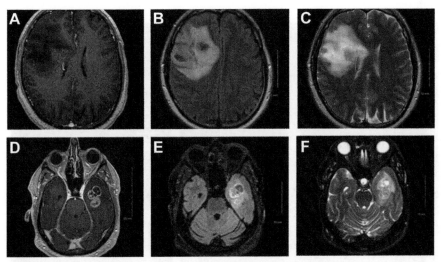

Fig. 1. MRI showing differences between low-grade and high-grade gliomas. (*A*) Axial T1 with contrast, (*B*) axial FLAIR, and (*C*) axial T2 show a nonenhancing right frontal lesion. (*D*) Axial T1 with contrast, (*E*) axial FLAIR, and (*F*) axial T2 show a ring-enhancing left temporal lesion.

Although fMRI can be very helpful for preoperative evaluation and surgical planning, the data do not yet support its use over intraoperative direct cortical stimulation (DCS) for functional mapping.[11] The largest study to evaluate the accuracy of fMRI in mapping language and motor functions in patients with focal masses adjacent to eloquent cortex (34 total, 28 glioma) reported an overall sensitivity of 83% and specificity of 82%.[15] Notably, the authors also found that sensitivity and specificity varied with respect to glioma grade.[14] Across the literature, accuracy is reported to range from 66% to 100%.[11]

MR tractography uses diffusion tensor imaging (DTI) to visualize the anatomic location of white matter tracts.[11] A randomized controlled trial comparing resection of gliomas involving the pyramidal tracts with and without preoperative DTI in 214 patients demonstrated that the use of DTI is associated with decreased postoperative motor deficits and improved 6-month Karnofsky performance score in both LGG and HGG patients. In addition, the use of DTI was associated with an increased rate of complete resection (74.4% vs 33.3%, $P<.001$) and improved median survival (21.2 vs 14.0 months, $P = .048$) in patients undergoing resection for HGGs[16] (**Fig. 2**).

Preoperative imaging plays a critical role not only for diagnosis but is also used routinely in the form of stereotactic navigation system for planning incision and guiding surgical resection. With respect to image-guided navigation system, T2/FLAIR imaging is the current standard for nonenhancing lesions, whereas contrast-enhanced T1-weighted sequences are preferred for enhancing tumors.[11]

Monitoring response to treatment and recurrence

MRI is the modality of choice for monitoring response to treatment and tumor recurrence, but this is not without limitations. Postcontrast enhancement on T1-weighted imaging reflects nonspecific impairment of the blood-brain barrier (BBB) and as such is not necessarily representative of active disease.[17] This is particularly important with respect to monitoring the malignant progression of LGGs as the development or evolution of focal enhancement on imaging often precedes clinical changes.[17]

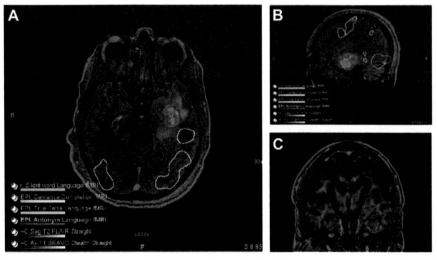

Fig. 2. fMRI and DTI imaging. (*A*) Axial and (*B*) sagittal FLAIR sequencing demonstrating left temporal lesion with functional mapping. (*C*) Tractography shows the relationship of major tracts in relation to the lesion.

Although reduction or lack of enhancement can occur due to tumor shrinkage, it may also occur secondary to treatment with steroids or antiangiogenic therapy and the resultant vascular normalization in areas adjacent to tumor infiltration (pseudoresponse).[17] Alternatively, pseudoprogression, an early subacute reaction to treatment (eg, radiotherapy), is associated with findings seen in true progression such as contrast enhancement, edema, and mass effect. In some cases, associated clinical symptoms may also initially suggest tumor progression, but these subsequently resolve without any further treatment.[9,17] Although T2 and FLAIR hyperintensity can be suggestive of tumor infiltration, it is also indicative of edema, ischemia, gliosis, demyelination, and inflammation. In particular, inflammation may mimic radiological features of tumor progression and this ambiguity can often delay the diagnosis of true disease progression.[10] To address the challenges of distinguishing treatment-related changes from tumor progression, The Response Assessment in Neuro-Oncology (RANO) criteria were developed as an objective tool for radiologic assessment of treatment response for both LGG and HGG (**Table 3**).[7,18–20]

MANAGEMENT

The management of glioma patients is best executed through a multidisciplinary approach with the involvement of specialists from neurosurgery as well as neuro-oncology and radiation oncology. Initial management should first address urgent clinical symptoms and establish a comprehensive molecular diagnosis. Although surgery is an essential component of the management of gliomas, the highly infiltrative nature of these tumors means that surgical resection alone, even when complete, is not typically curative. Adjuvant therapy is therefore of the utmost importance in extending progression-free survival (PFS) and OS (**Box 2**).

Table 3
RANO criteria for evaluation of glioma recurrence

	Response Criteria		
RANO Guidelines	Complete	Partial	Progression Criteria
RANO-LGG • PMID: 21474379	Requires all of the following: Complete disappearance of all T2/FLAIR disease for ≥4 wk New or increased enhancement No new T2/FLAIR abnormalities other than what is attributable to treatment effects No more than physiologic steroids, clinically stable or improved	Requires all of the following: ≥50% decrease in the sum of perpendicular diameters of T2/FLAIR disease for ≥4 wk; No new or increased enhancement, No new T2/FLAIR abnormalities other than what is attributable to treatment effects, No more steroids than at the time of the baseline scan, clinically stable or improved	Defined by any of the following: Development of new lesions or increase of enhancement; ≥25% increase in size of the T2/FLAIR abnormality on stable or increased doses of steroids and not attributable to radiation effect or comorbid events Definite clinical deterioration, death or loss to follow-up

(continued on next page)

	Response Criteria		
Table 3 **(continued)**			
RANO Guidelines	**Complete**	**Partial**	**Progression Criteria**
RANO-HGG • PMID: 20231676	Requires all of the following: Complete disappearance of all enhancing measurable and nonmeasurable disease sustained for at least 4 wk No new lesions Stable or improved nonenhancing (T2/FLAIR) lesions Patients must be off corticosteroids (or on physiologic replacement doses only) And stable or improved clinically. Note: Patients with nonmeasurable disease only cannot have achieved CR; the best response possible is stable disease	Requires all of the following: ≥50% decrease compared with baseline in the sum of products of perpendicular diameters of all measurable enhancing lesions sustained for at least 4 wk No progression of nonmeasurable disease No new lesions; stable or improved nonenhancing (T2/FLAIR) lesions on same or lower dose of corticosteroids compared with baseline scan The corticosteroid dose at the time of scan evaluation should be no greater than the dose at time of baseline scan And stable or improved clinically	Defined by any of the following: ≥25% increase in the sum of the products of perpendicular diameters of enhancing lesions (compared with baseline if no decrease) on stable or increasing doses of corticosteroids; Significant increase in T2/FLAIR nonenhancing lesions on stable or increasing doses of corticosteroids compared with the baseline scan or the best response after initiation of therapy, not due to comorbid events; The appearance of any new lesions; Clear progression of nonmeasurable lesions; or definite clinical deterioration not attributable to other causes apart from the tumor or to a decrease in the corticosteroid dose

SURGICAL MANAGEMENT

Indications for surgery include the need to obtain tissue for diagnosis, cytoreduction, relief of mass effect with potential for symptom improvement, and to improve survival and quality of life (QOL). In most patients, surgical intervention is warranted for the acquisition of tissue alone.

Biopsy

Stereotactic needle biopsy is recommended in patients with deep lesions or those within eloquent structures where surgical resection carries an unacceptably high

---

Box 2
Standard of care for glioma

Standard of Care for High-Grade Glioma for Patients with Good Performance Scale:

- Surgery
- Chemotherapy with Temozolomide (TMZ) (75 mg/m^2 per day 7 days per week during radiotherapy followed by maintenance dosing of 150–200 mg/m^2 for 5 days on 2 off in a 28-day cycle)
- Radiation to the resection 60 Gy 6 weeks (fractionated at 2 Gy given 5× per week)
- Tumor Treating Fields (TTF)

Standard of Care for High-Grade Glioma for Patients with Poor Performance Scale:

- Surgery/Biopsy for tissue diagnosis
- Chemotherapy with TMZ (75 mg/m^2 per day 7 days per week during radiotherapy followed by maintenance dosing of 150–200 mg/m^2 for 5 days on 2 off in a 28-day cycle)
- Palliative radiation (30 Gy whole brain)

---

risk of morbidity or mortality.[21] Furthermore, as the degree of surgical resection may be dependent on the specific glioma subtype, patients may need to undergo a biopsy before more extensive surgical resection.[22] Needle biopsies are targeted, where possible, to the portion of the lesion that appears the highest grade on imaging—an enhancing area. Several biopsy specimens are obtained to allow for accurate diagnosis as a sampling bias can lead to nondiagnostic biopsies or biopsies of a lower grade.[2] Stereotactic navigation is required for this procedure and can be frame-based or non–frame-based. The use of frozen section analysis can help ensure the presence of lesioned tissue in the samples before completion of the procedure. Despite proper planning and surgical technique, the risk of catastrophic hemorrhage with sampling is 1% per procedure.[23]

Surgical Resection

For both LGG and HGG, the primary goals of surgery are the acquisition of tissue for accurate diagnostics and improving patient survival.[22] With respect to LGGs, the resection threshold associated with improved survival is dependent on the specific subtype.[22,24] Data currently support maximum total resection of enhancing tumor components for IDH-*wt* LGGs and both the enhancing and nonenhancing components in IDH-*mutant* astrocytomas.[22,25] In addition, a recent meta-analysis of grade I/II gliomas suggests that extensive resection is associated with improved OS and PFS at 2, 5, and 10 years compared with subtotal resection.[26] Maximum resection can also delay the progression of LGGs to malignant tumors and is the preferred approach in the treatment of all LGGs as well as diffuse gliomas regardless of grade.[27,28]

Although achieving maximum resection is important for improving PFS and OS, this must be accomplished without compromising the integrity of the surrounding normal tissue. Recent advances in technology have led to improvements in patient safety and outcomes while enabling the maximum tumor resection. The use of iMRI guides resection in "real-time" by permitting evaluation of residual tumor volume while accounting for intraoperative anatomic changes and is associated with increased rate of complete tumor resection, without increased postoperative rates of new neurologic deficits.[29,30]

In patients where preservation of motor function is the primary objective, motor evoked potentials may also be used to determine the integrity of the motor pathways, instead of performing an awake craniotomy[31] (**Fig. 3**).

Awake craniotomies may be performed to allow for the protection of key motor and speech functions when tumors are located in eloquent regions.[32] Under these conditions, the patient is not intubated or placed under general anesthesia. He or she is then able to cooperate with an examiner during the procedure, which allows for early identification of any decrease in function and alerts the surgeon that they are approaching an area of functional importance.[30] In addition, intraoperative neurophysiological monitoring with DCS may also allow for maximal resection of tumors deemed inoperable on imaging by permitting accurate localization of functional areas intraoperatively.[28]

In patients with HGGs, gross total resection (GTR) is associated with both a survival benefit and improved QOL.[33] As such achieving GTR is particularly important in these patients and several techniques can be used for optimization. The use of fluorescent agents such as 5-aminolevulinic acid (5-ALA) and sodium fluorescein (SF) can assist the surgeon by allowing for improved visualization of the tumor.[11] 5-ALA is a nonfluorescent prodrug that causes an intracellular accumulation of fluorescent porphyrins and gives the tumor a pink appearance when visualized using a special filter on the operating microscope.[11] In clinical trials, the use of 5-ALA has been shown to improve rates of GTR of contrast-enhancing material and prolong 6-month PFS in patients with HGGs.[34] Alternatively, SF is a fluorescent dye that is injected intravenously during surgery and accumulates in malignant cells as a result of BBB disruption.[11] In contrast to 5-ALA, SF tumors appear yellow when visualized on the operating microscope.[11] Support for the use of SF comes from a prospective, multicenter phase II trial in which 82% of patients received GTR of contrast enhancement.[34] Results from biopsies collected from areas with and without fluorescence suggest the sensitivity and specificity of SF in identifying tumor-containing tissues to be 80%.[34] Although there has yet to be a prospective study comparing the efficacy of 5-ALA and SF, a recent retrospective study found no difference between the two, suggesting that SF may be a viable alternative to 5-ALA.[35]

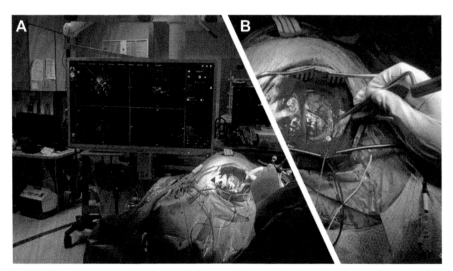

Fig. 3. Intraoperative monitoring. (*A*) Intraoperative monitoring of motor evoked potential. (*B*) Intraoperative strip placement for motor mapping via DCS.

Raman spectroscopy is another emerging technology that may be used to optimize GTR in glioma patients. This is a nondestructive vibrational spectroscopy technique that provides structural and chemical information based on the distinct composition and structure of specific samples.[36] Studies have shown that Raman spectroscopy is capable of differentiating between normal brain, brain tumors, and necrosis across a range of tissue preservation methods.[36] In addition, when used intraoperatively, this technique demonstrates a high degree of accuracy (92%), sensitivity (93%), and specificity (91%) in distinguishing normal brain from both tumor bulk and tumor infiltration.[37]

Accessing and resecting HGGs located deep to critical cortical and subcortical structures has historically been associated with significant morbidity.[38] However, the use of a tubular retractor system with exoscopic visualization can provide access to these deep-seated tumors by displacing rather than disrupting the fibers of critical pathways.[38,39]

Surgical intervention also provides a direct means of delivering therapeutics in the resection cavity and bypasses BBB. The first-in-human, phase 1, dose-escalation trial of NSC-CRAd-S-pk7f, an engineered oncolytic adenovirus delivered by neural stem cells to the glioma resection cavity, was recently completed in patients with newly diagnosed HGGs.[40] There were no treatment-related deaths and the median PFS and OS were 9.1 and 18.4 months, respectively.[40] The intraoperative placement of GammaTile cesium-131 (131Cs), a permanent brachytherapy brain implant, allows for irradiation to begin immediately after tumor resection.[41] 131Cs has recently received FDA approval for the use outside of clinical trials, and a multicenter observational study (NCT04427384) is currently recruiting patients who have undergone GammaTile placement to evaluate patient outcomes.[41] To optimize drug delivery for gliomas, the use of ultrasound-mediated disruption of the BBB through the physical interactions of ultrasonic waves and microbubbles that are administered systemically is also currently being evaluated for HGG.[42] There are several open clinical trials assessing the innovative role of surgery in glioma management (**Table 4**).

MANAGEMENT OF RECURRENCE/PROGRESSION

Even with aggressive multimodal treatment, most gliomas will recur or progress. Time to recurrence is significantly shorter for HGG compared with LGG and there is great variability in the management of recurrence.

Management of Recurrence for LGG

Recurrence in LGG may be treated with repeat resection, radiation, or re-irradiation depending on initial treatment and recurrence pattern. A study analyzing tumor recurrence patterns after surgical resection of LGG found that recurrence patterns differ based on the molecular subtype of LGG with the initial extent of resection less than 90%; however, with the extent of resection $\geq$ 90%, no differences in recurrence characteristics were found between 3 molecularly defined groups of LGG. In addition, the study showed that early onset of recurrence, fast radiological progression, and nonlocal site of relapse have a significant negative impact on OS and are often associated with malignant transformation.[43] Thus, surgical intervention in the setting of recurrence provides another opportunity to analyze the tissue for malignant transformation. However, a systematic review of recent literature on the benefits of re-resection of LGG found insufficient evidence to make any specific recommendations. Rather, they recommended that individuals with recurrent LGGs be enrolled in a properly designed clinical trial to assess the role of surgery at recurrence.[44]

Table 4
Innovative surgical clinical trials for glioma

PI	Jian Campian	Michael Vogelbaum	Josh Rubin	John Boockvar	John Boockvar	Adam Sonabend
Identifier	NCT02311582	NCT04608812	NCT02372409	NCT04222309	NCT03630289	NCT04528680
Beginning year	2014	2020	2015	2020	2018	2020
Estimated completion	2021	2021	2028	2021	2021	2024
Trial phase	Phase I/II	Phase I	Phase II	Phase I	Phase I	Phase I/II
Age range (y)	18+	18+	3–21	18+	18+	18+
Trial N	58	24	12	10	10	39
Primary outcome measure	Maximal Tolerated Dose of MK-3475 when combined with MRI guided laser ablation	Treatment emergent adverse events or dose limiting toxicities	Progression Free Survival	Proportion of patients reporting rapidly progressing disease	Proportion of patients reporting rapidly progressing disease	Dose limiting toxicity
Surgical intervention	MRI guided laser ablation for BBB disruption to administer MK-3475	Convection Enhanced Delivery for OS2966	MRI guided laser ablation for BBB disruption and administration of doxorubicin or etoposide	Omental Free Tissue Autograft to Bypass BBB	Tissue Autograft of pericranial flap to bypass BBB	Sonication for opening of BBB to deliver paclitaxel

Management of Recurrence for HGG

For highly aggressive HGG, local recurrence is an inevitable event with most patients experiencing recurrence after 6 to 9 months of initial treatment.[22] GBM recurrence often accompanies new neurologic symptoms/deficits and in many cases, the new deficits are due to tumor infiltration into critical eloquent structure making the recurrence less conducive to further surgical or radiotherapy intervention. Even in the most optimistic studies, the rate of re-resection for GBM is less than 40%.[45] Although re-resection is of uncertain clinical benefit for a focal, local recurrence in patients with good performance status, repeat resection may be a reasonable option.[46]

As an alternative to surgery, laser interstitial thermal therapy (LITT) is an emerging technology that allows for laser ablation of tumors that could otherwise not be removed either due to deep location or involvement of an eloquent area. The laser fiber is passed to the tumor using stereotactic navigation. The laser is then used to heat the tissue surrounding the tip to a temperature causing cytolysis. One single-institution study of using LITT for 8 newly diagnosed GBM and 13 recurrent GBM showed that in the setting of recurrent disease, 5 patients showed response to LITT with radiographical shrinkage of the tumor, which was not seen in any of the newly diagnosed patients. The study concluded that in carefully selected patients with recurrent GBM, LITT may be an effective alternative to surgery as a salvage treatment; however, its role in the treatment of newly diagnosed, unresectable GBMs is not yet established.[47]

Regardless of operative management, following recurrence, additional adjuvant treatments must be considered to optimize clinical benefit. McBain and colleagues performed a network meta-analysis to evaluate the most effective treatment option for progressive or recurrent GBM after initial treatment with standard of care. They concluded that for treatment of first recurrence of GBM, lomustine appears to be the most effective chemotherapy treatment and other combination therapies tested had a higher risk of serious side effects. A second operation or radiotherapy, or both, may be of value in selected individuals. For second recurrence, radiotherapy with or without bevacizumab may have a role but more evidence is needed.[48] In a small, multi-institution, randomized clinical trial of involving 35 patients, Cloughesy and colleagues found that neoadjuvant administration of immune checkpoint PD-1 blockade followed by surgical re-resection for recurrent GBM enhances local and systemic antitumor immune response, suggesting that timing of repeat surgery in combination with multimodal innovative therapeutics will possibly direct future clinical trials in this arena.[49]

SUMMARY

Neurosurgical oncology plays a central role in the management of glioma patients by aiding with diagnosis, symptom control as well as providing an avenue for direct delivery of therapeutics that bypasses BBB. GTR is typically curative for grade I lesions, whereas more infiltrative gliomas (grades II-IV) typically require maximal safe resection and potential adjuvant therapy with radiation and/or chemotherapy depending on the specific histologic and molecular diagnosis. Grade IV gliomas carry a particularly dismal prognosis and significant research efforts are underway worldwide to improve patient outcomes.

CLINICS CARE POINTS

- There is class IIB evidence to suggest that "gross total resection" in glioblastoma should be replaced by the more precise term "complete resection of enhancing tumor"[50]

- There is class III evidence to suggest that supramaximal resection beyond enhancing tumor borders might be beneficial in terms of survival for HGG[51]
- There is class II evidence to suggest that surgical resection, in general, is associated with improved survival in gliomas WHO grades 2 and 3[52,53]

ACKNOWLEDGEMENT

This work was supported by the NINDS K08NS092895 Grant (MD).

DISCLOSURE

The authors have nothing to disclose.

REFERENCES

1. Ostrom QT, Cioffi G, Gittleman H, et al. CBTRUS Statistical report: Primary brain and other Central Nervous system tumors diagnosed in the United States in 2012–2016. Neuro Oncol 2019;21. v1–100.
2. Louis DN, Perry A, Reifenberger G, et al. The 2016 World health Organization Classification of tumors of the Central Nervous system: a summary. Acta Neuropathol 2016;131:803–20.
3. Network CGAR, Brat DJ, Verhaak RGW, et al. Comprehensive, Integrative Genomic analysis of diffuse lower-grade gliomas. N Engl J Med 2015;372:2481–98.
4. Yan H, Parsons DW, Jin G, et al. IDH1 and IDH2 mutations in gliomas. N Engl J Med 2009;360:765–73.
5. Yao J, Hagiwara A, Raymond C, et al. Human IDH mutant 1p/19q co-deleted gliomas have low tumor acidity as evidenced by molecular MRI and PET: a retrospective study. Sci Rep 2020;10:11922.
6. Hegi ME, Diserens A-C, Gorlia T, et al. MGMT Gene Silencing and benefit from Temozolomide in glioblastoma. N Engl J Med 2005;352:997–1003.
7. Cairncross G, Wang M, Shaw E, et al. Phase III trial of Chemoradiotherapy for Anaplastic Oligodendroglioma: long-term results of RTOG 9402. J Clin Oncol 2012;31:337–43.
8. van den Bent MJ, Brandes AA, Taphoorn MJB, et al. Adjuvant Procarbazine, Lomustine, and Vincristine Chemotherapy in newly diagnosed Anaplastic Oligodendroglioma: long-term Follow-up of EORTC brain tumor group study 26951. J Clin Oncol 2012;31:344–50.
9. Liu X-Y, Gerges N, Korshunov A, et al. Frequent ATRX mutations and loss of expression in adult diffuse astrocytic tumors carrying IDH1/IDH2 and TP53 mutations. Acta Neuropathol 2012;124:615–25.
10. Killela PJ, Reitman ZJ, Jiao Y, et al. TERT promoter mutations occur frequently in gliomas and a subset of tumors derived from cells with low rates of self-renewal. Proc Natl Acad Sci U S A 2013;110:6021–6.
11. Verburg N, Hamer PC de W. State-of-the-art imaging for glioma surgery. Neurosurg Rev 2021;44:1331–43.
12. Guillevin R, Herpe G, Verdier M, et al. Low-grade gliomas: the challenges of imaging. Diagn Interv Imag 2014;95:957–63.
13. Bai J, Varghese J, Jain R. Adult glioma WHO Classification Update, Genomics, and imaging: what the Radiologists need to Know. Top Magn Reson Imag 2020;29:71–82.

14. Pamir MN, Özduman K, Yıldız E, et al. Intraoperative magnetic resonance spectroscopy for identification of residual tumor during low-grade glioma surgery: clinical article. J Neurosurg 2013;118:1191–8.

15. Bizzi A, Blasi V, Falini A, et al. Presurgical functional MR imaging of Language and Motor functions: Validation with intraoperative Electrocortical mapping. Radiology 2008;248:579–89.

16. Wu J-S, Zhou L-F, Tang W-J, et al. Clinical evaluation and Follow-up outcome of Diffusion Tensor imaging-Based functional Neuronavigation: a Prospective, controlled study in patients with gliomas Involving Pyramidal Tracts. Neurosurgery 2007;61:935–49.

17. Upadhyay N, Waldman AD. Conventional MRI evaluation of gliomas. Br J Radiol 2011;84:S107–11.

18. Chukwueke UN, Wen PY. Use of the Response Assessment in Neuro-Oncology (RANO) criteria in clinical trials and clinical practice. CNS Oncol 2019;8:CNS28.

19. Wen PY, Macdonald DR, Reardon DA, et al. Updated Response assessment criteria for high-grade gliomas: Response assessment in neuro-oncology Working group. J Clin Oncol 2010;28:1963–72.

20. van den Bent M, Wefel J, Schiff D, et al. Response assessment in neuro-oncology (a report of the RANO group): assessment of outcome in trials of diffuse low-grade gliomas. Lancet Oncol 2011;12:583–93.

21. Akshulakov SK, Kerimbayev TT, Biryuchkov MY, et al. Current Trends for Improving Safety of Stereotactic brain Biopsies: Advanced Optical methods for Vessel Avoidance and tumor detection. Front Oncol 2019;9:947.

22. Stupp R, Mason WP, van den Bent MJ, et al. Radiotherapy plus Concomitant and Adjuvant Temozolomide for glioblastoma. N Engl J Med 2005;352:987–96.

23. Kreth FW, Muacevic A, Medele R, et al. The risk of Haemorrhage after image guided Stereotactic biopsy of intra-axial brain tumours – a Prospective study. Acta Neurochir 2001;143:539–46.

24. Pope WB, Sayre J, Perlina A, et al. MR imaging correlates of survival in patients with high-grade gliomas. AJNR Am J Neuroradiol 2005;26:2466–74.

25. Rasmussen BK, Hansen S, Laursen RJ, et al. Epidemiology of glioma: clinical characteristics, symptoms, and predictors of glioma patients grade I–IV in the the Danish Neuro-Oncology Registry. J Neuro Oncol 2017;135:571–9.

26. Lapointe S, Perry A, Butowski NA. Primary brain tumours in adults. Lancet 2018;392:432–46.

27. Kim M, Jung SY, Park JE, et al. Diffusion- and perfusion-weighted MRI radiomics model may predict isocitrate dehydrogenase (IDH) mutation and tumor aggressiveness in diffuse lower grade glioma. Eur Radiol 2020;30:2142–51.

28. Qin J, Liu Z, Zhang H, et al. Grading of gliomas by Using Radiomic Features on Multiple magnetic resonance imaging (MRI) Sequences. Med Sci Monit Int Med J Exp Clin Res 2017;23:2168–78.

29. Fahlbusch R, Nimsky C. Intraoperative MRI developments. Neurosurg Clin N Am 2005;16. xi–xiii.

30. Duffau H, Capelle L, Denvil D, et al. Usefulness of intraoperative electrical subcortical mapping during surgery for low-grade gliomas located within eloquent brain regions: functional results in a consecutive series of 103 patients. J Neurosurg 2003;98:764–78.

31. Zhou HH, Kelly PJ. Transcranial electrical Motor Evoked Potential Monitoring for brain tumor resection. Neurosurgery 2001;48:1075.

32. Li Y-C, Chiu H-Y, Lin Y-J, et al. The Merits of Awake Craniotomy for glioblastoma in the Left Hemispheric eloquent Area: one Institution experience. Clin Neurol Neurosurg 2021;200:106343.

33. Brown PD, Maurer MJ, Rummans TA, et al. A Prospective study of quality of life in adults with newly diagnosed high-grade gliomas: the impact of the Extent of resection on quality of life and survival. Neurosurgery 2005;57:495–504.

34. Stummer W, Pichlmeier U, Meinel T, et al. Fluorescence-guided surgery with 5-aminolevulinic acid for resection of malignant glioma: a randomised controlled multicentre phase III trial. Lancet Oncol 2006;7:392–401.

35. Hansen RW, Pedersen CB, Halle B, et al. Comparison of 5-aminolevulinic acid and sodium fluorescein for intraoperative tumor visualization in patients with high-grade gliomas: a single-center retrospective study. J Neurosurg 2020;133: 1324–31.

36. Livermore LJ, Isabelle M, Bell IM, et al. Raman spectroscopy to differentiate between fresh tissue samples of glioma and normal brain: a comparison with 5-ALA–induced fluorescence-guided surgery. J Neurosurg 2020;1–11. https://doi.org/10.3171/2020.5.jns20376.

37. Jermyn M, Mok K, Mercier J, et al. Intraoperative brain cancer detection with Raman spectroscopy in humans. Sci Transl Med 2015;7:274ra19.

38. Iyer R, Chaichana K. Minimally invasive resection of Deep-seated high-grade gliomas Using tubular Retractors and Exoscopic visualization. J Neurol Surg Part Cent Eur Neurosurg 2018;79:330–6.

39. Gassie K, Wijesekera O, Chaichana KL. Minimally invasive tubular retractor-assisted biopsy and resection of subcortical intra-axial gliomas and other neoplasms. J Neurosurg Sci 2018;62. https://doi.org/10.23736/s0390-5616.18.04466-1.

40. Fares J, Ahmed AU, Ulasov IV, et al. Neural stem cell delivery of an oncolytic adenovirus in newly diagnosed malignant glioma: a first-in-human, phase 1, dose-escalation trial. Lancet Oncol 2021;22:1103–14.

41. Ferreira C, Sterling D, Reynolds M, et al. First clinical implementation of Gamma-Tile permanent brain implants after FDA clearance. Brachytherapy 2021;20: 673–85.

42. Zhang DY, Dmello C, Chen L, et al. Ultrasound-mediated delivery of Paclitaxel for glioma: a Comparative study of Distribution, Toxicity, and Efficacy of Albumin-bound versus Cremophor Formulations. Clin Cancer Res 2020;26:477–86.

43. Fukuya Y, Ikuta S, Maruyama T, et al. Tumor recurrence patterns after surgical resection of intracranial low-grade gliomas. J Neuro Oncol 2019;144:519–28.

44. Nahed BV, Redjal N, Brat DJ, et al. Management of patients with recurrence of diffuse low grade glioma. J Neuro Oncol 2015;125:609–30.

45. Chaichana KL, Zadnik P, Weingart JD, et al. Multiple resections for patients with glioblastoma: prolonging survival: clinical article. J Neurosurg 2013;118:812–20.

46. Patel M, Au K, Davis FG, et al. Clinical Uncertainty and Equipoise in the management of recurrent glioblastoma. Am J Clin Oncol 2021;44:258–63.

47. Thomas JG, Rao G, Kew Y, et al. Laser interstitial thermal therapy for newly diagnosed and recurrent glioblastoma. Neurosurg Focus 2016;41:E12.

48. Lawrie TA, McBain C, Rogozińska E, et al. Treatment options for recurrent glioblastoma: a network meta-analysis. Cochrane Database Syst Rev 2020. https://doi.org/10.1002/14651858.cd013579.

49. Cloughesy TF, Mochizuki AY, Orpilla JR, et al. Neoadjuvant anti-PD-1 immunotherapy promotes a survival benefit with intratumoral and systemic immune responses in recurrent glioblastoma. Nat Med 2019;25:477–86.

50. Group A-GS, Stummer W, Reulen H-J, et al. Extent of resection and survival in glioblastoma Multiforme: identification of and Adjustment for Bias. Neurosurgery 2008;62:564–76.
51. Eyüpoglu IY, Hore N, Merkel A, et al. Supra-complete surgery via dual intraoperative visualization approach (DiVA) prolongs patient survival in glioblastoma. Oncotarget 2015;7:25755–68.
52. Jakola AS, Skjulsvik AJ, Myrmel KS, et al. Surgical resection versus watchful waiting in low-grade gliomas. Ann Oncol 2017;28:1942–8.
53. Roelz R, Strohmaier D, Jabbarli R, et al. Residual tumor Volume as best outcome Predictor in low Grade glioma – a Nine-Years Near-Randomized Survey of surgery vs. Biopsy. Sci Rep 2016;6:32286.

Neurosurgical Mimics

Robert J. Rothrock, MD[a], Turki Elarjani, MD[b], Allan D. Levi, MD, PhD[b],*

KEYWORDS

- Multiple sclerosis • Ring enhancing lesion • Amyotrophic lateral sclerosis
- Subacute combined degeneration • Parsonage turner syndrome

KEY POINTS

- The goal of the following article is to help the practicing physician learn to recognize conditions that mimic conditions requiring neurosurgical intervention.
- Each case vignette is presented with relevant clinical history and examination, imaging studies and findings as well as other testing results.
- The management for the corresponding diagnosis is presented.
- Finally, the relevant mimics and differentiating features are discussed.

INTRODUCTION: GENERAL APPROACH TO CASES

Practicing neurologists and neurosurgeons are often confronted with diagnostically complex cases presenting with focal symptoms that seem to be surgical, both in outpatient and inpatient hospital settings. Although certain cases may at first seem amenable to surgical intervention, they may in fact be not helped or even harmed by surgical intervention. Cases that do not meet the expected constellation of symptoms should give at least pause for further consideration.

In approaching any potentially surgical case, the clinical history is of critical importance. In weighing the following cases, the determination that the case is not surgical can be made through careful examination of the clinical history and physical examination. In the age of image-guided surgical decision-making, it can be tempting to intervene based on imaging triggers, but in some of the following presented cases, doing so would harm the patient, more than benefit.

The goal of the following article is to help the practicing physician learn to recognize conditions that mimic conditions requiring neurosurgical intervention. Each case vignette is presented with relevant clinical history and examination, imaging studies and findings, as well as other testing results. The management for the corresponding diagnosis is presented. Finally, the relevant mimics and differentiating features are discussed.

[a] Herbert Wertheim College of Medicine, Florida International University, Baptist Health South Florida, 8950 North Kendall Drive, Suite 410W Miami, FL 33176, USA; [b] Department of Neurological Surgery, University of Miami Miller School of Medicine, Second Floor, 1095 NW 14th Terrace, Miami, FL 33136, USA
* Corresponding author.
E-mail address: alevi@med.miami.edu

Neurol Clin 40 (2022) 455–469
https://doi.org/10.1016/j.ncl.2021.11.013
0733-8619/22/© 2021 Elsevier Inc. All rights reserved.
neurologic.theclinics.com

CENTRAL NERVOUS SYSTEM
Brain

Case 1: a 36-year-old woman with subacute agraphia

Clinical history. A 36-year-old female young professional with no stated past medical history presents with 1 month of difficulty writing at work. She then developed 1 week of difficulty seeing objects in the right visual field while driving. She endorses mild hemisensory loss on the right side. She denies headache, weakness of the upper or lower extremity, or bowel or bladder incontinence. On physical examination she has difficulty with speech, especially understanding complex commands and with appropriate responses. She has a right homonymous hemianopsia. Motor strength is full 5/5 throughout. On further history, she complained of acute visual loss and blurriness in the left eye 1 year ago that resolved spontaneously.

Imaging. MRI reveals a left parietal lesion extending to the splenium of the corpus callosum and the ependyma of the atrium of the left lateral ventricle. There is minimal surrounding edema. There is peripheral contrast enhancement of the lesion in an open ring pattern (**Fig. 1**).

Diagnosis. This case illustrates the typical presentation of tumefactive multiple sclerosis (MS). The patient is a woman in the third to fourth decade of life with a previous history suspicious for optic neuritis,[1] and this should raise a red flag to the possibility of MS. The clinical history and examination localize a lesion to the left (dominant) parietal lobe. The MRI reveals a solid, infiltrative appearing lesion, but without large surrounding vasogenic edema that would be expected from a malignant or infiltrative glioma or lymphoma.[1,2] In addition, the "open-ring" contrast enhancement is typical of tumefactive MS and should at least raise suspicion for diagnosis other than lymphoma (also periventricular) or glioma.[1,2] Computed tomography (CT)-PET can be used to help differentiate tumefactive MS from malignancy, given that tumefactive demyelinating lesions are usually hypometabolic or minimally hypermetabolic on CT-PET, whereas high-grade neoplasms have greater uptake and activity.[3] Magnetic resonance spectroscopy can also be helpful in differentiating these lesions, as tumefactive MS demonstrates a higher glutamine/glutamate peak, indicating an active inflammatory process.[4] The NAA/Cho ratio can also differentiate high-grade gliomas from tumefactive MS, with NAA/Cho ratio greater than 1.72 indicating high-grade glioma.[5]

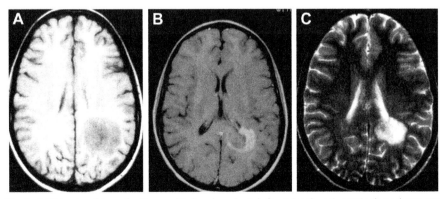

Fig. 1. MRI brain of tumefactive multiple sclerosis. A left parietal periventricular edema surrounding a mass lesion can be appreciated on T1-weighted image (see **Figs. 1**A & B). The mass lesion and vasogenic edema can be further appreciated on a T2-weighted image (see **Fig. 1**C).

Given the clinical suspicion for MS, further workup should start with noninvasive testing such as CT-PET or MRI of the cervical and thoracic spine, which may reveal other demyelinating lesions consistent with MS. If the brain lesion is not obstructive of cerebrospinal fluid (CSF) flow, diagnostic lumbar puncture can be performed. The presence of oligoclonal bands (OCBs) of immunoglobulin G (IgG) in the CSF is diagnostic of MS. Interestingly, however, isolated tumefactive MS lesions less commonly have positive OCBs in the CSF compared with more conventional MS.[6] If a tumefactive demyelinating lesion is highly suspected based on imaging characteristics alone, serial MRI scans showing improvement can reinforce the diagnosis.[7]

If all of these less invasive testing options are nondiagnostic, and the patient is severely symptomatic (more common with larger lesions), there is always a role for MS treatment and taking on a careful wait-and-see attitude with frequent neurologic and imaging follow-up. Given the possibility of surgical morbidity, biopsy or resection of lesion should be avoided at all costs if MS is suspected.[7]

Management. Specific management of MS depends on the subtype, but generally first-line therapy is corticosteroids.[6] Acute plasma exchange is considered for diagnostically confirmed patients with severely symptomatic lesions.[8] Most of the patients (90%) who present with a tumefactive demyelinating lesion will go on to develop MS.[9] Disease-modifying therapy (usually immunotherapy) can help decrease the frequency of relapsing MS attacks in these patients.[6] Glatiramer acetate (Copaxone) is a synthetic protein that modifies helper T-cell activity and helps reduce inflammation.[10] Glatiramer acetate was approved by the Food and Drug Administration having been shown to reduce the relapse rate of MS by 33% and preserve ambulation in approximately 80% of patients after 20 years of follow-up.[11]

Mimic. Differential diagnosis for this lesion involves primary intrinsic brain tumors such as glioma, lymphoma, brain abscess, and other demyelinating processes such as progressive multifocal leukoencephalopathy.

What sets it apart. The elements in this case that suggest MS are a young female patient with a past history of monocular visual deficit consistent with optic neuritis and an open-ring enhancing lesion without significant surrounding vasogenic edema. Fundoscopy should be used, as it can reveal optic disc pallor as opposed to optic disc edema. Most importantly, the rapidity of onset of her symptoms makes one suspect demyelination as opposed to a tumor. Without the stereotypical open-ring enhancement and history of optic neuritis, it would be difficult to differentiate this lesion from the others mentioned in the aforementioned differential diagnosis without further supplied diagnostic testing.

Case 2: headache in a young man
Clinical history. A 21-year-old undomiciled man presents to the emergency department with complaints of a worsening headache. He complains of previous fever, chills, unintentional weight loss, and loss of appetite. On physical examination, he seems malnourished with many visible punctures and abrasions on his arms and legs. He is oriented to person and place, but not time, and he displays poor insight. He has no other focal neurologic deficits on examination. Rapid human immunodeficiency virus (HIV) testing in the emergency department is positive, and cell counts are pending. The patient admits to intravenous drug use.

Imaging. CT head reveals a left periventricular hypodensity. MRI brain with and without contrast reveals a 3-cm ring enhancing lesion of the right basal ganglia with restricted diffusion and a surrounding edema (**Fig. 2**).

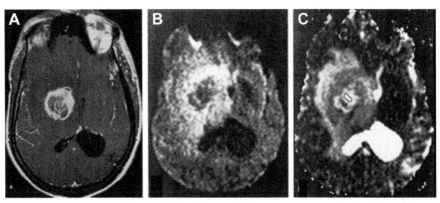

Fig. 2. MRI postcontrast (*A*), DWI (*B*), and ADC (*C*) demonstrates a right basal ganglia ring enhancing lesion with diffusion restriction. ADC, apparent diffusion coefficient; DWI, diffusion-weighted imaging.

Diagnosis. The differential diagnosis of a single ring enhancing basal ganglia lesion in a patient with untreated HIV and likely AIDS remains broad and includes primary central nervous system (CNS) lymphoma, toxoplasmosis, pyogenic abscess (bacterial or fungal), metastatic tumor, primary brain tumor, and less likely cerebral infarction or demyelinating process. This patient's case is particularly difficult, given that he has risk factors for multiple of these entities. His HIV status increases risk for both primary CNS lymphoma and opportunistic infection such as toxoplasmosis. His active intravenous drug abuse increases the risk for pyogenic abscess. In addition, the restricted diffusion does not narrow the differential diagnosis, because both abscess and lymphoma lead to a high degree of cellularity and diffusion restriction.[12]

If there is concern for metastatic disease, body CT scan or CT-PET can be used for screening. In this case, given the wide differential diagnosis, expeditious stereotactic brain biopsy will likely yield the fastest definitive diagnosis.[13] Given the size of the lesion, needle aspiration would also offer direct treatment if consistent with pyogenic abscess. Diagnostic and treatment paradigm depends partially on access to expeditious brain biopsy. In centers without this capability, empirical treatment with broad spectrum antibiotics, antifungals, and antiretrovirals would be prioritized.

Toxoplasmosis is an opportunistic infection and one of the most common infectious causes of brain abscesses in immunocompromised hosts.[14] *Toxoplasma gondii* colonize approximately one-third of humans but extremely rarely cause severe human infection outside of an immunocompromised state.[15] Diagnosis can be made in the setting of an immunocompromised patient with low CD4 cell count, ring enhancing lesion on MRI brain, and CSF polymerase chain reaction studies positive for toxoplasma.[14] If obtaining CSF is not possible and suspicion is high, then the presence of IgG antibodies in the serum can aid diagnosis. Diagnosis is also sometimes confirmed with response to empirical treatment.[16] Empirical treatment consists of pyrimethamine plus sulfadiazine, which has been used since the first described cases of cerebral toxoplasmosis.[17] In patients with HIV-related toxoplasma infection, 86% will show clinical improvement within 7 days of starting empirical therapy.[18]

Primary CNS lymphoma accounts for approximately 4% of brain tumors in the United States, and its incidence has increased with that of HIV/AIDS infection worldwide.[19] Most are diffuse B-cell lymphoma and are fairly responsive to steroids and chemotherapy compared with other non-Hodgkin lymphomas, although with worse overall survival.[20] The classic presentation is a single periventricular, ring enhancing lesion with diffusion restriction.[12] The presence of HIV coinfection increases the likelihood of diagnosis.

In the present case, expeditious brain biopsy is performed, and pathology is consistent with primary CNS lymphoma.

Management. Treatment of primary CNS lymphoma in the setting of HIV infection is focused on chemotherapy, usually with high-dose methotrexate and antiretroviral therapy. Antiretroviral therapy has been shown to improve overall survival in this patient population.[21] Whole brain radiation therapy is also sometimes used but often carries concerns of worsened neurologic outcomes in patients with concomitant HIV infection.[22] Brain biopsy is usually required, as CSF studies rarely result in definitive diagnosis on cytology.[13]

Mimic. There are several causes in the differential diagnosis of a ring enhancing lesion in a patient with AIDS and CD4 count less than 200. These include CNS lymphoma, toxoplasmosis, spontaneous intracerebral abscess, and less likely high-grade glioma, cavernous malformation, or subacute infarction.

What sets it apart. CNS lymphoma is typically represented by a single periventricular, diffusion-restricted lesion in a patient with HIV. Multiple ring enhancing lesions in a patient with HIV and low CD4 cell count is more suggestive of toxoplasmosis. A single ring enhancing lesion in a patient with untreated HIV/AIDS has a wider differential diagnosis that includes primary CNS Lymphoma, toxoplasmosis, pyogenic abscess (bacterial or fungal), metastatic tumor, primary brain tumor, and less likely infarction or demyelinating process. Given this wide differential diagnosis, brain biopsy is often required for definitive diagnosis.

Spinal Cord

Case 3: a 54-year-old man with right hand weakness
Clinical history. A 53-year-old man presents to his primary care doctor with 5 months of progressive right hand weakness. He denies any numbness, pain, or recent trauma. His past medical history is only significant for hypertension, which is well controlled on medication. His neurologic examination is significant for 4/5 weakness of hand grip and finger extension. There is atrophy of the first dorsal web space in the right hand associated with some fasciculations. The bilateral biceps are areflexic. His examination is otherwise intact with normal reflexes and strength throughout the bilateral upper and lower extremities. He is able to walk independently.

Imaging. MRI of the brain is unremarkable. MRI of the cervical spine reveals a mild right-sided disc bulge at C4-C5, without other abnormality. MRI of the brachial plexus is unremarkable (**Fig. 3**).

Diagnosis. This presentation of painless, hand weakness in a middle-aged man without any gross correlated abnormalities on MRI studies is suspicious for amyotrophic lateral sclerosis (ALS). The fasciculations on physical examination are also indicative. A mild C4/C5 disc herniation would not correlate with the deficit in this case (intrinsic hand weakness would localize to a C8 vs T1 radiculopathy). The clinical phenotype of ALS is marked by both upper and lower motor neuron signs.[23] Upper motor neuron signs include spasticity and hyperreflexia, whereas lower motor neuron signs include muscle atrophy and fasciculations. Most of the ALS cases (70%) present as limb onset, with symptoms in one extremity, such as in this case.[24] Most of the cases are sporadic (90%–95%), and the disease is rare with case incidence estimated to be 1 in 100,000 persons.[25]

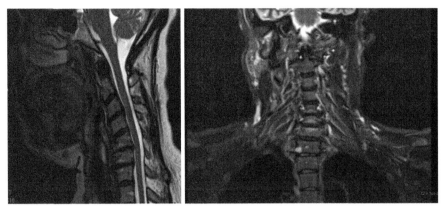

Fig. 3. MRI T2-weighted image of cervical spine and brachial plexus demonstrating degenerative cervical spine disease.

The next step in diagnosis would be electromyography (EMG) and nerve conduction studies. Nerve conduction study should reveal decreased amplitudes of the median and ulnar nerves without decreased velocities and importantly normal sensory responses.[26] EMG studies should reveal fasciculations and sharp wave fibrillations and large complex motor unit potentials in the hand. These findings may also be demonstrated in other muscle groups in the body that are not yet clinically symptomatic. The key elements of ALS diagnosis are evidence of both upper and lower motor neuron degeneration, coupled with clinical progression of symptoms. Once the diagnosis has been made clinically and corroborated by EMG, genetic testing is often offered for C9ORF72D and SOD1 mutations.[27]

Management. Unfortunately, there are not many effective options for the management of ALS at this time. Treatment is mainly focused on alleviation of symptoms and interdisciplinary/occupational therapy to help patients functionally adjust to new deficits.[28]

Riluzole is a sodium channel blocker that is thought to reduce glutamate-induced excitotoxicity and has demonstrated improved overall survival in clinical trials.[28] The median survival from the time of diagnosis in ALS is 3 to 5 years, with only 10% to 20% of patients surviving greater than 10 years from diagnosis.[29]

Mimic. ALS can mimic cervical or thoracic myelopathy, along with radiculopathy. It can also mimic numerous degenerative neurologic disorders such as myopathies, myositis, myasthenia gravis, poliomyelitis, and spinal muscular atrophy.

What sets it apart. The absence of sensory changes in the presence of weakness should raise suspicion for ALS, given that it is a purely motor disease. The presence of both upper and lower motor neuron findings such as hyperreflexia with atrophy and fasciculations is typical. Tongue fasciculations are often diagnostic. If multiple areas of the body are affected, and on both sides of the body, this should also raise suspicion, for instance, right hand and left foot changes would suggest a multifocal process such as ALS. Diagnosis can then be confirmed with EMG/nerve conduction studies.

Case 4: a 60-year-old man with progressive ataxia

Clinical history. A 60-year-old male auto mechanic presents to the clinic with complaints of decreased ability to walk. He states that over the last several years he has been having difficulty feeling and sensing his feet. He was told this was an idiopathic neuropathy. Five years ago he switched to a vegan vegetarian diet for heart health. For the last 2 months, he has been having trouble ambulating and has had 2 falls at work. He denies any back or neck pain, inciting trauma, or other changes. On physical examination, there is decreased position and vibratory sensation in both lower extremities; there is bilateral clonus in the feet and bilateral upgoing toes. There is no sensory level.

Imaging. MRI of the cervical spine reveals no compressive lesion. There are T2 signal changes throughout the dorsal aspect of the cervical spinal cord (**Fig. 4**).

Diagnosis. The clinical presentation and imaging are consistent with a lesion of the dorsal and lateral columns of the spinal cord and the condition of subacute combined degeneration, a later stage result of chronic vitamin B12 deficiency.[30] This condition develops over 5 to 10 years and can result from multiple causes including dietary vitamin B12 deficiency (ie, vegan without supplementation), gastrointestinal malabsorption (ie, pernicious anemia, postsurgical), or medication-based blocked absorption/metabolism.[31] Cobalamin (vitamin B12) is a water-soluble vitamin stored in large quantities in the liver. It cannot, however, be synthesized by the body. It is found primarily in animal meat as well as eggs and often added to fortified foods. Persons who follow a strictly plant-based vegan vegetarian diet without proper supplementation are at risk for dietary vitamin B12 deficiency.[32] Patients such as those with autoimmune pernicious anemia and postsurgical malabsorption are unable to physiologically absorb dietary B12 even with a plentiful diet.[33,34] Some medications and therapeutic agents such as the diabetic medication metformin and the anesthetic

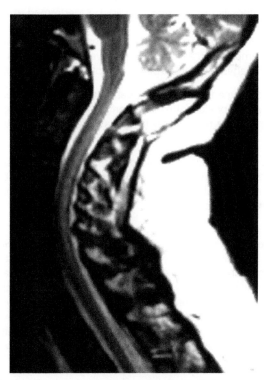

Fig. 4. Cervical T2 sagittal MRI demonstrating cord signal change.

nitrous oxide gas are known to interfere with absorption and metabolism of vitamin B12.[35]

Symptomatic cobalamin deficiency is most common in the elderly population and most frequently due to malabsorption and pernicious anemia.[36] Neurologic symptoms are often the presenting feature of B12 deficiency, given that the onset is insidious, and often at a later stage by the time of diagnosis. Neurologic symptoms can occur before hematological findings and anemia.[37] Clinical findings are often symmetric due to dorsal column involvement, spinocerebellar tracts, and lateral corticospinal tracts.[30] Classic neurologic findings with compromise of the dorsal columns includes impaired light touch sensation, proprioception, and vibration sense, usually starting in the lower extremities, and this can present as difficulty with balance ambulating, especially in the dark (Rhomberg). Further degeneration can result in involvement of the lateral corticospinal tracts, leading to diffuse hyperreflexia and clonus, and eventually spastic quadriparesis. This portrait is clinically similar to advanced degenerative cervical myelopathy.

The diagnosis of vitamin B12 deficiency can be made with multiple hematological assessments. Serum B12 measurement is a useful screening test with reported 95% sensitivity.[38] Methylmalonic acid and homocysteine are intermediates of cobalamin metabolism and if elevated, confirm B12 deficiency (more specific). Imaging with MRI often reveals focal changes in the dorsal and/or lateral columns of the spinal cord and likely in the absence of severe compressive disease.[39]

Management. Once vitamin B12 deficiency is demonstrated via laboratory testing, supplementation can be performed, often via intramuscular or subcutaneous administration to avoid malabsorption-related issues. Vitamin B12 levels are usually monitored at regular intervals. Monitoring should be performed more frequently in patients with subacute combined degeneration compared with anemia alone. The clinical improvement for neurologic symptoms takes at least 3 to 12 months, and patient's neurologic symptoms may not fully improve. Importantly, once the condition progresses to later stages (dementia, ocular symptoms), it is difficult to reverse.[40]

Mimic. Subacute combined degeneration can mimic cervical myelopathy and also normal pressure hydrocephalus (ataxia, dementia). From a radiographic perspective, it can also mimic infectious myelopathy (ie, transverse myelitis) and/or demyelinating disease.

What sets it apart. Isolated loss of proprioception and vibration is suspicious for isolated lesion of the dorsal columns. This sort of isolated deficit would be uncommon for cervical myelopathy, which should also exhibit other upper motor neuron signs such as hyperreflexia and/or clonus.

Case 5: a 35-year-old man with progressive lower extremity weakness

Clinical history. A 35-year-old man with a known history of cervical spinal stenosis presents to the emergency department with 24 hours of new ataxia. He denies preceding trauma or new neck pain. He endorses numbness in the hands and feet. On physical examination, his sensation of the hands and feet are preserved. He has weakness of bilateral dorsiflexion and plantar flexion in the feet and now is beginning to complain of weakness of bilateral hip flexion. Bilateral lower extremities are areflexic. He endorses a diarrheal illness 3 weeks ago that resolved on its own.

Imaging. MRI of the cervical spine demonstrates chronic cervical spondylosis and stenosis without new disc herniation or compressive lesion (**Fig. 5**).

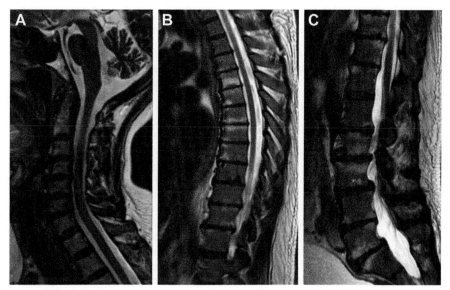

Fig. 5. MRI T2 weighted images of cervical (A), thoracic (B), and lumbar (C) spine demonstrating degenerative spine disease.

Diagnosis. The patient presented with bilateral paresthesia of the hands and feet, distal lower limb weakness that is starting to involve the proximal muscle groups, areflexia of the lower limbs, and ataxia after a diarrheal episode 3 weeks prior, which suggests Guillain-Barre syndrome (GBS).[41] GBS is an autoimmune disease in response to a recent infection, most commonly diarrhea or pneumonia, caused primarily by *Campylobacter jejuni* (25%–50%), cytomegalovirus, or Epstein-Barr virus.[42] The estimated incidence is 0.8 to 1.9/100,000, and the risk increases with advancing age.[42,43] It is known that molecular mimicry of microbial and myelin sheath/axon antigens is the inciting factor of the antibody mediated disease process.[42,44]

GBS has diverse clinical phenotypes and depends on axonal or myelin sheath involvement. The most common variant is acute inflammatory demyelinating polyneuropathy.[45] The average symptom onset is within 2 weeks of infection, and usually manifest with distal symmetric ascending lower limb weakness and areflexia; however, it can present initially with proximal lower limb weakness.[41,42] In addition, paresthesia of the distal limbs and ataxia may manifest.[41,42] Approximately 50% of patients develop oropharyngeal weakness, and others may develop bilateral facial palsy, autonomic dysfunction (labile blood pressure and arrhythmia), and respiratory failure (20%).[42,46] Interestingly, some patients may present with lower back pain or lumbar radiculopathy.[41]

Several diagnostic modalities are used to aid physicians. Most notable is CSF analysis that demonstrates albuminocytologic dissociation, with elevated protein and normal white cell count.[47] Electrodiagnostic studies are important in aiding diagnosis of GBS. Nerve conduction study may reveal prolonged latency, decreased velocity, and the appearance of F waves. EMG also shows fibrillation patterns.[41,45]

Management. Treatment of Guillain-Barre syndrome relies on plasma exchange to remove the offending antibodies and administration of intravenous IgG (IVIG) to bind autoantibodies.[41,46] There is no difference in treatment efficacy between IVIG and plasma exchange.[41] Importantly, steroids, such as methylprednisolone, do not affect the course and outcome of GBS.[46] Recovery is usually 2 to 3 weeks after starting therapy and may take years for complete independence.[41,46]

Mimic. Presenting with ataxia, paresthesia, and symmetric motor weakness can mimic spinal cord compression. Meticulous clinical history, physical examination, and imaging should be performed to distinguish a compressive lesion from GBS.

What sets it apart. Weakness with areflexia differentiates Guillain-Barre from an upper motor neuron injury such as spinal cord compression. Involvement of cranial nerve VII and oropharyngeal muscles would also preclude a spinal cord compression cause.

Peripheral Nervous System

Case 6: a 45-year-old man with severe shoulder pain and now deltoid and biceps and triceps weakness

Clinical history. A 45-year-old man presents to his primary care doctor with complaints of 3 days of left shoulder pain. He is prescribed ibuprofen and asked to monitor his symptoms. His shoulder pain worsens and begins to affect his arm as well. After 2 weeks, he sees an orthopedist, and on examination he now has 4/5 weakness of the deltoid, biceps, and triceps along with numbness throughout the arm. Left-sided biceps and triceps reflexes are absent. He endorses paresthesias of the thumb and index finger.

Imaging. MRI of the cervical spine reveals mild degenerative changes. MRI of the left brachial plexus shows some nonspecific changes, but no tumor, avulsion, or compressive lesion (**Fig. 6**).

Diagnosis. Parsonage-Turner syndrome (PTS) is an uncommon entity that usually presents with pain in the upper extremity that subsequently develops into sensory deficits and motor weakness, with main involvement of the brachial plexus's upper trunk. It can present with various synonyms, such as neuralgic amyotrophy.[48] The incidence is controversial and reported as widely as 1.64/100,000 to 1/1000 due to underrecognition and missed diagnosis.[49,50] The commonly affected age group ranges between 20 and

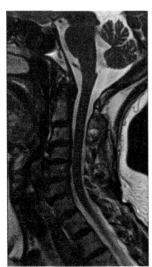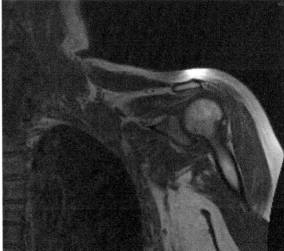

Fig. 6. MRI of the cervical spine and brachial plexus demonstrating degenerative spine disease.

60 years, with a male predilection.[51] An inciting factor is found in up to 70% of patients, with infection and autoimmune diseases as frequent elements.[48] Various other factors have been identified, such as vaccinations, surgery, exercise, or stretch injuries.[48]

Almost 95% of patients present with severe pain involving the upper limb that may radiate to the neck, shoulder, and scapula.[52] The pain is usually nocturnal and lasts for 1 to 2 week.[53] Patients may develop an excruciating neuropathic pain once the acute pain resolves.[48] Concomitantly, weakness and atrophy of the upper limb and shoulder occurs within 1 to 2 week of the acute pain episode, and patients may have a concurrent sensory abnormalities, commonly paresthesias or numbness.[48,52] It is important to note that motor and sensory symptoms are patchy in distribution, following a mononeuritis-like picture.[54]

Diagnosis is largely depending on history and physical examination. MRI may reveal some findings, such as focal intrinsic constriction and T2 hyperintensity of the nerves or brachial plexus.[55] Electrodiagnostic studies are nonspecific and may not reveal pathologic findings, especially during the early phase (within 6 weeks) of PTS.[48] Generally, delayed conduction velocity and lower amplitude could be seen in nerve conduction studies. EMG may reveal denervation and reinnervation patterns, such as fibrillation patterns, decreased muscle recruitment, and large amplitude and duration polyphasic patterns.[48]

Management. Generally, there is no specific treatment paradigm that improves the symptoms and outcome of PTS. However, studies have explored pharmacologic, nonpharmacologic, and surgical treatment modalities.[48,56] Pharmacologic treatments include corticosteroids (prednisolone), opioids, nonsteroidal antiinflammatory medication, and neuropathic pain medications (gabapentin, pregabalin, and tricyclic antidepressants).[48,56] Nonpharmacologic management includes physical therapy and psychotherapy (desensitization).[48,57,58] Surgery is controversial and is reserved for resistant cases; approaches include neurolysis, transposition, or nerve grafting.[48]

The time course for neurologic improvement is variable, with some patients having motor improvement after 1 month (66%), but others with a more prolonged recovery period. In one series, 89% of patients reported complete neurologic improvement by 3 years.[51] In another series, 6% of patients had severe weakness and 69% had mild weakness after 3 years of follow-up.[52] Up to 33% of patients may have persistent pain, despite motor improvement.[48] Patients should be counseled accordingly regarding the variable clinical course and recovery period.

Mimic. PTS can mimic cervical radiculopathy. However, a key finding in PTS is the patchy distribution of sensory and motor symptoms, with multiple nerve roots involved, the rapidity of onset, and the relative profoundness of weakness typically not seen in cervical radiculopathy. Cervical radiculopathy generally follows a single dermatome and myotome. In addition, neck examination, such as a positive Spurling test, may favor the diagnosis of cervical radiculopathy.

What sets it apart. Patients with Parsonage-Turner syndrome present with severe pain involving the upper limb, neck, and shoulder followed by a progressive course of patchy numbness, paresthesia, weakness, and atrophy. Cervical radiculopathy generally presents following the distribution of a single nerve distribution.

CLINICS CARE POINTS

- Typical findings in multiple sclerosis include a young female patient with a past history of monocular visual deficit consistent with optic neuritis and an open-ring enhancing lesion without significant surrounding vasogenic edema. Fundoscopy should be used, as it can reveal optic disc pallor as opposed to optic disc edema. Most importantly, the rapidity of onset of symptoms makes one suspect demyelination as opposed to a tumor.

- CNS lymphoma is typically represented by a single periventricular, diffusion-restricted lesion in a patient with HIV. Multiple ring enhancing lesions in a patient with HIV and low CD4 cell count is more suggestive of toxoplasmosis. A single ring enhancing lesion in a patient with untreated HIV/AIDS has a wider differential diagnosis that includes primary CNS Lymphoma, toxoplasmosis, pyogenic abscess (bacterial or fungal), metastatic tumor, primary brain tumor, and less likely infarction or demyelinating process. Given this wide differential diagnosis, brain biopsy is often required for definitive diagnosis.

- The absence of sensory changes in the presence of weakness should raise suspicion for ALS, given that it is a purely motor disease. The presence of both upper and lower motor neuron findings such as hyperreflexia with atrophy and fasciculations is typical. Tongue fasciculations are often diagnostic. If multiple areas of the body are affected, and on both sides of the body, this should also raise suspicion, for instance, right hand and left foot changes would suggest a multifocal process such as ALS. Diagnosis can then be confirmed with EMG/nerve conduction studies.

- Isolated loss of proprioception and vibration is suspicious for isolated lesion of the dorsal columns. This sort of isolated deficit would be uncommon for cervical myelopathy, which should also exhibit other upper motor neuron signs such as hyperreflexia and/or clonus.

- Weakness with areflexia differentiates Guillain-Barre from an upper motor neuron injury such as spinal cord compression. Involvement of cranial nerve VII and oropharyngeal muscles would also preclude a spinal cord compression cause.

- Patients with Parsonage-Turner syndrome present with severe pain involving the upper limb, neck, and shoulder followed by a progressive course of patchy numbness, paresthesia, weakness, and atrophy. Cervical radiculopathy generally presents following the distribution of a single nerve distribution.

REFERENCES

1. Lucchinetti CF, Gavrilova RH, Metz I, et al. Clinical and radiographic spectrum of pathologically confirmed tumefactive multiple sclerosis. Brain 2008;131(7): 1759–75.
2. Kiriyama T, Kataoka H, Taoka T, et al. Characteristic neuroimaging in patients with tumefactive demyelinating lesions exceeding 30 mm. J Neuroimaging 2011; 21(2):e69–77.
3. Takenaka S, Shinoda J, Asano Y, et al. Metabolic assessment of monofocal acute inflammatory demyelination using MR spectroscopy and (11)C-methionine-, (11) C-choline-, and (18)F-fluorodeoxyglucose-PET. Brain Tumor Pathol 2011;28(3): 229–38.
4. Malhotra HS, Jain KK, Agarwal A, et al. Characterization of tumefactive demyelinating lesions using MR imaging and in-vivo proton MR spectroscopy. Mult Scler 2009;15(2):193–203.
5. Ikeguchi R, Shimizu Y, Abe K, et al. Proton magnetic resonance spectroscopy differentiates tumefactive demyelinating lesions from gliomas. Mult Scler Relat Disord 2018;26:77–84.
6. Altintas A, Petek B, Isik N, et al. Clinical and radiological characteristics of tumefactive demyelinating lesions: follow-up study. Mult Scler 2012;18(10): 1448–53.
7. Hardy TA. Pseudotumoral demyelinating lesions: diagnostic approach and long-term outcome. Curr Opin Neurol 2019;32(3):467–74.

8. Weinshenker BG, O'Brien PC, Petterson TM, et al. A randomized trial of plasma exchange in acute central nervous system inflammatory demyelinating disease. Ann Neurol 1999;46(6):878–86.

9. Balloy G, On behalf of the Société Francophone de la Sclérose en Plaques, Pelletier J, et al. Inaugural tumor-like multiple sclerosis: clinical presentation and medium-term outcome in 87 patients. J Neurol 2018;265(10):2251–9.

10. Weber MS, Hohlfeld R, Zamvil SS. Mechanism of action of glatiramer acetate in treatment of multiple sclerosis. Neurotherapeutics 2007;4(4):647–53.

11. Wynn DR. Enduring Clinical Value of Copaxone® (Glatiramer Acetate) in Multiple Sclerosis after 20 Years of Use. Mult Scler Int 2019;2019:7151685.

12. Haldorsen IS, Espeland A, Larsson E-M. Central Nervous System Lymphoma: Characteristic Findings on Traditional and Advanced Imaging. Am J Neuroradiology 2011;32(6):984–92.

13. Morell AA, Shah AH, Cavallo C, et al. Diagnosis of primary central nervous system lymphoma: a systematic review of the utility of CSF screening and the role of early brain biopsy. Neuro-Oncology Pract 2019;6(6):415–23.

14. Vidal JE. HIV-Related Cerebral Toxoplasmosis Revisited: Current Concepts and Controversies of an Old Disease. J Int Assoc Provid AIDS Care 2019;18. 2325958219867315.

15. Dunay IR, Gajurel K, Dhakal R, et al. Treatment of Toxoplasmosis: Historical Perspective, Animal Models, and Current Clinical Practice. Clin Microbiol Rev 2018;31(4). https://doi.org/10.1128/CMR.00057-17.

16. Pellegrino D, Gryschek R, de Oliveira ACP, et al. Efficacy and safety of trimethoprim-sulfamethoxazole in HIV-infected patients with cerebral toxoplasmosis in Brazil: a single-arm open-label clinical trial. Int J STD AIDS 2019; 30(12):1156–62.

17. Luft BJ, Conley F, Remington JS, et al. Outbreak of central-nervous-system toxoplasmosis in western Europe and North America. Lancet 1983;1(8328):781–4.

18. Porter SB, Sande MA. Toxoplasmosis of the Central Nervous System in the Acquired Immunodeficiency Syndrome. N Engl J Med 1992;327(23):1643–8.

19. Welch K. Autopsy findings in the acquired immune deficiency syndrome. JAMA 1984;252(9):1152–9.

20. Grommes C, Nayak L, Tun HW, et al. Introduction of novel agents in the treatment of primary CNS lymphoma. Neuro Oncol 2019;21(3):306–13.

21. Hoffmann C, Tabrizian S, Wolf E, et al. Survival of AIDS patients with primary central nervous system lymphoma is dramatically improved by HAART-induced immune recovery. AIDS 2001;15(16):2119–27.

22. Glass J, Gruber ML, Cher L, et al. Preirradiation methotrexate chemotherapy of primary central nervous system lymphoma: long-term outcome. J Neurosurg 1994;81(2):188–95.

23. Brotman RG, Moreno-Escobar MC, Joseph J, et al. Amyotrophic lateral sclerosis. In: StatPearls. Treasure Island (FL): StatPearls Publishing; 2020.

24. Couratier P, Truong C, Khalil M, et al. Clinical features of flail arm syndrome. Muscle Nerve 2000;23(4):646–8.

25. Jordan H, Rechtman L, Wagner L, et al. Amyotrophic lateral sclerosis surveillance in Baltimore and Philadelphia. Muscle & Nerve 2015;51(6):815–21.

26. Krivickas LS. Amyotrophic lateral sclerosis and other motor neuron diseases. Phys Med Rehabil Clin N Am 2003;14(2):327–45.

27. Agudelo A, St Amand V, Grissom L, et al. Age-dependent degeneration of an identified adult leg motor neuron in a SOD1 model of ALS. Biol Open 2020; 9(10). https://doi.org/10.1242/bio.049692.

28. Miller RG, Jackson CE, Kasarskis EJ, et al. Practice parameter update: the care of the patient with amyotrophic lateral sclerosis: multidisciplinary care, symptom management, and cognitive/behavioral impairment (an evidence-based review): report of the Quality Standards Subcommittee of the American Academy of Neurology. Neurology 2009;73(15):1227–33.

29. Limousin N, Blasco H, Corcia P, et al. Malnutrition at the time of diagnosis is associated with a shorter disease duration in ALS. J Neurol Sci 2010;297(1–2):36–9.

30. Qudsiya Z, De Jesus O. Subacute combined degeneration of the spinal cord. In: StatPearls. Treasure Island (FL): StatPearls Publishing; 2020.

31. Bi Z, Cao J, Shang K, et al. Correlation between anemia and clinical severity in subacute combined degeneration patients. J Clin Neurosci 2020;80:11–5.

32. Wolffenbuttel BHR, Wouters HJCM, Heiner-Fokkema MR, et al. The Many Faces of Cobalamin (Vitamin B) Deficiency. Mayo Clin Proc Innov Qual Outcomes 2019;3(2):200–14.

33. Marcuard SP, Sinar DR, Swanson MS, et al. Absence of luminal intrinsic factor after gastric bypass surgery for morbid obesity. Dig Dis Sci 1989;34(8):1238–42.

34. Zhang N, Li R-H, Ma L, et al. Subacute Combined Degeneration, Pernicious Anemia and Gastric Neuroendocrine Tumor Occurred Simultaneously Caused by Autoimmune Gastritis. Front Neurosci 2019;13:1.

35. Bauman WA, Shaw S, Jayatilleke E, et al. Increased intake of calcium reverses vitamin B12 malabsorption induced by metformin. Diabetes Care 2000;23(9):1227–31.

36. Bizzaro N, Antico A. Diagnosis and classification of pernicious anemia. Autoimmun Rev 2014;13(4–5):565–8.

37. Lindenbaum J, Rosenberg IH, Wilson PW, et al. Prevalence of cobalamin deficiency in the Framingham elderly population. Am J Clin Nutr 1994;60(1):2–11.

38. Devalia V, Hamilton MS, Molloy AM, British Committee for Standards in Haematology. Guidelines for the diagnosis and treatment of cobalamin and folate disorders. Br J Haematol 2014;166(4):496–513.

39. Sun HY, Lee JW, Park KS, et al. Spine MR imaging features of subacute combined degeneration patients. Eur Spine J 2014;23(5):1052–8.

40. Stabler SP. Clinical practice. Vitamin B12 deficiency. N Engl J Med 2013;368(2):149–60.

41. Wijdicks EF, Klein CJ. Guillain-Barre Syndrome. Mayo Clin Proc 2017;92(3):467–79.

42. Willison HJ, Jacobs BC, van Doorn PA. Guillain-Barré syndrome. Lancet 2016;388(10045):717–27.

43. Sejvar JJ, Baughman AL, Wise M, et al. Population incidence of Guillain-Barré syndrome: a systematic review and meta-analysis. Neuroepidemiology 2011;36(2):123–33.

44. Willison HJ, Yuki N. Peripheral neuropathies and anti-glycolipid antibodies. Brain 2002;125(Pt 12):2591–625.

45. Levin KH. Variants and mimics of Guillain Barré Syndrome. Neurologist 2004;10(2):61–74.

46. Yuki N, Hartung H-P. Guillain-Barré syndrome. N Engl J Med 2012;366(24):2294–304.

47. van den Berg B, Walgaard C, Drenthen J, et al. Guillain-Barré syndrome: pathogenesis, diagnosis, treatment and prognosis. Nat Rev Neurol 2014;10(8):469–82.

48. Smith CC, Bevelaqua A-C. Challenging pain syndromes: Parsonage-Turner syndrome. Phys Med Rehabil Clin N Am 2014;25(2):265–77.

49. Beghi E, Kurland LT, Mulder DW, et al. Brachial plexus neuropathy in the population of Rochester, Minnesota, 1970-1981. Ann Neurol 1985;18(3):320–3.
50. van Alfen N, van Eijk JJJ, Ennik T, et al. Incidence of neuralgic amyotrophy (Parsonage Turner syndrome) in a primary care setting–a prospective cohort study. PLoS One 2015;10(5):e0128361.
51. Tsairis P, Dyck PJ, Mulder DW. Natural history of brachial plexus neuropathy. Report on 99 patients. Arch Neurol 1972;27(2):109–17.
52. van Alfen N, van Engelen BGM. The clinical spectrum of neuralgic amyotrophy in 246 cases. Brain 2006;129(2):438–50.
53. Feinberg JH, Radecki J. Parsonage-turner syndrome. HSS J 2010;6(2):199–205.
54. Feinberg JH, Nguyen ET, Boachie-Adjei K, et al. The electrodiagnostic natural history of parsonage-turner syndrome. Muscle Nerve 2017;56(4):737–43.
55. Sneag DB, Rancy SK, Wolfe SW, et al. Brachial plexitis or neuritis? MRI features of lesion distribution in Parsonage-Turner syndrome. Muscle Nerve 2018;58(3):359–66.
56. Finnerup NB, Otto M, McQuay HJ, et al. Algorithm for neuropathic pain treatment: an evidence based proposal. Pain 2005;118(3):289–305.
57. van Alfen N, van Engelen BGM, Hughes RAC. Treatment for idiopathic and hereditary neuralgic amyotrophy (brachial neuritis). Cochrane Database Syst Rev 2009;3:CD006976.
58. Tjoumakaris FP, Anakwenze OA, Kancherla V, et al. Neuralgic amyotrophy (Parsonage-Turner syndrome). J Am Acad Orthop Surg 2012;20(7):443–9.

Moving?

Make sure your subscription moves with you!

To notify us of your new address, find your **Clinics Account Number** (located on your mailing label above your name), and contact customer service at:

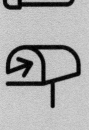

Email: **journalscustomerservice-usa@elsevier.com**

800-654-2452 (subscribers in the U.S. & Canada)
314-447-8871 (subscribers outside of the U.S. & Canada)

Fax number: 314-447-8029

Elsevier Health Sciences Division
Subscription Customer Service
3251 Riverport Lane
Maryland Heights, MO 63043

ELSEVIER

Printed and bound by CPI Group (UK) Ltd, Croydon, CR0 4YY

03/10/2024

01040468-0005